T0205925

# Challenge and Innovation

# Social Aspects of AIDS

*Series Editor:* Peter Aggleton, Goldsmiths' College, University of London

# Challenge and Innovation:
## Methodological Advances in Social Research on HIV/AIDS

Edited by
## Mary Boulton

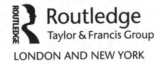

Routledge
Taylor & Francis Group

LONDON AND NEW YORK

First published 1994 by Taylor & Francis

Published 2013 by Routledge
4 Park Square, Milton Park, Abingdon, Oxon OX14 4RN
605 Third Avenue, New York, NY 10017

*Routledge is an imprint of the Taylor & Francis Group, an informa business*

ISBN 13: 978-0-7484-0198-7 (pbk)

**A Catalogue Record for this book is available from the British Library**

**Library of Congress Cataloging-in-Publication Data are available on request**

Series cover design by Barking Dog Art.

Typeset in 10/12 pt CG Baskerville
by RGM Associates, Lord Street, Southport, England

# Contents

List of Figures     vii
List of Tables     viii
List of Acronyms     ix
Series Editor's Preface     x
Preface     xi

Chapter 1    The Methodological Imagination     1
               *Mary Boulton*

**Research Design, Theoretical Frameworks and the Research Question**    23

Chapter 2    Using Longitudinal Cohort-Sequential Designs to Study    25
               Changes in Sexual Behaviour
               *Glynis M. Breakwell and Chris R. Fife-Schaw*
Chapter 3    Monitoring Behavioural Change in the Population: A    39
               Continuous Data Collection Approach
               *David McQueen and Stefano Campostrini*
Chapter 4    Acts, Sessions and Individuals: A Model for Analysing    57
               Sexual Behaviour
               *Peter Davies*
Chapter 5    Analysing Naturally-Occurring Data on AIDS    69
               Counselling: Some Methodological and Practical Issues
               *David Silverman*

**Samples and Populations**    95

Chapter 6    Some Methodological and Practical Implications of    97
               Employing Drug Users as Indigenous Fieldworkers
               *Robert Power*
Chapter 7    How Many Prostitutes? Epidemiology out of    111
               Ethnography
               *Neil McKeganey, Marina Barnard and Michael Bloor*

**Methods of Data Collection**                                                           123

Chapter 8      Diaries and Sexual Behaviour: The Use of Sexual Diaries      125
               as Method and Substance in Researching Gay Men's
               Response to HIV/AIDS
               *Anthony P. M. Coxon*
Chapter 9      Social Science Methods Used in a Study of Prostitutes in      149
               the Gambia
               *Helen Pickering*
Chapter 10     Focus Groups: Methods or Madness?                            159
               *Jenny Kitzinger*

**Evaluating Health Education Interventions**                                           177

Chapter 11     Theory, Utility and Stakeholders: Methodological Issues      179
               in Evaluating a Community Project on HIV/AIDS
               *Ian S. Peers and Margaret Johnston*
Chapter 12     Assessing AIDS Preventive Strategies in Europe               199
               *Kaye Wellings*

**A Feminist Approach to Social Research on HIV/AIDS**                                   217

Chapter 13     Methodological Issues in Researching Young Women's           219
               Sexuality
               *Janet Holland, Caroline Ramazanoglu, Sue Scott, Sue Sharpe and
               Rachel Thomson*

**Looking Forward**                                                                     241

Chapter 14     Towards the Mainstreaming of HIV Research                    243
               *Mildred Blaxter*

Notes on Contributors                                                       253
Index                                                                      259

# List of Figures

2.1 The Longitudinal Cohort — Sequential Design Used in the
    Survey of Young People                                           26
2.2 The Pure Form of the Longitudinal Cohort — Sequential Design     27
3.1 Four variable types — nature over time                           43
3.2 Basic ordering and structure of lifestyle and health questionnaire  44
3.3 Knowledge about AIDS stability over time — Scottish data using
    a five-item scale                                                45
3.4 Per cent of respondents reporting talking about AIDS with family
    and friends over time                                           46
3.5 Stable AIDS item over time — good agreement with two versions
    of question on difficulty of getting AIDS                       47
3.6 Less stable AIDS item over time — agreement with question on
    whether AIDS spread in general population                       48
3.7 Agreement with two versions of a statement on employer being
    able to dismiss employee with AIDS                              48
3.8 Question item showing both instability over time and sensitivity to
    change in question polarity                                     49
5.1 Objectivism and subjectivism                                    86
7.1 Working habits of female prostitutes                            114
8.1 Aggregate diary vs. interview estimates of sexual behaviour     137
8.2 Alternatives for destination of ejaculation                    140
8.3 Unprotected anal intercourse by type                           142
10.1 Types of groups involved in the study                          161
12.1 HIV antibody tests in England and Wales — January 1985 to July
     1988                                                           203
12.2 Practice of condom use in the UK                               208
12.3 Condom usage in Netherlands                                    209
12.4 Knowledge and practice of condom use amongst Swiss youth       210
12.5 Calls taken per week by Belgian AIDS helpline                  211

# List of Tables

3.1 Possible risk in behaviour by gender, age and marital status 52
5.1 Standard expectations about HIV counselling 72
5.2 Form of advice and degree of uptake 80
8.1 Destination of ejaculate in anal intercourse 141
8.2 Percentage of acts where anal intercourse involves a condom (c) or is unprotected (h and m) by wave 141
8.3 Percentage of unprotected acts of anal intercourse, by age and relationship type 143
8.4 Median polish of percentage of unprotected acts of anal intercourse, by age and relationship 143
12.1 Knowledge of ways in which HIV is transmitted, UK, January 1987 213
12.2 Knowledge of transmission routes in selected European countries 214

# List of Acronyms

Acquired Immune Deficiency Syndrome (AIDS)
Advisory Council on the Misuse of Drugs (ACMD)
Behavioural Risk Factor Surveillance System (BRFSS)
British Social Attitudes (BSA)
Centre for Research on Drugs and Health Behaviour (CRDHB)
Computer Assisted Telephone Interviewing (CATI)
Conversation Analysis (CA)
Council of American Survey Research Organization (CASRO)
Economic and Social Research Council (ESRC)
Health Belief Model (HBM)
Health Education Authority (HEA)
Health Education Board for Scotland (HEBS)
Human Immuno-deficiency Virus (HIV)
Inventory of Sexual Behaviour (ISB)
Joint Council on Standards for Educational Evaluation (JCSE)
Knowledge, Attitudes, Beliefs and Practice (KABP)
Longitudinal Cohort-Sequential Design (LCSD)
Medical Research Council (MRC)
National Associations for the Care or Resettlement of Offenders (NACRO)
Research Unit in Health and Behaviour Change (RUHBC)
Scottish Associations for the Care and Resettlement of Offenders (SACRO)
Scottish Home and Health Department (SHHD)
Sexually Transmitted Disease (STD)
Socio-sexual Investigations of Gay Men and Aids (SIGMA)
Women Risk and AIDS Project (WRAP)
World Health Organization (WHO)

# Series Editor's Preface

The advent of HIV and AIDS issued a challenge to social and behavioural researchers globally — that of generating knowledge and understanding for the development of effective interventions, in the fields of prevention, care, counselling and community support. It encouraged too an in-depth exploration of aspects of life which had hitherto been left unexamined: sex between men, sex work, injecting drug use, each became an important research area in its own right. Such enquiry called for the use of research techniques which were both sensitive and specific to the issue in question. Only rarely were existing methodologies adequate for the challenge.

Some ten years into the epidemic, it is appropriate to pause and consider what was achieved by this first wave of social scientific endeavour. Numerous publications in this series and elsewhere do so from the point of view of what has been learned substantively in the fields of sociology, psychology, anthropology and education. Rather less often do we have the opportunity to assess what has been learned methodologically. *Challenge and Innovation: Methodoloical Advances in Social Research on HIV/AIDS* is unique in bringing together papers which reflect on these concerns. It examines questions of research design, sampling, data collection and evaluation, whilst focusing too on the adequacy of existing conceptual and explanatory frameworks. The contributors describe their own experiences working on HIV and AIDS with freshness and candour, highlighting as much the deficiencies that exist, as the methodological advances that have been made. Of relevance to those seeking insight into the contribution that social research can make to the epidemic, this book is essential reading for all concerned with the social dimensions of health.

Peter Aggleton

# Preface

This volume arises largely out of a meeting with the same title which was sponsored by the Economic and Social Research Councill (ESRC) as part of efforts to disseminate the work of its AIDS Initiative. The meeting, held in Harrogate in May 1992, brought together over forty British, European and American researchers in the social and behavioural sciences, as well as those involved in policy, planning and evaluation, to discuss methodological aspects of social research in relation to HIV/AIDS. A version of nine of the papers were presented at that time and five were later commissioned from other participants. They describe work that was funded by the ESRC but also by other funding agencies including the Department of Health, the Health Education Authority and the Medical Research Council.

A number of people have contributed to the success of the Harrogate meeting and hence to this volume. First, I would like to thank all those who took part in the meeting for their lively debate — particularly the Discussants, whose critical perspective helped focus the discussion and sharpen the papers collected here: Theo Sandfort, Pam Gillies, Sally McIntyre, Roger Ingham, Peter Aggleton, and Helen Ward. I would also like to thank the Steering Committee of the ESRC AIDS Initiative for their imagination in suggesting the theme of the meeting and their support in funding it. Peter Linthwaite and Margaret Edmonds deserve special thanks for their many and varied efforts. Finally, my thanks to David Miller for comments on the manuscript and Mary Egan for help in producing it.

Mary Boulton
London, 1993

Chapter 1

# The Methodological Imagination

*Mary Boulton*

In the early 1980s, Human Immuno-deficiency Virus (HIV) infection and Acquired Immune Deficiency Syndrome (AIDS) were recognized as threatening the most devastating infectious disease epidemic of the twentieth century. It was soon realized that an enormous effort would be needed to understand the disease, to provide care and treatment for those affected by it and to limit its spread within the population. While biological scientists and the medical profession began the hard drive towards finding effective treatments and vaccines, it was recognized that for the foreseeable future, the only effective way to combat the epidemic was through understanding and altering the behaviours by which it was transmitted. Social scientists were called upon to contribute to this enterprise, providing information on patterns of risk behaviours and how and why they were changing and, more recently, on the experience of those who have been affected by HIV/AIDS and the services they receive.

Those engaged in research on the social dimensions of HIV/AIDS have had to face new and exceptionally difficult challenges in conducting their investigations (Ankrah, 1989; Kaplan, 1989; Catania *et al.*, 1990a; Schoepf, 1991; Samuels *et al.*, 1992; Standing, 1992; Boulton, 1993). Many of the behaviours thought to transmit HIV are private and hence difficult to investigate. Many of the people considered to be at highest risk of HIV infection are also amongst the least accessible to social research. The urgent need for detailed and accurate information to guide AIDS prevention programmes and plan appropriate services, however, has provided the impetus — and the necessary funds — to tackle these difficulties and to devise new and imaginative strategies for conducting research.

This book brings together some of the most interesting advances in research methods that have been developed by those working in the United Kingdom. The aim is to draw attention to these advances and make them more widely accessible to those working in this area and in the field of health more generally.

The chapters are drawn from the work of twelve research groups who, in response to the challenge of HIV/AIDS research, have developed the tools of social research to new degrees of sophistication, or put them to use in novel and imaginative ways.

The papers are grouped under five headings according to the area of research methods in which they have made their most significant contribution. This is for organizational convenience only: the many areas of research strategy are inevitably interdependent. Thus, imaginative methods of data collection may allow researchers to develop more sophisticated research designs. Similarly, studies which develop more effective ways of accessing 'hidden' groups in the population may contribute to improvements in the reliability and validity of the data collected. Moreover, research methods cannot be divorced from questions of theory: the researchers' stance with regard to potential explanations, whether implicit or explicit, shapes the way their research questions are framed and the way in which their data are interpreted and generalized. Finally, it should be remembered that the ultimate test of the value of a research method is in the quality of data it generates, the analysis it allows and the insights it facilitates (Albrecht, 1989). Thus, while the emphasis in this book is on the *methods* the researchers have developed, it is often in the substantive findings of their studies, and their contribution to our understanding of the epidemic, that the methods have proved their worth.

This introductory chapter is intended to provide a context for the work described in the following chapters by examining the methodological debates and developments which have characterized research on the social aspects of HIV/AIDS. Its focus is largely methodological. In the final chapter, Mildred Blaxter takes a more outward-looking view, considering the value of these developments for research on health and illness more generally.

## Research Design, Theoretical Frameworks and the Research Question

Early in the AIDS epidemic, little was known about patterns of knowledge, attitudes or behaviour relevant to the transmission of HIV in the population or about the effects of efforts to change them. Media coverage of HIV infection and its modes of transmission also meant that the situation was changing rapidly and in unforseeable ways. Those concerned with planning for and preventing the epidemic needed accurate and up-to-date descriptions of social responses to HIV/AIDS as well as clear and theoretically-informed explanations for how and why they were changing. To be able to provide this information, social scientists needed to give careful attention to the design of their studies, the conceptual models underlying them and the way they framed their research questions.

*Measuring Behaviour and Explaining Change*

Cross-sectional design has long been the mainstay of social research and has been perhaps the most commonly used design in empirical studies of social aspects of HIV/AIDS (e.g., Bowie and Ford, 1989; Fitzpatrick *et al.*, 1990a; Johnson *et al.*, 1992; Richardson *et al.*, 1993; Ward *et al.*, 1993). These studies have produced baseline descriptions of the frequency and distribution of many behaviours of concern for the epidemic. Traditional cross-sectional surveys, however, provide only a static picture of attitudes and behaviour and, given the volatility of publicity surrounding HIV/AIDS, one which is likely to be quickly out of date. In order to measure change over time, researchers have increasingly turned to prospective cohort designs. A number of large scale, multi-site cohort studies have been established, most notably for research on gay men (e.g., Joseph *et al.*, 1987; McKusick *et al.*, 1990; Davies *et al.*, 1993; Kippax *et al.*, 1993). These studies have been invaluable in monitoring patterns of risk behaviour and the effects of particular interventions. However, while the nature of the research design allows change to be measured and causal ordering to be established, prospective cohort studies have other problems, most notably those of sampling bias and the effects of repeated measurements. The limitations of both cross sectional and prospective cohort designs have encouraged researchers to turn to more sophisticated designs to address questions of specific concern in predicting and controling the AIDS epidemic.

Two such designs are described in Chapters 2 and 3. Breakwell and Fife-Schaw describe a research design which is particularly useful in addressing some of the fundamental questions in HIV/AIDS research — how do risk behaviours change over time and what factors contribute to this — in their chapter, 'Using Longitudinal Cohort-Sequential Designs to Study Changes in Sexual Behaviour'. They point out that three types of factors may influence age-related behaviour change and that it is difficult to disentangle their effects in a study which uses a traditional design. The strength of a longitudinal cohort-sequential design is in allowing them to distinguish the contribution of each type factor individually and in interaction.

In Chapter 3, 'Monitoring Behavioural Change in the Population', McQueen and Campostrini describe a research design which allows a similar set of questions to be addressed in a very different way. This design has been described as a type of interrupted time series in which repeated samples are drawn from the general population to examine changes in patterns of behaviour as they occurr at the population level (Uitenbroek and McQueen, 1992). Behavioural variables are viewed as dynamic, and how they appear in population data collected over several years is examined. This has allowed them not only to measure the extent of change but also to identify the *characteristics* of the change, for example, stable or fluctuating rapidly.

### *Models of Behaviour and Behaviour Change*

Implicit in a research design is a theoretical model which defines the variables of interest and the expected relationships amongst them. The value of empirical research is thus circumscribed by the theoretical model on which it is based. Prior to the AIDS epidemic, the Health Belief Model (HBM) and its variants and elaborations (e.g., Becker, 1974; Bandura, 1977; Ajzen and Fishbein, 1980) had long dominated research in the field of health behaviour, and thus provided the theoretical foundation for most of the early studies of behaviour change in relation to HIV/AIDS (e.g., Kotarba and Lang, 1986; Joseph *et al.*, 1987; Fitzpatrick *et al.*, 1989; Fitzpatrick *et al.*, 1990b). Although many of these studies obtained findings that were consistent with aspects of the HBM at one time, they were not noted for their success in predicting behaviour at another time. This has given rise to considerable dissatisfaction with the HBM as a framework for research and the development of alternative models specifically in relation to the AIDS epidemic (e.g., Catania *et al.*, 1990b).

In the third chapter in this section, 'Acts, Sessions and Individuals', Peter Davies makes the case for one such alternative model, based on an analysis of the structure of sexual behaviour. Using this model to look at sexual behaviour in relation to HIV infection, researchers would adopt a radically different research design, with the sexual session replacing the sexual individual as the unit for recording detailed information and with attention shifting from the characteristics of the respondent to the process of sexual interaction between partners in explaining risk behaviours. This approach is taken up in Chapter 8, where Tony Coxon describes the use of sexual diaries to collect information on sexual behaviour from gay men. Because a different model is used, different types of data are collected and different types of analyses are possible, for example, in terms of the structure of sexual sessions and the volume of sexual acts.

### *Framing the Research Question*

Chapter 5 takes us one step further back in the research process and considers the fundamental issue of how the basic research question should be framed. In 'Analyzing Naturally-Occurring Data on AIDS Counselling', David Silverman argues that research should be informed not by 'social problems' but by clear analytical issues. His argument is that before we can ask *why* a social phenomenon is occurring or how we can *change* it, we need to understand the phenomenon itself. This means concentrating research interest on the phenomenon rather than on what preceeds or follows it, the failing of research designs — whether experimental or non-experimental, quantitative or qualitative — defined by social problems. Silverman illustrates the value of framing research questions in terms of analytic issues by showing how common assumptions about what makes for effective counselling are challenged by his analysis of the local organization of counselling for safer sex, and by showing how such an analysis provides further insights which, in turn, can lead to unexpected policy recommendations.

In the context of social research on HIV and AIDS, Silverman's paper is a timely reminder of the need to give careful thought to the way in which research is conceived. Because the epidemic poses such a problem, most research has been couched in problem-oriented terms. The danger he draws attention to is of losing sight of analytical issues in designing research to address practical or policy-oriented issues, hence losing the power of sociological analysis.

## Sampling: Accessing 'Hard to Reach' Populations

A key aspect of research design is the definition of the appropriate population in which to conduct the research and the recruitment of an adequate sample of respondents. From the beginning of the AIDS epidemic, the need was recognized for both large-scale probability surveys of the general population and for more targeted surveys amongst groups practising high-risk behaviours to provide the range of information required for both predictive and preventive purposes. The recruitment of appropriate samples, however, has posed considerable problems. It was widely believed that it would be difficult to conduct population surveys on risk behaviours because the general public would resist the invasion of their privacy and refuse to answer questions on such personal and sensitive topics (Wellings *et al.*, 1990a). Similarly, more targeted studies were expected to face difficulties in identifying and recruiting members of groups practising high-risk behaviours. These challenges have required the development of a variety of sampling strategies designed for the particular objectives of individual studies.

### General Population Surveys

Because a primary aim of general population surveys is to provide baseline information on the prevalence and distribution of risk behaviours in the population, the representativeness of the sample is particularly important (Sundet *et al.*, 1990; Fife-Schaw and Breakwell, 1992). Considerable attention has therefore been given to developing strategies both for drawing representative samples and for achieving high participation rates. In a review of fifteen major surveys using probability sampling, Miller and her colleagues (Miller *et al.*, 1990) found that relatively high rates of participation could be achieved when targets were set high and attention was given to training and supporting interviewers. McQueen and Campostrini (Chapter 3) describe the use of two further strategies which have been found to be particularly effective in ensuring a high response rate in surveys amongst the general population: they included their questions on sexual behaviour in a broader survey of health related behaviours and they preceded these questions with an 'informed consent' statement specifying the nature of the questions to follow. Evidence of respect for the privacy and sensibilities of the respondent through procedures such as this, and through mechanisms which allow the respondent to reveal information without embarrassment or threat, appear to be crucial in achieving a high response rate.

High response rates, however, do not themselves guarantee the representativeness of a sample. While comparisons with census data can give some assurance of minimal bias with respect to demographic characteristics, they can give no indication of the bias regarding the parameters of interest in AIDS-related research (Wadsworth and Johnson, 1991). The sampling frames used in household and telephone surveys systematically exclude the homeless and institutionalized, groups with potentially high rates of risk behaviours, while involvement in covert activities may themselves reduce the likelihood of participating (Mays and Jackson, 1991). The accuracy of estimates of the prevalence of risk behaviours derived from general population surveys therefore remains problematic. One response to this has been the more imaginative use of descriptive statistics. In Chapter 2, Breakwell and Fife-Schaw describe the use of 'lower bound estimates' in their survey of risk behaviours amongst teenagers. Although their response rate was less than ideal, they argue that their findings provide an accurate estimate of the minimum proportion of their target population who engage in risk behaviours.

### Groups Practising High-Risk Behaviour

While researchers concerned with specific groups practising high-risk behaviours were aware of the technical problems of sampling error and non-participation bias, most were more concerned with the prior problem of generating a sample at all. Because they are socially stigmatized or illegal, many behaviours associated with HIV transmission are driven underground. Those involved in buying or selling sex, in injecting drugs and in homosexual activity are generally wary of outsiders and suspicious of those asking questions. The communities surrounding them also tend to be exclusive, and further shelter those participating from outside view. The sampling problems for studies of these groups therefore arose in relation to the practical difficulties entailed in identifying potential respondents and in gaining their co-operation in research.

Institutional settings have provided the most convenient sites for recruitment and many studies have obtained their samples through medical agencies (Coleman and Curtis, 1988; Donoghoe *et al.*, 1989; Evans *et al.*, 1989; Ostrow *et al.*, 1991) or legal institutions (Power *et al.*, 1992). This method has advantages in gaining access to large numbers of individuals, a defined sampling frame and the sponsorship of the agency. High response rates have been achieved and it has been possible to maintain continuity of contact for follow-up studies (Robertson *et al.*, 1988). However, it is well known that those who are in contact with official agencies are only a proportion of those who are involved in similar activities and that they differ from those not in contact with the agencies in many characteristics of interest to researchers (Lampinen *et al.*, 1992; Haw *et al.*, 1992).

In their attempts to reach beyond institutional settings and recruit individuals in the community, researchers have shown considerable imagination and resourcefulness (Watters and Biernacki, 1989). A variety of approaches have been used, including enlisting the co-operation of community organizations, advertising in relevant newspapers, distributing leaflets at special events and going out to the places where people congregate, such as pubs, clubs, poolrooms, toilets, bathhouses, drop-in centres, 'red light districts' or 'cruising sites' (Bennett *et al.*, 1989; Connell *et al.*, 1989; Day and Ward, 1990; Fitzpatrick *et al.*, 1990b; Hays *et al.*, 1990; Klee *et al.*, 1990; Myers *et al.*, 1992; Davies *et al.*, 1993). Most community-based studies have used several of these approaches in order to contact people in a wide variety of contexts and hence have recruited a greater diversity of respondents than are seen in agency-based studies.

Perhaps the most innovative development, however, has been the use of *indigenous workers* — current or former members of covert communities such as sex workers or injecting drug users — as temporary research staff to work amongst those most resistant to contact with official agencies (Morgan Thomas *et al.*, 1989; Power *et al.*, 1991, 1992). In Chapter 6, 'Methodological and Practical Implications of Employing Drug Users as Indigenous Interviewers', Power describes the methodological, ethical and practical issues surrounding this practice. Their drug using experience means indigenous workers have a knowledge of the local network and access to individuals within it which would take an outside researcher a considerable time to acquire and also ensures that they feel at ease in the fieldwork context and are accepted by the community they work in. Familiarity with the culture of the respondents also reduces misunderstandings in data collection and the likelihood that false information is provided. However, Power also points to a number of questions about the use of indigenous workers, in terms of both methodological and ethical issues. Because they do not have formal skills as researchers, they require considerable training in techniques of interviewing and data recording, as well as continuous supervision and debriefing in the course of fieldwork. Safeguards must also be provided to counter the opportunities and pressures to exploit their position.

*Estimating Hidden Populations*

A major difficulty in interpreting the findings of research on groups practicing high-risk behaviours is the lack of information on the population from which study samples are drawn. While official statistics or commissioned surveys may provide figures on the size of some populations, they cannot do so for hidden populations. This has prompted researchers to develop their own methods for estimating the size of such populations.

A particularly fruitful approach developed by researchers in the drugs field has entailed the adaptation of the capture/recapture method used by ecologists who are concerned with estimating the size of animal populations in the wild. Two or more partial and independent samples of drug users, contacted by different agencies, are compared and the overlap between them used as a multiplier for estimating the overall drug using population in a defined area (Hartnoll *et al.*, 1985; Frischer *et al.*, 1991). McKeganey, Barnard and Bloor have developed a further variant for fieldwork situations, based on the observation that, over the course of fieldwork, an increasing proportion of contacts are with people who have been contacted before (McKeganey *et al.*, 1990). In Chapter 7, 'How Many Prostitutes? Epidemiology out of Ethnography', they describe their study of Glasgow prostitutes where, combining ethnographic fieldwork with outreach service provision, they were able to keep a record of each woman contacted during each fieldwork period. On the basis of the 'capture history' for each woman, they were able to estimate the number of women working on the streets in Glasgow and the proportion who were HIV positive. However, they also note a number of methodological and ethical caveats to this approach in terms of the assumptions on which the estimates are based and the conflicts arising from the combination of research and service-provider roles (Barnard, 1992).

## Data Collection and Measurement: Reliability and Validity

Because of cultural taboos and legal restrictions on observing sexual behaviour directly, most studies rely on the respondents' own reports of their activities. While injecting drug use and needle sharing are more easily observed by researchers, the majority of studies again rely on respondents' own accounts of their behaviour. The accuracy of reports of such behaviours, which are intensely personal, heavily value laden and sometimes illegal, however, has inevitably been questioned. Embarrassment, shame or fear may lead to distortions in reports, while misunderstandings, difficulties in recall and impaired cognitive function due to HIV disease may also contribute to discrepancies between 'actual' and 'self-reported' behaviour. These problems introduce considerable uncertainty into the interpretation of survey data in social research on HIV/AIDS.

Nevertheless, evidence is accumulating that it is possible to collect reliable and valid data on sexual behaviour and injecting drug use. In relation to reliability, studies amongst a variety of populations have shown that respondents give *generally* consistent accounts of sexual behaviour at different points in time, although there is considerable variability in relation to specific areas of information (Coates *et al.*, 1986; Saltzman *et al.*, 1987; James *et al*, 1991; Hartgers, 1992). The question of reliability has become increasingly important as the focus of research has moved from behaviour to *behaviour change* (Stall *et al.*,

1990; Adib *et al.*, 1991; Hart *et al.*, 1992; McCusker *et al.*, 1992). The confounding effect of unreliable measures may go some way towards accounting for the difficulties which have been encountered in longitudinal studies in explaining and predicting behaviour change.

The validity of data collected in survey research is much more difficult to establish. Amongst drug users, accounts of injecting and needle sharing have been compared with a range of alternative measures, including urinalysis (Magura *et al.*, 1987), observation of puncture marks (Anthony *et al.*, 1991), and forensic testing of used injecting equipment (Gibson *et al.*, 1991). Power reviews some of the research evidence in Chapter 6. Moderately good agreement has been found between different types of measures which tends to support the validity of self-reports of drug injecting activities. Self-reports of sexual behaviour are more difficult to validate. Such observations as the consistency between men and women's self-reports of heterosexual behaviour (Johnson *et al.*, 1990) and the parallel declines amongst gay men in sexually transmitted disease (STD) rates and self-reports of unsafe sexual activities (Johnson and Gill, 1989) provide only indirect support for validity. More direct evidence is the degree of concordance between reports of sexual partners (Coates *et al*, 1988; Upchurch *et al.*, 1991; Seage *et al.*, 1992). Once again, however, there is considerable variability in relation to specific questions, particularly amongst the sexually most active (Coxon, 1988a) and amongst heavy substance users (Seage *et al.*, 1992). Since these individuals may play a disproportionately important role in the epidemic, this is a particular cause for concern.

Because of scepticism about the reliability and validity of self-reports of risk behaviours, researchers have paid particular attention to the methods they use to collect data. Considerable effort has been put into refining and improving traditional methods and considerable imagination into developing new ones.

### Questionnaires

The accuracy of data gathered by standardized questionnaire — which remains the most common method of data collection — is influenced both by the design of the schedule and by the way it is administered. Since the language used in questions is fundamental, considerable attention has been paid to the phrasing of questions on both sexual behaviour and injecting drug use (Spencer *et al.*, 1988). Terms like *sexual partner* (Day, 1990) and *pumping* (Smith *et al.*, 1992) have been shown to have variable meanings to respondents which could contribute to substantial measurement error, and the importance of defining terms clearly has been well established. Debate continues, however, about what type of terms should be used to describe sexual activities. Those who advocate vernacular terms argue that rapport and understanding are best established when words familiar to the respondents are used (Mays and Jackson, 1991). Those who advocate the use of more formal terms argue that lay terms vary between geographical, ethnic and subcultural groups and that respondents can be embarrassed or offended by the use of street language in interviews (Wellings *et al.*, 1990b). While allowing respondents themselves to choose the terms they prefer to use may appear to offer a helpful compromise, this may introduce further variability into questioning and be difficult to administer.

The most common mode of administering questionnaires is the face-to-face interview, sometimes incorporating a self-administered questionnaire as well. Face-to-face interviews allow some opportunity for clarification of questions but introduce the element of interviewer effects (Davies and Baker, 1987). While interviewer effects are generally seen as problematic, Power (Chapter 6) argues that the effect of indigenous interviewers is to enhance the quality of data collected by reassuring the respondents and reducing misunderstandings. Self-administered questionnaires eliminate the need to verbalize responses to sensitive questions and hence may elicit more candid answers. However, respondents may have difficulty in reading or understanding questionnaires and so leave questions unanswered, or they may simply lack the interest to complete them.

Of particular significance in AIDS-related research has been the increasing use of telephone interviews as an alternative to face-to-face interviews in community surveys of risk behaviours (McQueen *et al.*, 1987; Tielman, 1990; ASCF Principal Investigators, 1992; Stall *et al.*, 1992; Davis *et al.*, 1993). Telephone interviews combine the advantages of an interviewer for clarification and motivation with those of increased anonymity for reducing embarrassment or anxiety. Reservations about their use have turned largely on concerns that sexual behaviour and injecting drug use are different from other forms of behaviour and that those contacted will feel offended or threatened by questions from an unseen caller (McQueen, 1992). However, as the study reported by McQueen and Campostrini (Chapter 3) found, people are willing to answer questions on sensitive topics over the telephone, so long as safeguards are included to assure them of the legitimacy of the research and the confidentiality of their responses. The fact that socially stigmatized behaviour is reported in telephone interviews also suggests that this form of contact facilitates openness and honesty in responses. Comparisons between telephone and face-to-face interviews suggest that each has different strengths in collecting reliable and valid data and that neither is inherently superior (McQueen, 1989; ASCF Principal Investigators, 1992). Financial consideration are therefore likely to encourage the use of telephone interviews in the future.

### Diaries

Dissatisfaction with questionnaires has led to increased interest in diaries as a means of collecting information, particularly on sexual behaviour (Coxon, 1988b; Pickering, 1988; McLaws *et al.*, 1990; Pickering *et al.*, 1992). Diaries are designed to collect data on a daily basis over an extended period of time but there are wide variations as to what data are collected, how and by whom. Two contrasting ways of using diaries are described in Chapters 8 and 9. In his chapter, 'Diaries and Sexual Behaviour', Coxon compares diaries with other methods of data collection and sets out their advantages and disadvantages. Diaries are used to collect data in a naturalistic way, to minimize recall error and to provide data which can be directly quantified. They have a distinct advantage in the potential they offer for recording more detailed information than can generally be collected in retrospective interviews or questionnaires (Coxon *et al.*, 1992; Coxon *et al*, 1993). However, keeping a diary requires a substantial commitment, whether the diarist is recording his own or someone else's behaviour, and this is likely to lead to either a biased or a very small sample of completed diaries. In addition, diary data may be difficult to analyse: the very advantages which diaries offer for recording detailed descriptions may be seen as disadvantages when it comes to analysing them.

In advocating the use of sexual diaries, both Coxon (Chapter 8) and Pickering (Chapter 9) argue that the data collected through diaries are more reliable and valid than that collected in other ways. Coxon also illustrates the particular value of data collected by diary procedures by showing how they allow a more informative investigation of key research questions relating to the AIDS epidemic — for example, that of anal intercourse and risk. Because diarists record detailed, sequential descriptions of each sexual encounter over the course of the diary period, the data can be analysed to throw light on both the role of anal intercourse in the process of sexual interaction and on the proportion of acts that involve different degrees of risk.

### Observational Approaches

Direct observation of behaviour provides an alternative to respondents' reports as a method of data collection and has obvious advantages in relation to socially stigmatized or illegal behaviour (Power, 1989). By directly recording their own observations, researchers are able to avoid the potential biases of respondents' self-reports. Observational approaches range from the qualitative to the quantitative according to the researchers' involvement in the community or group they are concerned with. Participant observers become active members of the community and gather qualitative information from their own experience and from individuals who have come to accept them as part of the community (Bolton, 1992). Because of the nature of some risk behaviours for HIV/AIDS, fully participant observation is problematic and many researchers have adopted a non-participant observation approach, gathering information as accepted outsiders. These studies have provided a unique source of understanding of the experiences and practices of sex workers (Bloor *et al.*, 1990; McKeganey and Barnard, 1992) and injecting drug users (Grund *et al.*, 1991) in particular. Observations can also be made with minimal interaction with the community but such observations are usually limited to counting behaviours or their artefacts without exploring their meanings for those involved. Imaginative attempts to provide unobtrusive measures of risk behaviours have included counting the number of used condoms in selected motel rooms (Davey Smith *et al.*, 1991) and the number of marked needles returned to a needle exchange programme (Guydish *et al.*, 1991).

## Combined Methods

Observational methods have most frequently been used in conjunction with other methods of data gathering, particularly in ethnographic studies. In Chapter 6, Power suggests that, when indigenous interviewers are employed to conduct systematic interviews with individual drug users, full-time research staff should conduct participant observation and ethnographic research amongst the same drug-using networks. By understanding the social and cultural context of drug use, they are better able to interpret the responses given in the structured interviews and to assess the validity of the data they get.

In chapter 9, 'Social Science Methods Used in a Study of Prostitutes in the Gambia', Pickering describes another study which uses a variety of research methods, including standardized questionnaires, systematic observation, informal interviews, participant observation and economic monitoring. A key feature of anthropological research such as this is the relationship which develops between fieldworkers and the people they are studying as a result of the extended and multi-faceted interaction between them. Many of the research subjects thus become *informants*, giving the researchers access to more hidden areas of their lives and providing them with an insider's view of their social worlds. Traditionally, anthropologists have been more concerned with description and interpretation than with precise statistical analysis, concentrating on beliefs and meanings and extrapolating from observations of specific events to the underlying rules or norms which govern behaviour in a particular community (Herdt and Boxer, 1991; Kane, 1991; Magana, 1991; Parker, 1992). By contrast, Pickering's paper illustrates that there need not be a polarization between quantitative and qualitative research studies. In her study of female prostitutes in The Gambia, considerable quantitative data were collected using standardized questionnaires and observation sheets, in line with its initial epidemiological aims. Essential to the research, however, were the more informal, qualitative methods based on prolonged contact with prostitutes, their families, their clients and their boyfriends which produced crucial insights that lead to the modification of the standardized, quantitative methods of data collection and allowed the researchers to weigh up and interpret the meaning of the data gathered in this way.

*Focus Groups*

Focus groups, so called because group discussion is focused around a common task, are traditionally associated with market research more than with academic research. In relation to HIV/AIDS, they have been used in developing and piloting health education literature and media advertising (Warren, 1992; Cragg *et al.*, 1994) and in developing questionnaires for groups about whom researchers have limited knowledge.

However, the research potential of focus groups is much greater than that of establishing the acceptability and comprehensibility of representations or the themes and parameters for quantitative studies. In Chapter 10, 'Focus Groups: Method or Madness?', Kitzinger describes a study which makes particularly good use of the defining feature of focus groups — the interaction amongst members of the group — to explore research questions which are not easily investigated through more traditional methods of data collection. These include questions not only about the substance of their knowledge and opinions, but also about how people *use* knowledge or *form* and *change* opinions. Each small group of friends or colleagues is given a structured task to complete which generates a discussion of issues related to HIV/AIDS. The researcher can then observe directly the assumptions, moral values and models of thinking which the individual members bring to bear and the way they are used, challenged and confirmed or altered by the social processes within the group. Kitzinger contrasts focus-group data with that produced by questionnaires and interviews and argues that focus groups provide an ideal method for exploring communication issues and examining the cultural construction of experience.

## Evaluating Health Education Interventions

Perhaps the single most common type of empirical research in relation to the social aspects of HIV/AIDS has been evaluation research of health promotion interventions (Aggleton *et al.*, 1992; Paccaud *et al.*, 1992). Evaluations of one sort or another, albeit often limited and pragmatic, have been a part of most preventive interventions. Despite its long tradition in health promotion, however, evaluation research is inherently problematic (Aggleton, 1989; Tones *et al.*, 1990; Aggleton and Moody, 1992). Difficulties arise, for example, from tensions between the perceived needs of the health promotion activities and the demands of the evaluation, from conflicts between the differing aims of funders, managers, workers and recipients, or from clashes between differing interpretations of what constitutes evaluation, when it should be conducted and how its findings should be used. In relation to HIV/AIDS, the sensitivity of the subject matter, the vulnerability of the target groups and the urgency with which the interventions were planned and initiated has made evaluation even more problematic. Further difficulties have arisen from the need to find methods of evaluation which are appropriate to the more imaginative methods of health promotion which HIV/AIDS has encouraged.

One such imaginative method is that of *peer education*, a form of community health education which appeared to have the potential to influence individuals resistant to more traditional methods of health education. Because of its loosely defined aims and emergent activities, peer education is difficult to evaluate: evaluations run the risk of being seen as unfair, intrusive and irrelevant to those involved in the project or as vague, superficial and irrelevant to those ouside who fund it. In Chapter 11, 'Theory, Utility and Stakeholders', Ian Peers and Margaret Johnson describe the principles underlying their approach to evaluating a Community Youth Project on HIV/AIDS. In discussing their experience in applying these principles, they show how evaluation research has been taken forward by attempts to face the challenges presented by health promotion in the era of AIDS.

At the other end of the spectrum of health education, Kaye Wellings considers the difficulties involved in evaluating mass media campaigns in Chapter 12, 'Assessing AIDS Preventive Strategies in Europe'. Making a distinction between measuring the effects, effectiveness and efficacy of mass media campaigns, she discusses the particular difficulties associated with each level of evaluation in the context of campaigns which were mounted with varying degrees of urgency at varying stages of HIV/AIDS in different European countries. In identifying the sources of some of these difficulties and suggesting ways of dealing with them, she outlines a possible methodology for future efforts to evaluate national campaigns at a European-wide level.

### A Feminist Approach to Social Research on HIV/AIDS

In the penultimate chapter of this volume, Janet Holland and her colleagues in the Women, Risk and AIDS Project (WRAP) team give an overview of what it means to undertake a feminist study in relation to HIV/AIDS, in this case of young women's sexuality. It is one of the ironies of the AIDS epidemic that the need for information and insights relevant to its control has had some positive benefits for the development and wider acceptance of feminist analyses of social relations (e.g., Holland *et al.*, 1990; Richardson, 1990; Wilton and Aggleton, 1991). Nevertheless, the particular power of feminist analyses to illuminate the social processes, pressures and power relations which permeate heterosexual relationships and mediate against safer sex practices is now widely recognized.

What marks the feminist approach of the WRAP team as different from other approaches to young women's sexuality is the central role they give to gendered power relations as a structural feature of young women's sexual relationships and the value they place on women's lived experience of sexuality. In Chapter 13, 'Methodological Issues in Researching Young Women's Sexuality', they show how working within a framework of feminist assumptions affects all the aspects of research methods — the way questions are framed and the underlying explanatory models; how the population is defined and a sample recruited; methods of data collection and their ethical considerations as well as strategies for analysing and interpreting the data collected. The distinct contribution of this work is evident in the nature of the conclusions they are able to draw about the limited value of disseminating knowledge to reduce unsafe sexual practices, and the need for more fundamental changes in social and sexual relationships. In making explicit the links between theory, method, data and interpretation, the chapter also ties together the variety of themes which are considered throughout this volume.

### Looking Forward

In the last decade, social research on HIV/AIDS has made a major contribution to our understanding not only of behaviours associated with transmission of the virus, but also of fundamental aspects of social structure and social processes and of appropriate methods for investigating them. Its lasting significance, however, will depend to a great extent on how far the developments within HIV/AIDS research are taken up within the social sciences more generally.

It is this integration of HIV/AIDS social research with other fields of work in relevant disciplines that Mildred Blaxter urges in the concluding chapter of this volume, 'Towards the "Mainstreaming" of HIV/AIDS Research'. To situate the work described in the preceding chapters in a broader context, she speculates on the lessons it has for the sociology of health and illness more generally, making links with other areas of health behaviour which could benefit from the critical perspective developed in HIV/AIDS research and pointing to issues raised by HIV/AIDS research which deserve consideration in other contexts.

As Blaxter points out, HIV/AIDS has changed the rules for social research on health and illness. The urgency surrounding the epidemic has given rise to an openness to different disciplines and new approaches within the research community. New alliances have been formed, new perspectives have been legitimated. Not the least of the advances are those that have been made in relation to research methodology. The developments described in this volume represent the way social science has been taken forward by researchers who have confronted the new and exceptionally difficult challenges posed by research on the social dimensions of HIV/AIDS. The next set of challenges are in the 'mainstreaming' of these advances in social science more generally.

### References

ADIB, M., JOSEPH, J., OSTROW, D., TAL, M. and SCHWARTS, S. (1991) 'Relapse in sexual behaviour among homosexual men: a two-year follow-up from the Chical', MACS/CCS, *AIDS*, 5, pp. 757-60.

AGGLETON, P. (1989) 'Evaluating health education about AIDS', in AGGLETON, P. HART, G. and DAVIES, P. (Eds) *AIDS: Social Representations, Social Practices*, London: Falmer Press.

AGGLETON, P. and MOODY, D. (1992) 'Monitoring and evaluating HIV/AIDS health education and health promotion', in AGGLETON, P., YOUNG, A., MOODY, D., KAPILA, M. and PYE, M. (Eds) *Does It Work? Perspectives on the Evaluation of HIV/AIDS Health Promotion*, London: Health Education Authority.

AGGLETON, P., YOUNG, A., MOODY, D., KAPILA, M. and PYE, M. (Eds) (1992) *Does It Work? Perspectives on the Evaluation of HIV/AIDS Health Promotion*, London: Health Education Authority.

AJZEN, I. and FISHBEIN, M. (1980) *Understanding Attitudes and Predicting Social Behaviour*, Englewood Cliffs, NJ: Prentice-Hall.

ALBRECHT, G. (1989) 'The intelligent design of AIDS research strategies', in SECHREST, L., FREEMAN, H. and MULLEY, A. (Eds), *Health Services Research Methodology: A Focus on AIDS*, Washington, DC: NCHSR.

ANKRAH, M. (1989) 'AIDS: Methodological problems in studying its prevention and spread', *Social Science and Medicine*, 29, pp. 265–76.

ANTHONY, J., VLAHOV, D., CELENTANO, D., MENON, A., MARGOLICK, J., COHN, S., NELSON, K. and POLK, B. (1991) 'Self-report interview data for a study of HIV-1 infection among intravenous drug users: Description of methods and preliminary evidence on validity', *Journal of Drug Issues*, 21, pp. 739–57.

ASCF Principal Investigators and their Associates (1992) 'Analysis of sexual behaviour in France (ACSF). A comparison between two modes of investigation: telephone survey and face-to-face survey', *AIDS*, 6, pp. 315–23.

BANDURA, M. (1977) 'Self-Efficacy: Toward a unifying theory of behavioural change', *Psychological Review*, 84, pp. 191–215.

BARNARD, M. (1992) 'Working in the dark: Researching female prostitution', in *Women's Health Matters*, ROBERTS, H. (Ed.) London: Routledge.

BECKER, M. (1974) 'The health belief model and personal health behaviour', *Health Education Monographs*, 2, pp. 220–43.

BENNETT, G., CHAPMAN, S. and BRAY, F. (1989) 'Sexual practices and 'beats': AIDS-related sexual practices in a sample of homosexual and bisexual men in the western suburbs of Sydney', *Medical Journal of Australia*, 151, pp. 314–18.

BLOOR, M., MCKEGANEY, N. and BARNARD, M. (1990) 'An ethnographic study of HIV-related risk practices among Glasgow rent boys and their clients: Report of a pilot study', *AIDS Care*, 2, pp. 17–24.

BOLTON, R. (1992) 'Mapping terra incognita: Sex research for AIDS prevention — An urgent agenda for the 1990s', in HERDT, G., LINDENBAUM, S. (Eds) *The Time of AIDS: Social Analysis, Theory and Method*, London: Sage.

BOULTON, M. (1993) 'Methodological issues in HIV/AIDS social research: Recent debates, recent developments', *AIDS* 7 (suppl 1), pp. S249–S255.

BOWIE, C. and FORD, N. (1989) 'Sexual behaviour of young people and the risk of HIV infection', *Journal of Epidemiology and Community Health*, 43, pp. 61–5.

CATANIA, J., GIBSON, D., CHITWOOD, D. and COATES, T. (1990a) 'Methodological problems in AIDS behavioural research: Influences on measurement error and participation bias in studies of sexual behaviour', *Psychological Bulletin*, 108, pp. 339–62.

CATANIA, J., KEGELES, S. and COATES, T. (1990b) 'Towards an understanding of risk behaviour: an AIDS risk reduction model (ARRM)', *Health Education Quarterly*, 17, pp. 53–72.

COATES, R., SOSKOLNE, C. and CALZAVARA, L. (1986) 'The reliability of sexual histories in AIDS-related research: evaluation of an interview-administered questionnaire', *Canadian Journal of Public Health*, 17, pp. 343–8.

COATES, R., CALZAVARA, L., SOSKOLNE, C., READ, S., FANNING, M., SHEPHERD, F., LKEIN, M. and JOHNSON, K. (1988) 'Validity of sexual histories in a prospective study of male sexual contacts of men with AIDS or an AIDS-related condition', *American Journal of Epidemiology*, 128, pp. 719-28.

COLEMAN, R. and CURTIS, D. (1988) 'Distribution of risk behaviour for HIV infection amongst intravenous drug users, *British Journal of Addiction*, 83, pp. 1331-4.

CONNELL, R., CRAWFORD, J., KIPPAX, S., DOWSETT, G., BAXTER, D., WATSON, L. and BERG, R. (1989) 'Facing the epidemic: Changes in the sexual lives of gay and bisexual men in Australia and their implications for AIDS prevention strategies', *Social Problems*, 36, pp. 384-402.

COXON, A. (1988a) 'The numbers game: Gay lifestyles, epidemiology and social science', in AGGLETON, P. and HOMANS, H. (Eds) *Social Aspects of AIDS*, London: Falmer Press.

COXON, T. (1988b) 'Something sensational... The sexual diary as a tool for mapping detailed sexual behaviour', *Sociological Review*, 36, pp. 353-67.

COXON, A., COXON, H., WEATHERBURN, P., HUNT, A., HICKSON, F., DAVIES, P. and MCMANUS, T. (1993) 'Sex role separation in sexual diaries of homosexual men', *AIDS*, 7, pp. 877-82.

COXON, A., DAVIES, P., HUNT, A., WEATHERBURN, P., MCMANUS, T. and REES, C. (1992) 'The structure of sexual behaviour', *The Journal of Sex Research*, 29, pp. 61-83.

CRAGG, A., HAINGE, M., TAYLOR, C. and PORTER, T. (1994) 'Safer Sex and Sexual Health; Understanding Young People', in GLANZ, A., MCVEY, D. and GLASS, R. (Eds) *Talking About It: Sexually Active Young People and HIV*, London: Health Education Authority.

DAVEY SMITH, G., LOW, N., GORTER, A., MIRANDA, E. and ARAUZ, R. (1991) 'Condom use in motels in Managua: An opportunity for AIDS prevention', *35th Annual Scientific Meeting of the Society for Social Medicine*, Southampton, September 1991.

DAVIES, J. and BAKER, R. (1987) 'The impact of self-presentation and interviewer bias effects on self-reported heroin use', *British Journal of Addiction*, 82, pp. 907-12.

DAVIES, P., HICKSON, F., WEATHERBURN, P. and HUNT, A. (1993) *Sex, Gay Men and AIDS*, London: Falmer Press.

DAVIES, P., YEE, R. L., CHETWYND, J. and NATASHA MCMILLAN (1993) 'The New Zealand Partner Relations Survey: Methodological results of a national telephone survey', *AIDS*, 7, pp. 1509-16.

DAY, S. (1990) 'Anthropological perspectives on sexually transmitted diseases', in JOB-SPIRA, N., SPENCER, B., MOALTTI, J. and BOUVET, E. (Eds) *Saute Publique et Maladies a Transmission Sexuelle*, Paris: John Libbey Eurotext.

DAY, S. and WARD, H. (1990) 'The Praed Street project: A cohort of prostitute women in London', in PLANT, M. (Ed.) *AIDS, Drugs and Prostitution*, London: Routledge.

DONOGHOE, M., STIMSON, G., DOLAN, K. and ALLDRITT, L. (1989) 'Changes in HIV risk behaviours in clients of syringe-exchange schemes in England and Scotland', *AIDS*, 3, pp. 267-72.

EVANS, B., MCLEAN, K., DAWSON, S., TEECE, S., BOND, R., MACRAE, K. and THORP, R. (1989) 'Trends in sexual behaviour and risk factors for HIV infection among homosexual men', *British Medical Journal*, 298, pp. 215-18.

FIFE-SCHAW, C., and BREAKWELL, G. (1992) 'Estimating sexual behaviour parameters in the light of AIDS: a review of recent UK studies of young people', *AIDS Care*, 4, pp. 187-201.

FITZPATRICK, R., BOULTON, M. and HART, G. (1989) 'Gay men's sexual behaviour in response to AIDS: Insights and problems', in AGGLETON, P., HART, G. and DAVIES, P. (Eds), *AIDS: Social Representations, Social Practices*, London: Falmer Press.

FITZPATRICK, R., MCLEAN, J., DAWSON, J., BOULTON, M. and HART, G. (1990a) 'Factors influencing condom use in a sample of homosexually active men', *Genitourinary Medicine*, 66, pp. 346–50.

FITZPATRICK, R., MCLEAN, J., BOULTON, M., HART, G. and DAWSON, J. (1990b) 'Variation in sexual behaviour in gay men', in AGGLETON, P., DAVIES, P. and HART, G. (Eds) *AIDS: Individual, Cultural and Policy Dimensions*, London: Falmer Press.

FRISCHER, M., BLOOR, M., FINLAY, A., GOLDBERG, D., GREEN, S., HAW, S., MCKEGANEY, N. and PLATT, S. (1991) 'A new method for estimating prevalence of injecting drug use in an urban population: results from a Scottish city', *International Journal of Epidemiology*, 20, pp. 997–1000.

GIBSON, D., GUYDISH, J., WRAXAL, B., BLAKE, E. and CLARK, G. (1991) 'Using forensic techniques to verify self-reports of needle sharing', *AIDS*, 5, pp. 1149–50.

GRUND, J-P., KAPLAN, C. and ADRIAANS, N. (1991) 'Needle sharing in the Netherlands: An ethnographic analysis', *American Journal of Public Health*, 81, pp. 1602–7.

GUYDISH, J., CLARK, G., GARCIA, D., DOWNING, M., CASE, P. and SORENSEN, J. (1991) 'Evaluating needle exchange: Do distributed needles come back?', *American Journal of Public Health*, 81, pp. 617–19.

HART, G., BOULTON, M., FITZPATRICK, R., MCLEAN, J. and DAWSON, J. (1992) '"Relapse" to unsafe sexual behaviour among gay men: A critique of recent behavioural HIV/AIDS research', *Sociology of Health and Illness*, 14, pp. 216–32.

HARTGERS, C. (1992) *HIV Risk Behaviour Among Injecting Drug Users in Amsterdam*. Amsterdam: Rodopi.

HARTNOLL, R., LEWIS, R., MITCHESON, M. and BRYER, S. (1985) 'Estimating the prevalence of opioid dependence', *Lancet*, i, pp. 203–5.

HAW, S., FRISCHER, M., DONOGHOE, M., GREEN, S., CROSSIER, A., HUNTER, G., FINLAY, A., COVELL, R., ETTMORE, B., BLOOR, M., STEPHENS, S., GOLDBERG, D., STIMSON, G., MCKEGANEY, N., PLATT, S., TAYLOR, A., FOLLET, E. and PARRY, J. (1992) 'The importance of multisite sampling in determining the prevalence of HIV among drug injectors in Glasgow and London', *AIDS*, 6, pp. 517–18.

HAYS, R., KEGELES, S. and COATES, T. (1990) 'High HIV risk-taking among young gay men', *AIDS*, 4, pp. 901–7.

HERDT, G. and BOXER, A. (1991) 'Ethnographic issues in the study of AIDS', *The Journal of Sex Research*, 28, pp. 171–87.

HOLLAND, J., RAMAZANOGLU, C. and SCOTT, S. (1990) 'AIDS: From panic stations to power relations', *Sociology*, 24, pp. 499–518.

JAMES, N., BIGNELL, C. and GILLIES, P. (1991) 'The reliability of self-reported sexual behaviour', *AIDS*, 5, pp. 333–6.

JOHNSON, A. and GILL, N. (1989) 'Evidence for recent changes in sexual behaviour in homosexual men in England and Wales', *Philosophical Transactions of the Royal Society*, B325, pp. 153–61.

JOHNSON, A., WADSWORTH, J., FIELD, J., WELLINGS, K. and ANDERSON, R. (1990) 'Surveying sexual attitudes', *Nature*, 343, p. 109.

JOHNSON, A., WADSWORTH, J., WELLINGS, K., BRADSHAW, S. and FIELD, J. (1992) 'Sexual lifestyles and HIV risk', *Nature*, 360, pp. 410–12.

JOSEPH, J., MONTGOMERY, S., EMMONS, C., KESSLER, R., OSTROW, D., WORTMAN, C., O'BRIEN, K., ELLER, M. and ESHLEMAN, S. (1987) 'Magnitude and determinants of behaviour risk reduction: longitudinal analysis of a cohort at risk for AIDS', *Psychology and Health*, 1, pp. 73–96.

KANE, S. (1991) 'HIV, heroin and heterosexual relations', *Social Science and Medicine*, 32, pp. 1037–50.

KAPLAN, H. (1989) 'Methodological problems in the study of psychosocial influences on the AIDS process', *Social Science and Medicine*, 29, pp. 277–92.

KIPPAX, S., CRAWFORD, J., DAVIS, M., RODDEN, P. and DOWSETT, G. (1993) 'Sustaining safe sex: A longitudinal study of a sample of homosexual men', *AIDS*, 7, pp. 257–63.

KLEE, H., FAUGIER, J., HAYS, C., BOULTON, T. and MORRIS, J. (1990) 'Factors associated with risk behaviour among injecting drug users', *AIDS Care*, 2, pp. 133–45.

KOTARBA, J. and LANG, N. (1986) 'Gay lifestyles change and AIDS: Preventive health care'. In FELDMAN, D. and JOHNSON, T. (Eds) *The Social Dimensions of AIDS: Method and Theory*, New York, Praeger.

LAMPINEN, T., JOO, E., SEWERYN, S., HERSHOW, R. and WIEBEL, W. (1992) 'HIV seropositivity in community recruited and drug treatment samples of injecting samples of injecting drug users', *AIDS*, 6, pp. 123–6.

MCCUSKER, J., STODDARD, A., MCDONALD, M., ZAPKA, J. and MAYER, K. (1992) 'Maintenance of behavioural change in a cohort of homosexually active men', *AIDS*, 6, pp. 861–8.

MCKEGANEY, N. and BARNARD, M. (1992) *AIDS, Drugs and Sexual Risk: Lives in the Balance*, Buckingham: Open University Press.

MCKEGANEY, N., BARNARD, M., BLOOR, M. and LEYLAND, A. (1990) 'Injecting drug use and female street-working prostitution in Glasgow', *AIDS*, 4, pp. 1153–5.

MCKUSICK, L., COATES, T., MORIN, S., POLLACK, L. and HOFF, C. (1990) 'Longitudinal predictors of reductions in unprotected anal intercourse among gay men in San Francisco: The AIDS Behavioural Research Project', *American Journal of Public Health*, 80, pp. 978–83.

MCLAWS, M., OLDENBURG, B., ROSS, M. and COOPER, D. (1990) 'Sexual behaviour in AIDS-related research: Reliability and validity of recall and diary measures', *The Journal of Sex Research 1990*, 27, pp. 265–81.

MCQUEEN, D., ROBERTSON, B. and SMITH, R. (1987) *Computer Assisted Telephone Interviewing (CATI) - Reference Manual*, Edinburgh: Research Unit on Health and Behaviour Change.

MCQUEEN, D. (1989) 'Comparison of results of personal interview and telephone surveys of behaviour related to risk of AIDS: Advantages of telephone tehniques', in FOWLER, F. (ed.) *Health Survey Research Methods*, Rockville, MD: Department of Health & Human Services, pp. 247–52. [publication no. (PHS) 89-3447].

MCQUEEN, D. (1992) 'Understanding sexual behaviour', *AIDS*, 6, pp. 329–30.

MAGANA, R. (1991) 'Sex, drugs and HIV: An ethnographic approach', *Social Science and Medicine*, 33, pp. 5–9.

MAGURA, S., GOLDSMITH, D., CASRIEL, C., GOLDSTEIN, P. and LIPTON, D. (1987) 'The validity of methadone clients' self-reported drug use', *International Journal of the Addictions*, 22, pp. 727–49.

MAYS, V. and JACKSON, J. (1991) 'AIDS survey methodology with black Americans', *Social Science and Medicine*, 33, pp. 47–54.

MYERS, T., ROW, C., TUDIVER, G., KURTZ, R., JACKSON, E., ORR, K. and BULLOCK, S. (1992) 'HIV, substance use and related behaviour of gay and bisexual men: An examination of the talking sex project cohort', *British Journal of Addiction*, 87, pp. 207–14.

MILLER, H., TURNER, C. and MOSES, L. (1990) *AIDS: The Second Decade*, Washington, DC: National Academy Press.

MORGAN THOMAS, R., PLANT, M., PLANT, M. and SALES, D. (1989) 'Risk of AIDS among workers in the sex industry: some initial results from a Scottish study', *British Medical Journal*, 299, pp. 148–49.

OSTROW, D., WHITAKER, R., FRASIER, K., COHEN, C., WAN, J., FRANK, C. and
FISHER, E. (1991) 'Racial differences in social support and mental health in men
with HIV infection: a pilot study', *AIDS Care*, 3, pp. 55-62.

PACCAUD, F., VADER, J. and GUTZWILLER, F. (1992) *Assessing AIDS Prevention*, Basel:
Birkhauser Verlag.

PARKER, R. (1992) 'Sexual diversity, cultural analysis and AIDS education in Brazil', in
HERDT, G. and LINDENBAUM, S. (Eds) *The Time of AIDS: Social analysis, theory and
method*, London: Sage.

PICKERING, H. (1988) 'Asking questions on sexual behaviour . . . testing methods from
the social sciences', *Health Policy Planning*, 3, pp. 237-244.

PICKERING, H., TODD, J., DUNN, D., PEPIN, J. and WILKINS, A. (1992) 'Prostitutes and
their clients: A Gambian Survey', *Social Science and Medicine*, 34, pp. 75-88.

POWER, K., MARKOVA, ROWLANDS, A., MCKEE, K., ANSLWO, P., KILFEDDER, C.
(1992) 'Intravenous drug use and HIV transmission amongst inmates of Scottish
prisons', *British Journal of Addiction*, 87, pp. 35-45.

POWER, R. (1989) 'Participant observation and its place in the study of illicit drug abuse',
*British Journal of Addiction*, 84, pp. 43-52.

POWER, R., DALE, A. and JONES, S. (1991) 'Towards a process evaluation model for
community-based initiatives aimed at preventing the spread of HIV amongst
injecting drug users', *AIDS Care*, 3, pp. 123-35.

POWER, R., HARTNOLL, R. and CHALMERS, C. (1992) 'Help-seeking amongst illicit
drug users: Some differences between a treatment and non-treatment sample',
*International Journal of the Addictions*, 27, pp. 889-906.

RICHARDSON, C., ANCELL-PARK, R. and PAPAEVANGELOU, G., for the European
Community Study Group on HIV in Injecting Drug Users (1993) 'Factors
associated with HIV seropositivity in European injecting drug users', *AIDS*, 7,
pp. 1485-91.

RICHARDSON, D. (1990) 'AIDS education and women: Sexual and reproductive issues',
in AGGLETON, P., DAVIES, P. and HART, G. (Eds) *AIDS: Individual, Cultural and
Policy Dimensions*, London: Falmer.

ROBERTSON, J., SKIDMORE, C. and ROBERTS, J. (1988) 'HIV infection in intravenous
drug users: a follow-up study indicating changes in risk-taking behaviour', *British
Journal of Addiction*, 83, pp. 387-91.

SALTZMAN, S., STODDARD, A., MCCUSKER, J., MOON, M. and MAYER, K. (1987)
'Reliability of self-reported sexual behaviour risk factors for HIV infection in
homosexual men', *Public Health Reports*, 102, pp. 692-7.

SAMUELS, J., VLAHOV, D., ANTHONY, J. and CHAISSON, R. (1992) 'Measurement of
HIV risk behaviours among intravenous drug users', *British Journal of Addiction*, 87,
pp. 417-28.

SCHOEPF, B. (1991) 'Ethical, methodological and political issues of AIDS research in
Central Africa', *Social Science and Medicine*, 33, pp. 749-63.

SEAGE, G., MAYER, K., HORSBURGH, R., CAI, B. and LAMB, G. (1992) 'Corroboration
of sexual histories among male homosexual couples', *American Journal of
Epidemiology*, 135, pp. 79-84.

SMITH, A., VLAHOV, D., MENON, A. and ANTHONY, J. (1992) 'Terminology for drug
injection practices among intravenous drug users in Baltimore', *International Journal
of the Addictions*, 27, pp. 435-53.

SPENCER, L., FAULKNER, A. and KEEGAN, J. (1988) *Talking About Sex*, London: Social
and Community Planning Research.

STANDING, H. (1992) 'AIDS: Conceptual and methodological issues in researching sexual
behaviour in sub-Saharan Africa', *Social Science and Medicine*, 34, pp. 475-83.

STALL, R., BARRETT, D., BYE, L., CATANIA, J., FRUTCHEY, C., HENNE, J., LEMP, G.
and PAUL, J. (1992) 'A comparison of younger and older gay men's HIV risk-

taking behaviours: The communication technologies 1989 cross-sectional survey', *Journal of Acquired Immune Deficiency Syndromes*, 5, pp. 682–7.

STALL, R., EKSTRAND, M., POLLACK, L., MCKUSICK, L. and COATES, T. (1990) 'Relapse from safer sex: The next challenge for AIDS prevention efforts', *Journal of Acquired Immune Deficiency Syndromes*, 3, pp. 1181–87.

SUNDET, J., MAGNUS, P., KVALEM, I. and BAKKETEIG, L. (1990) 'Self-administered anonymous questionnaires in sexual behaviour research: the Norwegian experience', in HUBERT, M. (ed.) *Sexual Behaviour and Risks of HIV Infection*, Bruxelles: Facultes universitaires Saint-Louis.

TIELMAN, R. (1990) 'Telephone surveys in comparison with other methods in psycho-social AIDS research', in HUBERT, M. (ed.) *Sexual Behaviour and Risks of HIV Infection*, Bruxelles: Facultes universitaires Saint-Louis.

TONES, K., TILFORD, S. and KEELEY ROBINSON, Y. (1990) *Health Education: Effectiveness and Efficiency*, London: Chapman and Hall.

UITENBROEK, D. and MCQUEEN, D. (1992) 'Changing patterns in reported sexual practices in the population: Multiple partners and condom use', *AIDS*, 6, pp. 587–92.

UPCHURCH, D., WEISMAN, C., SHEPHER, M., BROOKMEYER, R., FOX, R., CELENTANO, D., COLLETTA, L. and HOOK, E. (1991) 'Interpartner reliability of reporting of recent sexual behaviours', *American Journal of Epidemiology*, 134, pp. 1159–65.

WADSWORTH, J. and JOHNSON, A. (1991) 'Editorial: Measuring sexual behaviour', *Journal of the Royal Statistical Society*, 154, pp. 367–70.

WARD, H., DAY, S., MEZZONE, J., DUNLOP, L., DONEGAN, C., FARRAR, S., WHITAKER, L., HARRIS, J. and MILLER, D. (1993) 'Prostitution and risk of HIV: Female prostitutes in London', *British Medical Journal*, 307, pp. 356–8.

WARREN, M. (1992) 'Another day, another debrief: The use and assessment of qualitative research', *Journal of the Market Research Society*, 33.

WATTERS, J. and BIERNACKI, P. (1989) 'Targeted sampling: Options for the study of hidden population', *Social Problems*, 36, pp. 416–30.

WELLINGS, K., FIELD, J., WADSWORTH, J., JOHNSON, A., ANDERSON, R. and BRADSHAW, S. (1990a) 'Sexual lifestyles under scrutiny', *Nature*, 348, pp. 276–8.

WELLINGS, K., FIELD, J., JOHNSON, A., WADSWORTH, J. and BRADSHAW, S. (1990b) 'Notes on the design and construction of a national survey of sexual attitudes and lifestyles', in HUBERT, M. (ed.) *Sexual Behaviour and Risks of HIV Infection*, Bruxelles: Facultes universitaires Saint-Louis.

WILTON, T. and AGGLETON, P. (1991) 'Condoms, coercion and control: Heterosexuality and the limits to HIV/AIDS education', in AGGLETON, P., HART, G. and DAVIES, P. (Eds) *AIDS: Responses, Interventions and Care*, London: Falmer Press.

*Research Design, Theoretical Frameworks and the Research Question*

*Chapter 2*

---

# Using Longitudinal Cohort-Sequential Designs to Study Changes in Sexual Behaviour

---

*Glynis M. Breakwell and Chris R. Fife-Schaw*

This chapter describes the advantages and disadvantages associated with using a longitudinal cohort-sequential research design to study age-related changes in sexual behaviour. The general arguments are illustrated with reference to a study of sexual activities, beliefs and attitudes amongst 16-21-year-olds in the UK which employed such a design (Breakwell and Fife-Schaw, 1992). In this research we were concerned to monitor changes in attitudes, beliefs and behaviours in the light of rapidly changing representations of HIV/AIDS in the media. In order to separate the effects of historical events from developmental changes the longitudinal cohort-sequential design seemed to be the most appropriate research strategy.

## What is a Longitudinal Cohort Sequential Design?

Researchers whose objective is to identify and explain changes in behaviour which are age-related have a choice of three main classes of data collection strategy: longitudinal, cross-sectional or sequential. A longitudinal design involves data being collected from the same sample of individuals on at least two occasions; the interval between data collections and the number of data collections varies greatly in longitudinal studies. So, for instance, a longitudinal design might involve surveying a sample of 16-year-olds initially in 1989 and recontacting the same individuals in 1990 and again in 1991. This would allow the researchers to establish changes in reported behaviour over time as the sample aged. A cross-sectional design involves eliciting information from a number of different age cohorts at a single time. The term age cohort refers to the total population of individuals born at approximately the same time which is usually taken to mean in the same calendar year. In the cross-sectional design, both the number of cohorts involved and the age differences between them vary considerably across studies. An example of a cross-sectional design might entail surveying samples of 16-year-olds, 17-year-olds and 18-year-olds in 1989. This permits age-related differences in behaviour to be gauged. A sequential design will choose samples of a specific age cohort but drawn at different times. The periodicity in sequential data gathering varies across studies. A simple sequential design might involve sampling the 16-year-old cohort of 1989, the 16-year-old cohort of 1990, and the 16-year-old cohort of 1991. This type of design is targeted at revealing whether the behaviour of a particular age group is affected by factors which are associated with their specific socio-historical era.

Figure 2.1 depicts the three types of design. The letters A–F symbolise six different age cohorts from 16-21-years-old. The subscripts reflect the age of each cohort at the various dates of data collection. Thus the diagram indicates that cohorts A–D are studied at three annual intervals. Cohort E is studied at two and cohort F only one time. Any column in the figure represents the structure of a cross-sectional design; any row (except the first) represents a longitudinal design; and a diagonal drawn from left to right upwards represents a sequential design.

| 1989 | 1990 | 1991 |
|---|---|---|
| | | $F_{16}$ |
| | $E_{16}$ | $E_{17}$ |
| $D_{16}$ | $D_{17}$ | $D_{18}$ |
| $C_{17}$ | $C_{18}$ | $C_{19}$ |
| $B_{18}$ | $B_{19}$ | $B_{20}$ |
| $A_{19}$ | $A_{20}$ | $A_{21}$ |

A–F represent Age Cohorts.
Subscript numbers represent actual age at data collection.

1  Any column represents a cross-sectional design.
2  Any row (except the first) represents a longitudinal design.
3  Top diagonal rising left to right represents a sequential design.

*Figure 2.1:   The Longitudinal Cohort-Sequential Design Used in the Survey of Young People.*

When studying age-related patterns in behaviour there are always three factors which could possibly explain the observed relationships: development tied to the ageing of the individual; characteristics associated with the particular age cohorts studied; and impact of the specific time of measurement. Time of measurement is the term suggested by Schaie (1965) to refer to the set of pressures upon the individual generated by the socio-environmental context at the point data is collected. The difficulty facing researchers interested in explained age-related changes in behaviour lies in establishing which of these three factors is the source of change. The strategy adopted by most researchers is to keep one of the factors constant. For instance, the longitudinal design keeps the cohort constant. The cross-sectional design keeps the time of measurement constant. The sequential design keeps the chronological age constant. Of course, this means that explanation of any observed age-related trend in behaviour remains problematic since these designs always leave two of the three explanatory factors to vary simultaneously. Irrespective of which of these three designs is adopted, two explanatory factors will be confounded. This represents the major methodological drawback in using such relatively simple designs. There is a secondary problem. By holding one factor constant, the design obviously rules out the possibility of exploring the effects of that factor in interaction with the others. Yet, in virtually all complex systems of behaviour, one would expect interaction effects between developmental, cohort and time of measurement factors. The solution to this fundamental methodological problem has been to integrate the three design types in what is known as a longitudinal cohort-sequential design.

The longitudinal cohort-sequential design (LCSD) requires all of the components of data-collection and sampling outlined in Figure 2.1. It combines the longitudinal follow-up of a series of cohorts first sampled simultaneously as in a cross-sectional study with the sequential addition of new cohorts of the same ages to the study at each subsequent data collection point. In fact, Figure 2.2 better represents the pure LCSD since it indicates the multiple samples needed from each cohort.

| 1989 | 1990 | 1991 |
|---|---|---|
| | | $F_{16x}$ |
| | $E_{16x}$ | $E_{17x}$ |
| | | $E_{17y}$ |
| $D_{16x}$ | $D_{17x}$ | $D_{18x}$ |
| | $D_{17y}$ | $D_{18z}$ |
| $C_{17x}$ | $C_{18x}$ | $C_{19x}$ |
| | $C_{18y}$ | $C_{19z}$ |
| $B_{18x}$ | $B_{19x}$ | $B_{20x}$ |
| | $B_{19y}$ | $B_{20z}$ |
| $A_{19x}$ | $A_{20x}$ | $A_{21x}$ |
| | $A_{20y}$ | $A_{21z}$ |

A–F represent Age Cohorts.
Subscript numbers represent actual age at data collection.

Subscript $x$ = first sample drawn from a cohort.
Subscript $y$ = second sample from a cohort.
Subscript $z$ = third sample drawn from a cohort.

*Figure 2.2: The Pure Form of the Longitudinal Cohort-Sequential Design.*

To avoid the possible biases introduced by comparing samples studied longitudinally with those studied only once when generating sequential comparisons, the full LCSD requires a new sample to be drawn from each cohort at each data point in addition to the sample established initially. Such a sampling strategy also has the advantage of allowing the researcher to estimate any differential effects across cohorts of the response biases introduced by repeated contacts with the respondents required by the longitudinal follow-up. However, it is rare indeed for such a full LCSD to be used. It is more frequently the case that a partial LCSD is used such as that depicted in Figure 2.1 where the only totally comparable sequential samples are drawn for one age group (in the figure, 16-year-olds). The other sequential comparisons in such a partial LCSD depend upon using samples which have been studied on one or more prior occasions and may consequently have been influenced by differential drop-out or by the growth of research fatigue and/or research sophistication during the period of the study. This curtailment of the LCSD certainly weakens the strength of any arguments which can be made about the influence of socio-historical context upon behavioural change. Yet, even in its abridged form, the LCSD is the best way to explore complex interactions between developmental, cohort and time of measurement effects.

## Methodological Issues using a Longitudinal Cohort-Sequential Design to Study Sexual Behaviour

The research used here to illustrate some of the issues arising when using a partial LCSD to study sexual behaviour was conducted as part of the Economic and Social Research Council (ESRC) Research Initiative on the Social and Behavioural Consequences of HIV/AIDS. The project started in 1989 with data collected by postal questionnaire from four cohorts (aged 16 through 19 years). These were followed annually for two further data collections. A new 16-year-old cohort sample was introduced in 1990 and followed up in 1991. A further new 16-year-old cohort was added in 1991. The design directly parallels that illustrated in Figure 2.1. Sampling was done randomly from lists made available by the local education authorities of individuals in the target age cohorts who had attended state sector schools. The details of the sample structure, which was stratified by sex and geographical area, are given elsewhere (Breakwell and Fife-Schaw, 1992). It is not our intention to go into any detail concerning the findings from this study. Our object is to use the study to exemplify some of the questions which must be addressed when using LCSD. It would be fair to say that it is only after completing the study that we became fully aware of how significant some of these questions can be.

### Choosing the Age Groups

An LCSD requires careful choice of age groups. The choice has three related components: the age range, the number of age cohorts, and the age difference between cohorts. The choice should obviously be determined by preconceptions, derived either empirically or theoretically, about the existence of age-related changes in behaviour. If theory or past research indicates that there are critical periods when the target behaviour pattern changes it would be foolish to ignore this in choosing an age-range for the LCSD. It should be added, however, that in any research which touches upon socially significant behaviours there are political and pragmatic determinants of choice of age groups in an LCSD. In the case of sexual behaviour, late adolescence is traditionally recognized by researchers as a time of significant change. To target 16–21 year olds would seem useful. It might have been even more useful to include younger age groups given the dearth of information available about them. However, doubts about the viability and morality of asking detailed questions about sexual attitudes and activities of individuals below the age of legal sexual consent were raised by the LEAs who were providing our sampling frame and by the research sponsors.

Within any chosen age range, the number of age cohorts studied, and consequently the age difference between them, should depend upon the expected rate of change in behaviour and the reasons for this change. It may be enough for certain purposes to have quite large age differences between the cohorts. For example, if the object was to plot changes in sexual courtship patterns over the lifespan, it might be enough to select cohorts at five-year intervals (15-, 20-, 25-year-olds, etc.). The point to remember in choosing the interval is that, if the study is to include a sequential component, the gap must not be so long that the overlap of longitudinal and sequential samples becomes impractical because it requires the study to continue for too many years. With a five-year gap in age cohorts, it would require a five-year study to generate a single overlap between sequential and longitudinal components of the study.

In our study we were explicitly concerned with young people who were developing their adult sexual identities and sexual careers. For pragmatic reasons we could not survey people under the legal age of consent for heterosexual intercourse, so our lower age limit was set at sixteen. The upper age limit was set at 21–22 since we were primarily concerned with the early phases of the sexual career. By 21, most people have at least begun sexual relationships. We therefore decided to draw samples from cohorts reflecting school-year group (i.e. 16–17, 17–18, 18–19 and 19–20-year-olds). This allowed the introduction of two 'new' 16–17-year-old cohorts within the period of the research.

### Periodicity of Data Collection

Periodicity of data collection refers to the frequency with which information is gathered. There is no reason why data should be collected only at annual intervals. The iteration of data collection can be much more rapid if the behaviours monitored are expected to change quickly; it can be slower, if behaviour fluctuations are rare. In designing a LCSD study there is always the problem of establishing before the study begins the likely rate of change in the target behaviour. This highlights the need when designing a LCSD for extensive preliminary pilot studies to ascertain the feasibility of monitoring change effectively.

The periodicity of data collection will also be influenced by the types of explanatory model to be used. Models which explain changes in the individual's sexual behaviour over time in terms of societal influences rather than developmental trends would prefer data collections to be timed to be contingent upon societal events. In terms of monitoring changes in relation to the development of the HIV/AIDS epidemic, it might be useful to have data collections following each major change in the disease's social representation (for example, due to the impact of advertising campaigns or significant single events, such as the death of a famous person). Models which explain changes in terms of maturation in the individual's physical or psychological capabilities will prefer data collection to be tied to identifiable personal life events. It might be valuable to have data collection linked with changes in sexual status (e.g., loss of virginity, first stable relationship, etc.). In practical terms, however, it is usually factors extraneous to the theoretical model deployed which determine periodicity of data collection. The administrative pressures in such complex research designs push towards less subtle reasons for choice of periodicity. If the samples are large, and they often are for reasons discussed below, mounting data collection more frequently than annually is expensive. Where the questions asked are targeted on intimate personal details, as in the case of sexual behaviour, frequent data collections over any extended period of time may be impossible because respondents tire of the study and drop out.

Allowing practical considerations in part to determine periodicity of data collection may not be such a weakness in any case. Periodicity determined by theoretical considerations will be likely to be unwieldy for such a complex design. For example, neither significant societal events nor personal life events happen sufficiently predictably to organize the design around them easily; most importantly, they would not happen for all members of the sample at the same time, in the same way. LCSD requires researchers to move away from a quasi-experimental way of conceiving of data collection. Even where periodicity of data collection is driven by pragmatic considerations, theoretical issues can be addressed effectively as long as the nature of the information gathered is appropriate. The very fact that individuals vary in their experience of different life events or exposure to particular societal events makes it possible, using multivariate statistical techniques, to assess the role of these events in explaining differences in behaviour. Given this, it becomes essential to incorporate adequate measures of both personal life events and societal events into any LCSD. For societal events, this means establishing subjective measures of their impact as well as objective measures of their occurrence.

Pragmatic influences upon timing decisions in LCSD studies may introduce inappropriate timeframes. The need for quick answers to policy-relevant questions has benefited research on sexual behaviour since the start of the

HIV/AIDS epidemic because it has released funds and has warranted studies which might otherwise have been seen as unnecessary intrusions into an area of people's lives which should be sacrosanct. The thirst for knowledge pertinent to finding some behavioural control of the spread of the virus opened avenues of research which had been blocked before. Yet, the urgency of the need for this knowledge has severely restricted the amount of time deemed necessary for any LCSD. The answers are needed sooner not later. The specific pressures from policymakers and research-sponsors may differ from one era to another but it is always likely to be true that LCSD studies, which are always expensive compared with other designs, will have shorter timeframes imposed than theory builders would recommend.

Though ideally we would have liked to have surveyed the people in our study every three or so months, financial limitations and likely problems with respondent fatigue led us to settle on surveying them at yearly intervals. This was essentially a compromise between losing sensitivity to historical changes and losing too many respondents to fatigue.

*Choosing Measurements*

In any LCSD it is vital that techniques used to measure any variable yield data which are genuinely comparable across age groups, cohorts and times of measurement. It is hardly necessary to say that questions must be repeated, without change in their overt form, across data collections. However, problems arise when questions asked, though remaining identical in their overt form, change their meaning according to age group, cohort or time of measurement. In relation to research on sexual behaviour, especially since the start of the HIV/AIDS epidemic, it has been clear that some questions have changed their meaning, particularly over time. Within a context where it has become more socially acceptable to ask about sexual behaviour, the meaning of questions related to condom use have markedly changed and certainly the significance of being willing to answer them has changed. Prior to the public awareness of HIV/AIDS, questions about condoms were seen to be related to contraception; subsequently, they are known to relate also to protection against STDs.

Some of the younger age groups in our study had no experience of sex prior to the outbreak of HIV/AIDS. Their whole understanding of questions regarding sexual promiscuity, homosexuality, condom use, and so on, has been acquired in the HIV/AIDS context. Their reports of behaviour but also their understanding of questions about their behaviour may be different from earlier generations. We can establish the former but only surmise the latter. Within any LCSD, the problem lies in proving the extent of differences in the meaning of measurements. Unless this can be done, it is always possible that differences between ages, cohorts or times of measurement are some artefact of the changing meaning of the measurement itself. This suggests that LCSD studies should take much greater care to assess the reliability of measurements than they do currently. This assessment needs not only to establish reliability in the measurement across age groups, cohorts and times of measurement, but also, given the longitudinal component of the design, across repeated measurements.

Studies of sexual behaviour are plagued with questions about the validity and reliability of measurements. Standard methods for establishing validity and reliability are not seen to be appropriate since not only is the objective (observational) evidence unlikely to be available but also many researchers assume that respondents are willing to lie systematically about their behaviour over long periods. As the body of studies of sexual behaviour grows some of the concerns about validity and reliability of data can be laid to rest. In a review of studies of late adolescent sexual activity, we were able to show that different studies by different researchers in different geographical areas are discovering similar patterns of reported sexual behaviour, and where there were differences they could generally be attributed to methodological artefacts such as vagueness in questions or sample biases (Fife-Schaw and Breakwell, 1992). Such similarities in the findings of independent studies are difficult to dismiss as the product of unreliable or invalid measurement procedures.

Perhaps equally importantly, the LCSD study allows for complex tests of respondents' consistency in self-report. In our own study, relatively few people can be shown to be providing inconsistent data even at annual intervals. If the data are consciously falsified by the respondents, they are remarkably coherent in their lies and remember them well. To give an example, in an analysis of 1151 people who had been questioned twice about their sexual activities only 111 (9.6 per cent) gave any logically inconsistent information about their past experience of a list of sexual acts.

In discussing choice of measurements, it should be stated explicitly that LCSD studies are not tied to any one mode of data elicitation. Our study used postal questionnaire surveys but it also employed in-depth interviews with some sub-sets of our sample. Many LCSD studies, especially with younger age groups, have used observational techniques. Whatever method of data elicitation is used, the reliability issues remain central. Even where observational techniques are used, it cannot be assumed that the measurement has the same meaning across age, cohort or time of measurement. The same observed behaviour can change its meaning. The meaning of kissing in public depends on the age of the actors, their cohort and the historical period when they are observed kissing.

### Some Implications of Sample Structures

The partial LCSD described in Figure 2.1 is subject to all of the sampling problems which affect simpler designs. First, the longitudinal element in the design will be affected by drop-out. Typically, longitudinal studies find that the greatest drop-out occurs between first and second data collections. The drop-out rate tapers off across data collections. Some researchers argue that this is a product of growing personal commitment to the study as time passes; others suggest that after a certain number of data collections, the sample is heavily biased towards the sort of people who are habitually compliant. Differential drop-out undoubtedly means that the sample available for longitudinal comparisons will be biased. Our own data show that the people who drop out are more likely to be more sexually active, risk takers, and, in common with the findings from other types of survey, have a lower educational attainment and lower socio-economic status. It seems likely that studies of longitudinal changes in sexual behaviour will be more likely to depict the less sexually active. They will tend to underestimate the amount and range of sexual activity. From the point of view of generating population estimates, this becomes important only if the longitudinal data is taken out of context of the whole LCSD. However, from the point of view of modelling developmental change, this bias is vital. It means that our models of developmental change are restricted to people within a limited band of sexual experience. Since estimates of developmental change have to be partialled out of estimates of cohort or era changes within the partial LCSD, this bias cannot be ignored or minimised. From the point of view of generating useful information for policymakers, this bias introduces significant limitations. In using such estimates, policymakers must understand that they are being provided with a very cautious estimate of the incidence and range of sexual activity.

Of course, there are other sample biases in such LCSD studies of sexual behaviour. There is always the more basic question of initial response rate. The object of all social researchers is to maximize response rate, since the lower the response rate, the greater the likelihood that the achieved sample will be biased. Response rates of 60 per cent are typically deemed acceptable for self-completion questionnaire studies. In fact, in a preliminary study to the one described above, Breakwell and Fife-Schaw (1991a) examined the impact upon return rates of including explicit questions about sexual activity in a postal questionnaire. Two forms of the questionnaire were sent out to two samples drawn randomly from the same population, one included explicit questions about sexual activity, the other was the same in other respects but the sexual activity questions were replaced with sexual attitude questions. The presence of sexual activity questions reduced the response rate by 5.1 per cent.

In the main study, we found that response rates were lower than we have achieved in other research on the social and political activities and attitudes of the same age group. For instance, in Swindon, our sexual behaviour survey achieved a return rate of 36.6 per cent. In contrast, another survey (Banks *et al.*, 1992) in the same area with the same age group, using similar postal strategies (though with the addition of interviewer follow-ups of non-responders which were thought to yield less than 10 per cent improvement on return) achieved a 74 per cent return rate.

It is particularly notable that females are more likely to respond than males, and younger cohorts more likely to respond than the older. Often in social research, response rates are improved by repeatedly contacting initial non-responders, sometimes sending people to their residences to pursue their assistance. We felt that such persistence could be justifiably considered intrusive. Two attempts at achieving a response, both by post, were made. Failure to return after the second contact was treated as a final non-response. It was not deemed appropriate to pursue non-responders further since it could be argued that the intimate nature of some of our questions might lead any respondent acting under the slightest hint of duress to misreport activities.

Recognizing the inherent limitations of a relatively low return rate when estimating population parameters has led us to recommend the use of lower bound incidence estimation procedures. This involves incorporating into any estimate of population parameters of sexual behaviour a weighting which takes account of the return rate. This method entails establishing 'lower bound estimates' (Breakwell and Fife-Schaw, 1991b). For instance, if one approached 1000 people and 500 agreed to participate in a survey and, of these, 100 (20 per cent) reported a certain behaviour then the lower bound prevalence estimate for the behaviour is 10 per cent. At least 10 per cent of the population (assuming a true random sampling frame, valid responses, and allowing for standard errors) have experienced the behaviour.

Ideally, whatever the non-response, all surveys should assess the representativeness of the achieved sample and identify the nature and extent of any bias. This can be done by direct or indirect methods (Moser and Kalton, 1971). Direct methods involve follow-up of non-responders. For instance very brief self-completion questionnaires can be sent to them requesting basic socio-demographic details. Extrapolations about the remainder of the non-respondents can then be made, though it is always questionable as to whether these two groups are comparable. Indirect methods involve comparing the sample against known population characteristics, such as age, sex or social class, obtained from the census or other government statistics. If significant under-representation is found in the sample for a particular group, the data from those in that group who did respond can be multiplied by the appropriate factor to recreate a sample matching the known population characteristics. This so-called weighting of data assumes non-responders in various identifiable subgroups are comparable with responders and this may not be the case. Remodelling of data is problematic in research on sexual behaviour because it is not established which population characteristics are particularly related to different patterns in sexual behaviour. So, for instance, in most research on sexual behaviour a good case might be made for weighting for non-response by age, socio-economic class, educational background, family structure, and so on. If all were adopted, given overall low response rates and the number of biases in the sample, any resemblance to original population parameter estimates would be lost. It would be very difficult to assess the degree of confidence with which any single estimate was made. In such a context, at this stage in our knowledge of patterns of sexual behaviour, it is our opinion that weighting to compensate for non-response must be done with caution. Our own reports of findings do not use weighted data. Since we are largely concerned with exploring relationships between variables as measured in our sample, the need for tendentious assumptions about the validity of weighting seems weak.

These concerns about non-response and how they should be handled in analysis are not peculiar to LCSD. There is a further problem which is rather more specific. A full LCSD, and the partial LCSD to a lesser extent, relies upon drawing new samples at time intervals. The logic of the design requires that the new samples drawn at each data collection be comparable to those at earlier points. Any disparities in response biases in each sample over data collection points will introduce error into estimates of change due to cohort or to time of measurement. Of course, it is possible to assess the extent of systematic differences in response for each new sample and, again, some weighting factor (based on the sample at first data collection) can be used to rectify any imbalance. If such corrections are used, however, there is a possibility that important differences on dependent variables between samples taken at different times will be obscured or introduced. In fact, in the partial LCSD used in our study, we found remarkable similarity across samples drawn to complete the sequential component of the design. The 16-year-old samples of 1989, 1990 and 1991 in terms of standard population characteristics were not significantly different.

## Analysing LCSD Data

The ultimate task in analysing data from an LCSD is to differentiate developmental, cohort and time of measurement sources of age-related trends of patterns of behaviour. Some statistical techniques necessary for establishing the nature of the complex interactions involved are now available (Hagenaars, 1990). As specified earlier, the use of a partial LCSD, such as that employed in our study, leads to great complexity in using such analyses to assess time of measurement effects. The full LCSD is better from the point of view of achieving a total analysis of these interacting determinants of age-related trends, requiring less questionable assumptions to be built into the adoption of the statistical models to be used.

In such complex designs, it is possibly useful to conduct basic exploratory analyses which fundamentally involve detecting the main effects of age, cohort, and time of measurement:

*Age Effects* can be assessed by comparing longitudinal changes in different cohorts. For instance, in Figure 2.1, is a change observed between $D_{16}$ and $D_{17}$ also present when $E_{16}$ is compared with $E_{17}$? The finding of similar changes of approximately equivalent magnitudes would suggest developmental rather than cohort effects or time of measurement effects. Differential levels of change indicate cohort and time of measurement effects cannot be ruled out.

In our study we found just such age effects for a number of reported sexual behaviours. For instance, among females in the equivalent of $D_{16}$, 52.8 per cent had experience of penetrative sexual intercourse. One year later ($D_{17}$) 71.1 per cent had had this experience. The equivalent figures for $E_{16}$ and $E_{17}$ were 55.2 and 76.0 per cent. Given the sizes of the standard errors associated with these percentages, we believe we are looking at a developmental trend here, around about 18–20 per cent of the 16-17-year-old female population will lose their virginity in the following year.

*Cohort Effects* are strongly indicated if, at all stages in the study, the rank ordering of cohorts on a particular measure remains the same. In practice, cohort effects may be less marked than this and their detection may depend upon establishing differences which clearly cannot be attributed to either developmental or time of measurement effects. In an ideal situation, sample sizes would be sufficiently large to exclude the possibility that apparent cohort differences are due in reality to chance variation.

*Time of Measurement Effects* can be estimated by comparing responses in cohorts across time. If some social event has a broad impact on the sample's responses, changes between, for instance, $D_{16}$ and $D_{17}$ should also be observed between $A_{19}$ and $A_{20}$ and, likewise, in cohorts B and C. One of the advantages of the LCSD is that there is the potential to show that a change between $D_{16}$ and $D_{17}$ which is mirrored in cohorts A, B, and C but not reflected in cohort E (between $E_{16}$ and $E_{17}$) is attributable to some event occurring in 1989/90 but not 1990/91. If the same pattern of change occurred for $E_{16}$ to $E_{17}$ it would be less clear that a time of measurement effect alone had been established. In such a case, a developmental trend may also be influencing responses.

In pursuing these analyses, some care must be taken in clarifying the exact nature of the population to which any conclusions apply. If, as in our example, there are three waves of questioning, these analyses could only possibly be applied to data from those people who are in the sample at all three data collections. As we discussed earlier, this could be a biased sample after differential drop-out.

Where the research is being used to estimate population parameters, rather than to test explanations for change, the data from first contacts with each respondent should be used so as to minimize the effects of sample biases. An advantage of the LCSD for these kinds of questions is that the addition of new cohorts (for example $E_{16}$ and $F_{16}$) allows the confirmation of estimates based on $D_{16}$. In the absence of independent corroboration of parameter estimates from other studies, these new cohorts can prove important in increasing (or decreasing) confidence in estimates.

Any summary of the strategies used in analysing LCSD, and particularly partial LCSD, designs indicate that the approach needs to be systematic and alert to deficits in the samples. This type of design is not susceptible to ritualistic statistical treatment: there is no recipe which will always work when analysing LCSD data. Firm conclusions can only be reached after rigorous and iterative statistical modelling. It is also our belief that such conclusions must be tested against the findings derived from other types of design which may have implemented other data elicitation techniques (many of which are described elsewhere in this book).

## Conclusions

Despite its complexities, the LCSD design is a precious research tool when examining sexual behaviour because it is unparalleled in allowing different explanations for change to be tested. In a context where most researchers are attempting to understand changes in sexual behaviour in order to influence those changes so as to improve the control of STDs, any research technique which unravels, even partially, the knotted web of factors which effect change is vital.

In our research we had hoped to detect the influence of changing representations of AIDS and education campaigns on sexual behaviours, however, the LCSD has led us to conclude that these historical changes have had relatively minor effects on behaviour. Though there are still many analyses to conduct, we have yet to find substantial time of measurement or cohort effects. What the design and sampling strategies have revealed are apparently regular developmental trends across a wide range of attitudes and behaviours. These suggest that the development of sexual identities went on largely uninfluenced by relatively short term social change in the period of our study. Whether patterns of behaviour were substantially different in the immediate pre-AIDS period we cannot tell from the present data. Our data and previous research, however, would suggest that most young people's sexual identities continued to develop much as before, despite AIDS.

## References

BANKS, M., BATES, I., BREAKWELL, G.M., BYNNER, J., EMLER, N., JAMIESON, L. and ROBERTS, K. (1992) *Careers and Identities*, Milton Keynes: Open University Press.

BREAKWELL, G.M. and FIFE-SCHAW, C.R. (1991a) Interim Report to the ESRC on Social and Behavioural Consequences of HIV/AIDS for 16–21 Year Olds Project, Swindon, Wiltshire: ESRC.

BREAKWELL, G.M. and FIFE-SCHAW, C.R. (1991b) 'Heterosexual anal intercourse and the risk of AIDS/HIV for 16–20-Year-Olds, *Health Education Journal*, 50, 4, pp. 166–9.

BREAKWELL, G.M. and FIFE-SCHAW, C.R. (1992) 'Sexual activities and preferences in a UK sample of 16–20-Year-Olds, *Archives of Sexual Behavior*, 21, 3, pp. 271–93.

FIFE-SCHAW, C.R. and BREAKWELL, G.M. (1992) 'Estimating sexual behaviour parameters in the light of AIDS: A review of recent UK studies of young people', *AIDS Care*, 4, 2, pp. 187–201.

HAGENAARS, J.A. (1990) *Categorical Longitudinal Data*, Newbury Park, CA: Sage.

MOSER, C.A. and KALTON, G. (1971) *Survey Methods in Social Investigation*, 2nd ed., London: Heinemann.
SCHAIE, K.W. (1965) 'A general model for the study of developmental problems', *Psychological Bulletin*, 64, pp. 92–107.

Chapter 3

# Monitoring Behavioural Change in the Population: A Continuous Data Collection Approach

*David McQueen and Stefano Campostrini*

The continuous collection of data from large samples represents one of the most robust research designs developed for assessing behavioural change in populations. It has been made possible by technical developments such as computer assisted telephone interviewing (CATI) which facilitates random sampling and allows the rapid collection and processing of questionnaire data. Continuous data collection in turn provides the foundation for further significant developments in research methodology. Behavioural variables can be viewed as dynamic, and innovative analytic techniques developed to uncover complex relationships within the data. Continuous data collection also provides the context for 'field' evaluation of questionnaire items and the investigation of several potential sources of measurement error in the survey.

This chapter considers the strengths and limitations of a continuous data collection research design in the context of studying AIDS-related knowledge, attitudes and behaviours in a lifestyle survey conducted by the Research Unit in Health and Behavioural Change (RUHBC) at the University of Edinburgh.

## Rationale

When this project was initiated (1987) the aims were to:

1 provide baseline data against which changes in health behaviour, particularly sexual behaviour, could be assessed;
2 evaluate a way of obtaining information about sensitive behaviours;
3 identify causal links between sociodemographic variables, social factors and behaviours;
4 suggest areas and strategies for future intervention;
5 seek compatibility with similar research in other countries.

Broadly considered, this project had two phases. The first phase placed emphasis on assessing the method used to collect information about health behaviour; and the second phase of the study emphasized the continuous monitoring of health behaviours over time with cost-efficiency and expediency in information gathering as a priority, particularly in the light of the dynamic growth of AIDS as a problem related to health behaviour.

The adequate measurement of sexual attitudes, behavioural intentions and actual practices was addressed in the first instance by the use of standardized items developed in English-speaking countries (Catania *et al.*, 1990). The argument was that if the US experience repeats itself in Britain, then one should expect a rapid change of opinion about the discussibility of the AIDS problem with all the consequences for a desensitization of the issues. The strategy was to 'bury' sexual behaviour questions within a questionnaire containing more 'acceptable' general health behaviour questions. The general lifestyle questions would be followed by an informed consent statement specifying the nature of the questions to follow. Termination of the interview at this point would still leave responses to the other questions intact.

The initial strategy was to design a dynamic method of data collection. In order to study short-term changes in behaviour and to account for temporal differences, data would be collected on a daily basis and aggregated monthly for analytic purposes. Unlike traditional survey research and in keeping with the continuous monitoring format of this study, interview processing and data management would be carried out daily. Regular reviews of the data at the end of each month would allow for strategic adjustments in data collection. The research would focus on changes in the attitudes and behaviours under study. Such an approach is analogous to taking an inventory, in this case an inventory of knowledge, attitudes, opinions and behaviours in the population.

Data collection began in July 1987 using a CATI-based system. The technical aspects on the CATI system are extensive; only a brief summary of the system is given here. The system resembles that used by the US Centers for Disease Control in Atlanta; their behavioural risk factor surveillance system (BRFSS) with CATI is an extension of their earlier behavioural risk factor (BRFS) monitoring system (Hogelin, 1988).

The questionnaire covered eleven topic areas:

1 safety;
2 environment;
3 exercise and fitness;
4 eating behaviour;
5 smoking;
6 alcohol use;
7 health practices;
8 health publicity;
9 HIV/AIDS-related attitudes, opinions and behaviours;

10   sexual behaviour;
11   demographic information about the respondent.

With regard to AIDS-specific topics the study collected:

a   information regarding transmission of the HIV virus;
b   information on 'safe sex' practices;
c   attitudes and emotional reactions of individuals to AIDS;
d   data on alcohol use in relation to health and sex;
e   information on homosexuality;
f   views and opinions on AIDS;
g   information on the maintenance of behavioural change with regard to sex;
h   information on trends in AIDS-related knowledge, opinions, and behaviours.

Between July 1987 and March 1991 a total of 27,712 interviews were completed. Of the completed interviews, 55.6 per cent were with women, 34.7 per cent were from London and the remainder from the Glasgow and Edinburgh areas. Approximately one-third of the participants were under 30 years of age, another 30 per cent were between 30 and 39. The monthly response rate calculated by the Council of American Survey Research Organizations (CASRO) method was in the 70–80 per cent range, with some variation by month and by area of data collection (CASRO, 1982). Scottish response rates are consistently higher than those for London.

Participants were selected randomly from adults, aged 18–60 years of age, resident in households with telephones. Prior to initiating the survey a pilot study examined the effect of coverage, differences between participants in households with and without phones on the key study variables (McQueen, 1989). These differences were minor and the results similar to those found elsewhere in such comparisons (Cannell *et al.*, 1987; Marcus and Crane, 1986; NCHS, 1987; Rogers, 1976). The monthly sample frame was selected by a multistage cluster procedure based on a random digit dialling procedure using a modified Waksberg method (Waksberg, 1978) as routinely used in other CATI surveys (Health and Welfare Canada, 1988, 1993). Following a household contact and determination of the number of eligible respondents within the household an adult was randomly selected by the computer and interviewed at the time or in a call back if the selected participant was not available.

In data collection, the CATI software presents the interviewer with the interview format on a personal computer monitor. It edits the questions and automatically checks answers for internal consistency, that is pre-cleaning of the data, and formats the questions and regulates question flow so that respondents are only read questions appropriate to them, for example, total abstainers would not be asked further questions about their drinking. It then codes the answers to questions directly into a data file, updates the data file by integrating the current interview, creates a SPSS-ready data file, and updates it automatically. It also provides a routine monitoring of interviewer efficiency, keeping track of average time taken in interviewing, repeated interviewer errors, and success in obtaining completed interviews, and automatically backs up the interview. In brief, the CATI system carries out many of the routinized tasks of data collection and management, but with relatively little chance for error and at considerable cost efficiency. Data are ready for analysis shortly after data collection.

## Methodological Issues and Theoretical Underpinnings

The cross-sectional survey has played a key role in sociomedical research for many years. For studying trends or monitoring changes over time a standard approach is a baseline survey followed by a series of widely spaced surveys conducted in a longitudinal design. This approach is built around many classical statistical assumptions, for example (i) known characteristics of the study population; (ii) data collection by some random sampling method; (iii) known characteristics of the measurement errors to be encountered; (iv) and many other ritualistically followed rules about how to carry out research. Like many assumptions in the pursuit of research, they are seldom challenged.

The theory underlying research on behaviour has changed over the past two decades. It has taken up the idea that behavioural variables are dynamic. This implies that studies of behaviour should contain a time component. Nonetheless, survey research designs used to study behaviour and behavioural processes have remained largely static, including the methods of sampling, data collection and assessment of error. This is not surprising because, in general, survey research is a cumbersome method of data collection. By its very nature it is difficult to collect and process data rapidly and in some kind of real time frame. The development of CATI has altered the data collection process, allowing the possibility for a more dynamic approach.

Once one considers the idea that behavioural variables are dynamic it is possible to hypothesize how they might appear in population data collected over time. Figure 3.1 shows four such hypothetical types of variables. The question of whether variables in the population behave in such a manner becomes an empirical question. One may conceptualize four primary types of variables: Type A: those which are relatively stable over time; show little variation over time; possess a slope, or change over a time by an increment which is largely determinable and relatively constant; Type B: those which are less stable over time; may show some broad over-time oscillatory behaviour and/or periods of reversals; the slope varies; Type C: those which are discrete, i.e. behaviour is either present or not at any given time; Type D: those which are markedly unstable over time; characterized by wide variance; marked rapid shifts in slope; quasi-regular patterns perhaps distinct over time, but catastrophic or chaotic

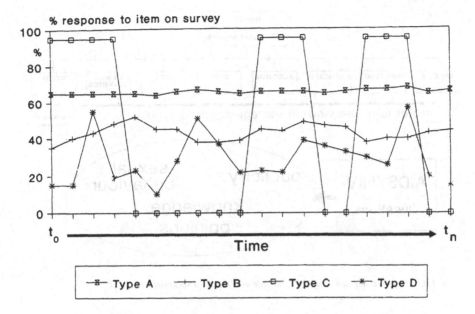

*Figure 3.1:   Four variable types — nature over time.*

behaviour possible. These are hypothetical types, but survey researchers should recognize these types of variables in their data, either in data collection or analysis. The logic of continuous data collection is quite clear: if you focus only on the analysis of cross-sectional data, these variable patterns are difficult to see because they are masked by the item variance within the cross-sectional data.

## Types of Variables and Questionnaire Development

Questionnaire development is a key component of a CATI-based survey which takes a continuous data collection strategy with a lifestyle perspective. In the history of risk-factor surveys, subsequent lifestyle surveys, and more recent surveys of sexual knowledge, attitudes and practices, a great amount of attention has been given to instrument development, notably questionnaire wording. The questionnaire in the RUHBC survey builds on this vast experience and many of the questions used are either similar or identical to questions used in other surveys. Nonetheless, static point-in-time surveys have to carry out their questionnaire development in advance of going into the field: they cannot test their questionnaire in the context of actual data collection. Continuous data collection as designed in the RUHBC project allows for a field evaluation of questionnaire characteristics. The resulting questionnaire structure of the survey is complex. What follows is a discussion of some aspects of question wording as an example of how emergent methodological issues may be addressed.

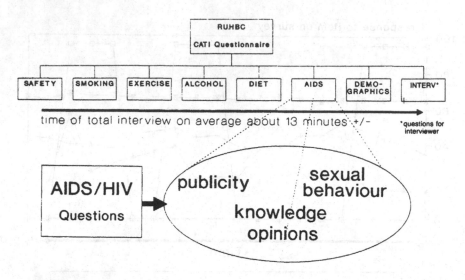

*Figure 3.2: Basic ordering and structure of lifestyle and health questionnaire*

Figure 3.2 shows the areas for question items relating to attitudes, opinions and behaviours related to AIDS as used in the RUHBC survey. The questions on AIDS enter after some general questions about publicity and health. Following a short introduction to the AIDS section the respondent is asked a series of questions on opinions about AIDS; this is followed by some questions to ascertain the respondent's knowledge about AIDS; the questions related to blood, (donation, transfusion, etc.) are designed to complement questions on blood donation practice asked earlier in the questionnaire in the health practices section; the questions on AIDS as a problem relate to the respondent's perception of AIDS as a problem at different levels of social organization (community, neighbourhood, country, area, etc.); the questions on talking about AIDS relate to family and friends; the questions on changes in behaviour relate to changes in sexual behaviour (use of condoms, fewer partners, etc.); those on intentions to change parallel those on reported changes; the questions on actual sexual practice follow after a brief reminder of the anonymity of the survey and statement of informed consent (these questions are asked only of respondents aged 18–50, 18–40 after July 1991). Asking this battery of questions on a daily basis since 1987 has allowed for an accurate mapping of these attitudes, opinions and behaviours as they occur in the sampled population.

As an example of stability in some variables measured over time, consider those related to AIDS knowledge. Five different items with 'correct' responses based on current medical opinion about AIDS make up a scale of knowledge about AIDS. The questions are standard; they ask if one can get AIDS from kissing with exchange of saliva, from donating blood, from insect bites, from eating food prepared by someone with AIDS, and by using public toilets. But the

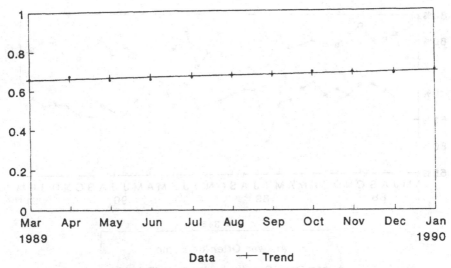

Data  ―+― Trend

• The knowledge about AIDS scale is constructed from five
items which have been dichotomized; scale ranges from 0 to 1

*Figure 3.3:   Knowledge about AIDS stability over time — Scottish data using a five-item scale.* *

stability and reliability of each of these items over time have given confidence in constructing a scale of knowledge about AIDS. As can be seen in Figure 3.3, the resulting index is stable and possesses a stable increment of change over time.

An example of variables which have not been constant over time but have shown a steady change are those measuring reported levels of talking about AIDS with friends and family. The percentages of respondents who report talking about AIDS have decreased steadily over time, with the percentage reporting that they talk about AIDS with their friends being consistently higher than with their families. Between April 1988 and March 1991 there was a decrease of around 10 per cent for those reporting that they had talked about AIDS with their family and a decrease of around 7 per cent in those reporting that they talked about AIDS with their friends, based on Scottish data (Figure 3.4).

Through continuous data collection it has been apparent that items which measure opinion are unstable over time. Fortunately, with respect to the issue of total survey error, continuous data collection allows for experimentation with each question so as to estimate the error or type of instability arising from wording effects. By reversing the direction of statements of some questions within the questionnaire, several phenomena can be studied which impinge on total survey error: (1) the problem of acquiescence; (2) the issue of validity; and (3) the issue of item consistency.

In the RUHBC survey, six questions on attitudes and opinions about AIDS were reversed for a period of eight months. That is, the polarity or direction of agreement was changed so that a person who 'disagreed' with the question as

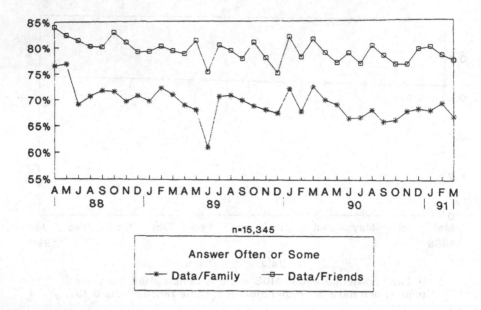

*Figure 3.4: Percent of respondents reporting talking about AIDS with family and friends over time.*

initially worded would 'agree' with the question as subsequently worded. In order to both observe and isolate the element of time, a probit analysis was carried out. Probit analysis considers the questionnaire items (after dichotomization) as dependent variables with time in months, and a dichotomous variable indicating the two different versions of the items as independent variables: the first (months) considered as the predictor while the second (the different versions) as a *grouping variable*. The main finding is that reversing the response direction of questions has different effects for different items. This illustrates, among other things, the effect of the type of variables with respect to stability over time. Traditionally, in cross-sectional surveys, one has been concerned with the problem of acquiescence. Nonetheless, a tendency to acquiesce has been found in only two of the six items considered, as opposed to an expectation of acquiescence in all these types of items. One explanation is that the problem of acquiescence is part of the problem of an item stabilizing over time, in conjunction with stability in the interviewers asking the question. That is, the error source is not in the respondent, but in the data collection process; continuous data collection serves to mitigate this source of error.

Probit analysis shows how the change of item polarity does not interrupt the time trend observed in answering those six questions. The only effect that the reversing of items has produced is a change of intercept in the probit model. In the questions analysed, acquiescence seems to be only one of the possible effects of the reversal of questionnaire items by rewording. There is a general tendency to answer statements posed in a positive or in a negative way in a slightly different manner. Where no acquiescence phenomenon is detectable, the differential answer tendency seems to increase with the level of the respondent's socio-economic status.

The following figures illustrate some of these points. Figure 3.5 shows an item which had very good stability in the data over time, that is stability in the response of respondents who agree with the statement that compared with most viruses AIDS is *difficult* to get (Version 1) and disagree with the statement that compared with most viruses AIDS is *easy* to get (Version 2); notable also, and revealed by the probit line, is the stability of the slope of the agreement over time. Figure 3.6 shows a less stable item related to the spread of AIDS in the general population; clearly this is a topic to which considerable attention has been paid in the media and it is not a very stable opinion over time. Once again the probit analysis helps to clarify the changing picture. Figure 3.7 probably illustrates an effect of data collection; that is, the change in direction of the question posed difficulties for the interviewers and it took some time for the reversed question to stabilize. Finally, Figure 3.8 illustrates a case where there is both instability in the data and a pronounced shift with the item reversal; the initial version was 'Everyone who carries the AIDS virus will eventually get AIDS'; the reversed version added the word 'not' to the beginning of the question.

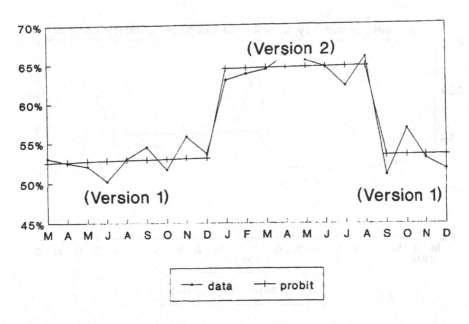

*Figure 3.5:   Stable AIDS item over time — good agreement with two versions of question on difficulty of getting AIDS.*

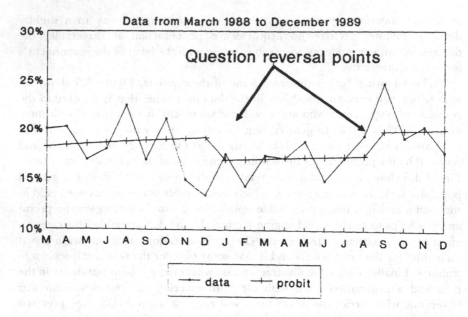

*Figure 3.6: Less stable AIDS item over time — agreement with question on whether AIDS will spread in general population.*

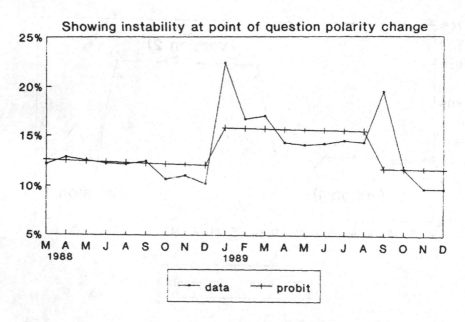

*Figure 3.7: Agreement with two versions of a statement on employer being able to dismiss employee with AIDS.*

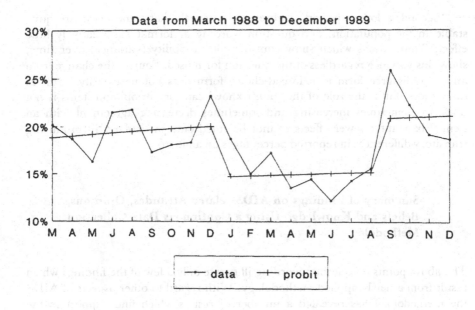

*Figure 3.8: Question item showing both instability over time and sensitivity to change in question polarity.*

## Effects of Changing Polarity of Statements on AIDS-related Opinions

Wording effects in questionnaires have long been considered a source of error in the collection of survey data, nevertheless the evidence for effects is largely taken from data collected cross-sectionally. This is particularly a problem for wording of AIDS related questions where the introduction of questions is recent and often *ad hoc*, that is, there is little experience with the use of questions on populations. The collection of data continuously offers evidence on wording effects from a different perspective and is therefore particularly useful with regard to the emerging questions related to HIV and AIDS. Examining wording effects through the use of three different versions of six AIDS-related questionnaire items over a period of three years, illustrates that questionnaire wording is a rather complex methodological issue. There are, however, several points which can be made and which are unique to an analysis of wording effects based on continuously collected data (Campostrini and McQueen, 1993).

First, question wording seems less of a problem for a time trend analysis. In none of the six cases did the changing of the polarity of a question alter the slope of the trend in the population; nor was the slope changed by adding a forced choice version of the question. This result, if confirmed in other studies, has implications for longitudinal/continuous survey methodology and particularly for the development of new questions in emerging areas of public health concern.

Second, a longer period of observation reveals that some items are quite stable in the population, and question wording or format has relatively little effect. Third, items which show considerable instability (variance) over time, show this variance regardless of the question form used. Fourth, the change from an agree/disagree form to a forced-choice form does not necessarily result in differences. Fifth, the role of the 'don't know' category in opinion items is not uniform, sometimes increasing and sometimes decreasing agreement with an item. Sixth, interviewer effects cannot be ruled out, particularly in producing transitory differences in reported percentages on an item.

## Summary of Findings on AIDS-related Attitudes, Opinions, Beliefs and Knowledge Using a Continuous Data Collection Methodology

The above points on question wording illustrate only a few of the findings which result from a newly applied methodology. With regard to other aspects of AIDS the methodology has revealed a number of results which find support in the general literature on AIDS-related population findings. For example, our results suggest that levels of knowledge about AIDS reached a plateau for most questions prior to April 1988. However, for some items there remains considerable uncertainty in the general public, particularly with reference to the unstable percentage of respondents who report that they think you can become infected with the 'AIDS virus' by giving blood.

As might be expected from the general finding in the social psychology literature, the relationship between knowledge and sexual behaviour is very weak. A knowledge scale constructed from several questionnaire items in the RUHBC survey has shown both consistency and stability over time, this holds largely within age, gender and class groups. Since knowledge has remained largely invariant, it explains little of the measured behavioural changes found over time. Nevertheless, even as the knowledge level remains fairly constant, the saliency of AIDS for the Scottish population appears to be declining if one assumes that respondents talk about an issue when they are unsure what they think about it, when they are concerned about the subject — that is when it is salient.

With regard to safer sexual practices, the data up to 1993 shows a small but gradual increase. Reported use of condoms and use of condoms as a protection against infection is increasing over time although it is not possible to state decisively that this increase is due to AIDS. However, this positive finding must be balanced against the small change in reported number of sexual partners, with young males reporting the highest number of partners. Respondents who are changing their behaviour are tending to use condoms rather than reduce their number of partners. This pattern is complex and discussed further below.

On the very negative side our findings reveal that personal perception of risk of AIDS is very low indeed, with only around 2 per cent of respondents reporting that there is anything they do in their daily life that puts them at risk of getting AIDS that is not related to their job. If respondents report that they are at risk, this is usually because of their job, for example, being a health care worker. Furthermore, the results obtained from applying our Risk Index suggest that there is a relatively high percentage of respondents in the general population who are at risk of AIDS because of their personal sexual behaviour (Campostrini and McQueen, 1993).

### Differences in Reported Sexual Behaviour by Population Characteristics

The relationship between sexual behaviour and population sociodemographic characteristics is complex. The understanding of the multi-factorial nature of this relationship requires many levels of analysis. It is probably premature to assert that AIDS-related research on sexual behaviour has sorted out the demographic parameters of 'safe' and 'unsafe' sex. Nonetheless, the RUHBC survey provides the opportunity to explore some of these dimensions in detail. What follows is a brief example of this relationship based on a summation of data presented in a series of reports on the project (McQueen *et al.*, 1989, 1990, 1991).

A large difference in reported number of partners between males and females is a common finding in surveys of sexual behaviour. Consequently, the distribution of risky sexual behaviour is seen as very different for males and females. Our data for the year 1990 are illustrative, based on over 7500 interviews. A three-point variable to assess possible risk on a scale of one (highest) to three (lowest) may be constructed, three being the roughly 87 per cent of respondents who reported less than four partners in the previous five years. Of those remaining 13 per cent with four or more partners in the previous five years roughly half (55 per cent) reported regularly using condoms always or nearly always. Those in the last category would appear to be at high risk because of multiple partners and low condom use and are assigned a risk level of one. Table 3.1 shows the relationship of gender, age and marital status to this possible risk level. In the analysis of the RUHBC data all other relevant socio-demographic factors and lifestyle behaviours were considered with regard to this possible risk level. In general, the findings on these other variables were un-remarkable.

Two broad conclusions can be drawn. First, there is a large gender difference in reported sexual behaviour which appears consistent across all sociodemographic groups. Second, there are only relatively weak relationships between indicators of socioeconomic status and sexual behaviour. Mainly the data show that risky sexual behaviour is strongly related to single status and has a strong inverse age gradient. Nonetheless, these complex relationships may

Table 3.1: *Possible risk in behaviour by gender, age and marital status*

| Risk Level | Males | | | Females | | |
|---|---|---|---|---|---|---|
| | One | Two | Three | One | Two | Three |
| | per cent | per cent | per cent | per cent | per cent | per cent |
| All Respondents | 11.6 | 10.0 | 78.4 | 3.1 | 2.3 | 94.6 |
| Age | | | | | | |
| 18–21 | 18.4 | 26.1 | 55.5 | 3.7 | 6.1 | 90.2 |
| 22–9 | 17.2 | 14.6 | 68.2 | 6.2 | 3.9 | 89.9 |
| 30–9 | 9.7 | 7.1 | 83.2 | 1.8 | 1.5 | 96.7 |
| 40–9 | 5.5 | 3.5 | 91.0 | 0.9 | 0.2 | 98.9 |
| Marital status | | | | | | |
| Married | 3.0 | 1.0 | 96.0 | 0.4 | 0.1 | 99.5 |
| Never married | 18.6 | 21.1 | 60.3 | 6.0 | 6.3 | 87.7 |
| Divorced | 28.4 | 12.1 | 59.6 | 3.5 | 2.6 | 93.9 |

(Based on data from RUHBC Lifestyle Survey collected in 1990)

emerge differently over time and the RUHBC data has the potential to take into account these changing patterns.

## Conclusions

AIDS is a recent phenomenon from a public health perspective. Furthermore, it is a complicated disease to study because of the powerful behavioural and cultural components embedded in its causation and prevention. Yet the demand for information about sexual attitudes, beliefs and behaviours which relate to the spread of this disease in the population far outpaces the ability of our current state of social science methodology to provide research designs, data collection strategies and appropriate analyses. The methodology developed at RUHBC is one attempt to provide a methodological answer to a number of the difficult questions raised by the AIDS epidemic. It provides rapid data collection at the population level of variables which are both little understood and subject to considerable fluctuation over time. It is methodologically stronger than any time survey approach.

The chief drawback of collecting data in this way is the attention which must be given to the technicalities of the data collection process. There is no time when the data collection may be considered to have ended, other than arbitrary periods assigned by the investigators. The result is less time for in-depth analysis of the data already collected. This problem is exacerbated at a small research unit like RUHBC by the necessity to supply fairly regular feedback analyses and reports and the need to respond to occasional requests for special analyses of the data. Furthermore, the resultant data set, with its added time dimension, is quite complex and presents considerable analytic challenges. It is relatively easy to break the data into cross-sections and analyse the data traditionally. Doing so yields much of the familiar cross-sectional output with regard to health-related attitudes, opinions, knowledge and behaviours. The challenge of these data is to apply more innovative analytical techniques in order to uncover relationships in the data. This task will take time and requires further efforts by a number of researchers.

In terms of general shortcomings this population survey approach suffers from the same drawbacks as any behavioural survey. First, the data are based entirely on self reports of participants; second, the ability to get in-depth responses on any topic area is very limited; and third, coverage is limited to the easy-to-reach part of the general population. This third drawback is an issue in telephone-based surveys where the households without telephones are generally found among poorer populations. Fortunately, studies have now shown that households without telephones in this stratum do not differ greatly from those with telephones. However, this lack of difference is found to be question or behaviour specific; thus, each question must be considerd in addressing the issue of sensitivity to coverage. Finally, it is now accepted that population surveys, whatever the mode of administration, fail to reach a significant number of the difficult to reach in the population. Unfortunately, these difficult to reach are often the subgroup most at risk for many behaviours leading to negative health outcomes.

It is important to emphasize that the survey is a population-based approach. While this may be self-evident, expectations are often placed upon surveys which are unreasonable and impossible. Surveys have three profound weaknesses: (1) they rely on self-reporting; (2) they tend to be very weak in obtaining samples which are representative of the very deprived or special groups which are a small subset of the general population; and (3) they collect information which rarely allows in-depth understanding of a specific issue. In studying sexual practices self-reporting is less an issue. Researchers have to rely on what they are told by a study participant, there are few alternatives which are not invasive of privacy. The second weakness is more serious in the study of AIDS-related behaviour, notably because the behaviour most likely to be causal in the transmission of AIDS may be found in difficult to reach subgroups. Finally, much speculation in the AIDS literature has centred around the complexities involved in negotiating safer sex in at-risk groups. These complexities are best explored with more ethnographic approaches.

### Acknowledgements

The authors wish to acknowledge that the data used and findings reported were obtained from the CATI-based lifestyle and health continuous data survey carried out from July 1987 to July 1992 at the Research Unit in Health and Behavioural Change (RUHBC), University of Edinburgh, Professor David V. McQueen, Principal Investigator. The following researchers had major responsibilities: Research Fellows, Daan Uitenbroek and Stefano Campostrini; Research Associates, Tessa Gorst, Lucy Nisbet, Beatrice Robertson, and Rebecca Smith; in addition we acknowledge the work of four supervisors, eighty-four interviewers and the following secretarial staff: Emanuelle Tulle Winton, Anna Sim and Sian Hay. RUHBC is funded by the Scottish Home and Health Department (SHHD), the Health Education Board for Scotland (HEBS) and the Economic and Social Research Council; however, the opinions expressed in this communication are solely those of the authors.

## References

CAMPOSTRINI, S. and MCQUEEN, D.V. (1993a) 'The wording of questions in a CATI-based lifestyle survey: Effects of reversing the polarity of AIDS-related questions in continuous data', *Quality and Quantity*, 27, pp. 157–170.

CAMPOSTRINI, S. and MCQUEEN, D.V. (1993b) 'Sexual behavior and exposure to HIV infection: Estimates from a general-population risk index', *AJPH*, 83, pp. 1139–43.

CANNELL, C.F., GROVES, R.M., MAGILAVY, L., MATHIOWETZ, N. and MILLER, P.V. (1987) *An Experimental Comparison of Telephone and Personal Health Survey*, US National Center for Health Statistics, Technical Series 2, 106.

CASRO (Council of American Survey Research Organizations) (1982) 'Report of the CASRO Completion Rates Task Force', unpublished reports, New York: Audits and Surveys Company, Inc.

CATANIA, J.A., GIBSON, D.R., CHITWOOD, D.D. and COATES, T.J. (1990) 'Methodological problems in AIDS behavioral research: Influences on measurement error and participation bias in studies of sexual behavior', *Psychol. Bulletin*, 108, pp. 339–62.

Health and Welfare Canada, ROOTMAN, I., WARREN, R., STEPHENS, T. and PETERS, L. (Eds) (1988) *Canada's Health Promotion Survey: Technical Report*, Ottawa: Minister of Supply and Services.

Health and Welfare Canada, STEPHENS, T. and FOWLER GRAHAM, D. (Eds) (1993) *Canada's Health Promotion Survey 1990: Technical Report*, Ottawa: Minister of Supply and Services.

HOGELIN, G. (1988) 'The behavioral risk factor surveys in the United States: 1981–1983', in ANDERSON, R., DAVIES, J.K., KICKBUSCH, I. and MCQUEEN, D.V., *Health Behaviour Research and Health Promotion*. Oxford: Oxford University Press, pp. 111–24.

MCQUEEN, D.V. (1989) 'Comparison of results of personal interview and telephone surveys of behavior related to risk of AIDS: Advantages of telephone techniques', in FOWLER, Jr., F.J. (Ed.) *Health Survey Research Methods*, pp. 247–52, Washington, DC: PHS, US Government Printing Office, September.

MCQUEEN, D.V., CAMPOSTRINI, S., GORST, T., NISBET, L., ROBERTSON, B.J., SMITH, R.J. and UITENBROEK, D. (1990) *A Study of Lifestyle and Health; Interim Report 2*, Edinburgh: RUHBC, Edinburgh University.

MCQUEEN, D.V., CAMPOSTRINI, S., ROBERTSON, B.J. and UITENBROEK, D. (1991) *A Study of Lifestyle and Health; Interim Report 3*, Edinburgh: RUHBC, Edinburgh University.

MCQUEEN, D.V., GORST, T., NISBET, L., ROBERTSON, B.J., SMITH, R.J. and UITENBROEK, D. (1989) *A Study of Lifestyle and Health: Interim Report No. 1*,

Edinburgh: RUHBC, (Research Unit in Health and Behavioural Change), Edinburgh University.

MARCUS, A.C. and CRANE, L.A. (1986) *The Validity and Value of Health Survey Research by Telephone*, New York: The Commonwealth Fund.

National Center for Health Statistics (NCHS) (1987) 'An experimental comparison of telephone and personal health interview surveys', THORNBERRY, O.T. (Ed.) *Vital and Health Statistics*, Series 2, 106, Washington, DC: PHS, US Government Printing Office.

ROGERS, T.F. (1976) 'Interviews by telephone and in person: Quality of responses and field performance', *Public Opinion Quarterly*, 40, 1, pp. 51–65.

WAKSBERG, J. (1978) 'Sampling methods for random digit dialling', *Journal of the American Statistical Association*, 73, 361, pp. 40-6.

*Chapter 4*

# Acts, Sessions and Individuals: A Model for Analysing Sexual Behaviour

*Peter Davies*

In the past decade, much has been written on the problem of the uptake and maintenance of safer sex among gay and bisexual men. There is, in this voluminous literature, a dominant paradigm that incorporates and empowers 'a particular discourse of sex and sexuality which is empirical, epidemiological and atomistic'. Project SIGMA's[1] work in this area has involved the development of an approach to the understanding of sexual behaviour in general, and unsafe behaviour in particular, which is theoretically informed, humanistic and holistic in scope and based on the simple insight that sex is interpersonal and interactive. In this chapter, the tenets of the traditional approach are briefly surveyed, together with some criticisms of it as applied to safer sex. The final section describes the interactional matrix within which safe and unsafe behaviour is negotiated and moulded.

## The Traditional Account

While it is not always possible to do so when considering specific pieces of research, it is possible and helpful to distinguish two broad families of theoretical model in the traditional account. The first is the Health Belief Model, a psychological formulation, widely used in the study of health promoting behaviour (Rosenstock, 1974a,b; Becker, 1974) The other is an approach deriving from the area of risk perception. These approaches are not logically incompatible and are often deployed in parallel (see for example, Fitzpatrick *et al.*, 1989).

### The Health Belief Model

The most influential of the theoretical approaches to the understanding of unsafe sexual behaviour has been the Health Belief Model (HBM) and its variants. The model seeks to predict whether people will make changes to their behaviour (such as accepting medical treatment, stopping smoking or taking up safe sex) by considering two broad groups of factors, first the individual's willingness, readiness or preparedness to change, and second a group of interactional factors. An individual's willingness to change is derived from knowledge (about the illness or condition involved), an assessment of its seriousness and of the costs involved in making the change. The interactional factors are those structural or other external factors which encourage or hinder the proposed changes, typically matters such as the cost of treatment or the level of peer support.

What we might term the basic model is typically augmented in various ways, most importantly by the introduction of the concept of self-efficacy (Bandura, 1977) or internal locus of control (Rotter, 1966). Noting that knowledge, attitudes and beliefs are not sufficient to predict behaviour change, researchers sought the mediating factors which enhanced or impeded their ability to act on their wishes. Noting that some people will always 'go with the herd' while others will persistently 'plough their own furrow', the researchers sought to quantify this ability in the concept of self-efficacy. The notion has some surface validity in the area of smoking. The decision not to smoke will be more difficult to put into practice if you are a herd follower and the herd is smoking.

### Risk Assessment

The second major strand of theoretical modelling of the uptake and maintenance of safer sex derives from ideas about subjective risk assessment (Kahnemann and Tversky, 1972; Tversky and Kahnemann, 1974). The assessment of risk, it is argued, is a complex but common facet of human experience, driven by fear and anxiety over uncertain outcomes. Fear and anxiety are biological mechanisms that generate motivation for coping actions. In this approach, the individual is seen to make an assessment of two things: the seriousness of the outcome — in this case, HIV infection — and the probability of infection. Both these processes are notoriously difficult to measure, not least because they often, in practice, affect one another in the sense that a particularly serious outcome will be seen as more likely than a less serious one.

There are, within this approach two broad schools. On the one hand, the straightforward risk assessment model sees the problem as one of convincing individuals that there is a real probability of infection. This focuses attention on 'perceived invulnerability' or denial. Implicit in this approach is the idea that the consequences of HIV infection are so bad that no-one would rationally discount them, though this may have to be re-assessed following the discovery of 'survivor guilt' (Odets, 1992).

The second broad strand of risk assessment models is the 'cost-benefit' analysis of sexual behaviour change. In this model, the costs of adopting safer sex, in terms of the loss of pleasure have to be counted against the benefits of non-infection. While there is much to be said for this approach, the way in which it has traditionally been used (see, for example, McKusick, 1985), is to call for the eroticization of safer sex — of condoms or of body rubbing for example — in an attempt to reduce the difference in pleasure to be gained from safe as opposed to unsafe behaviour.

## Problems with the Traditional Accounts

While a great deal of paper has been expended on considering the ability or failure of the various models, often entwined in differing degrees, to account for behaviour change or maintenance, we believe that the approaches are fundamentally misguided, based on two fallacious assumptions which render them at best partial, at worst simply misleading. These two assumptions we have elsewhere (Davies, 1992) termed the *individualist* and the *romantic fallacies*.

### The Individualist Fallacy

The vast majority of articles on unsafe sex among gay and bisexual men seek to elucidate the reasons why individuals continue to have unsafe sex. The aim of this literature is to enable the identification of individuals and groups who are in need of intervention, in the form of education, therapy or support. It is, we suggest, highly unlikely that this search will be particularly fruitful, and this for two reasons. First, the model, betraying its antecedents, implicitly assumes that the decision to have safe sex is one which is taken once and for all, when the constellation of knowledge, attitudes and beliefs comes into focus for an individual. This implicit characterization lies behind what we regard as the methodological artefact of 'relapse' (see Davies 1992; Davies *et al.*, 1993). While there is some validity in the idea that knowledge, attitude and behaviour have to be in agreement for the individual to decide to 'take up' safer sex, the putting of this intention into practice will involve a complex negotiation each and every time she or he has sex, a negotiation which is the more charged if the sexual partner is a new one. It seems misguided, therefore, to look for the causes of relapse only in the psychology of the individual rather than to take into account also the characteristics of the encounter. This refocusing of attention onto the encounter is not reducible to the measurement of interaction as prescribed by HBM. We do not regard individuals as carrying around with them fixed amounts of self-efficacy, for example. The ability to put into practice the good intention of having safe sex depends crucially on the person with whom that sex is happening.

Second, and most important, we note that sex is, after language, the most interactive of activities. We have written elsewhere (Davies *et al.*, 1993: 48): '[Sex] is, in its myriad diversities, an exchange of pleasure, a negotiation of desire, a sharing of self and body.' It is, admittedly, the case that the traditional models incorporate some measure of interaction, but two problems render this inclusion ultimately unhelpful. First, they usually assume (implicitly, in the main) that communication is verbal. Thus, communication skills are typically measured by questionnaire items such as 'I find it easy to tell my sexual partners that . . .'. Yet, the communication which goes on in sexual interaction is predominantly non-verbal. It is in the positioning of the body, in a set of non-verbal cues that intentions, preferences and desires are made known. Second, while it is clear that an individual can have good or poor communication skills, she or he will not always and in every situation be able to put these into good effect. Even a good conversationalist can be thrown by unforeseen circumstance or overshadowed by a better. With all this emphasis on interaction, communication and negotiation, it is also important to recognize that in many circumstances, there is little or no potential for an individual to make choices.

### The Romantic Fallacy

Implicit in much of the debate on safer sexual behaviour is the assumption that unsafe behaviour is the result of irrational, 'natural' drives, instincts or emotions overpowering or over-riding the rationally perceived need for safer sex. This perspective falls very straightforwardly out of two millennia of Western, particularly Christian, thought which has elaborated a dualistic and antagonistic view of humanity, one in which the (rational, spiritual, godlike) mind is in a battle for control of the individual's destiny with the (irrational, instinctual, base, animal) body. The language of Christian spirituality which extols the subservience of the bodily appetites to the needs of the spirit suffuses our language of sexuality.

The ramifications of this heritage are too wide to be discussed here, for what is at issue is the very particular way in which safer sex is presented and viewed as a means of rational control of sexual behaviour. This notion of rationality lies at the heart of the debate about safer sex. Yet, the concept is often used in a contradictory and confusing manner, which muddies the debate and is unhelpful in the urgent task of understanding, establishing and reinforcing safer sexual behaviour.

Perhaps the most insidious and pervasive misuse of the term *rational* is that which confuses the process of decision-making with the decision itself. When used correctly, the term refers to the process, not the outcome. Thus, a decision is rational if it is made after a consideration of the available evidence in the light of the circumstances pertaining at the time. By contrast, an irrational decision is one which ignores, dismisses or otherwise deems irrelevant available information.

The eventual decision — which we will take, for the sake of exemplar and without loss of generality, to be a decision to fuck — may, in addition, be right or wrong according to epidemiological or other criteria, but the rationality of the decision process is independent of the rightness of the outcome. Thus an individual can (a) rationally come to the right decision; (b) irrationally come to the right decision; (c) rationally come to the wrong decision; (d) irrationally come to the wrong decision. The criteria on which we decide whether a decision is right or wrong and the criteria by which we decide if a process is rational or irrational are distinct.

Even among those writers who use rational to refer to the process of decision-making, there is a tendency to use an unrealistically complex version of the decision making process. They regard individuals as making rational decisions on the basis of detailed epidemiological data and sophisticated models of contagion and infection which are simply outside the scope of the ordinary person in the street or bedroom. A common assumption of researchers using the rational model is that the utility of infection, or more accurately, its disutility, is so overwhelming that the transient pleasure of a mere fuck cannot, rationally, ever outweigh the potential devastation of infection. This is a bloodless and arrogant view, yet it underpins the agenda which sees the eradication of HIV transmission as following from the eradication of fucking among gay men.

Third, the failure of the model as a descriptive tool lies in its elision of the fact that individuals make choices, not on the basis of accurate information — the average man in the Cleethorpes omnibus does not anxiously peruse the British Medical Journal to assess the prevalence of HIV infection in his locality — but on the basis of heuristic rules (Tversky and Kahnemann, 1974; Weatherburn, 1990). Thus, the common decision in the early years of the epidemic in Britain not to fuck with Americans was a relatively good heuristic device which recognized the difference in prevalence between the two countries. On the other hand, cues such as the physical appearance of an individual or his perceived lifestyle are relatively poor heuristic devices and are rightly discouraged by health promotion interventions.

## The SIGMA Model

Sexual behaviour occurs in a wider, social context, within which it attains and creates meaning. No intervention can afford to ignore the implications of this cultural specificity. The following discussion is based on work carried out in Britain since 1986, which concentrates on gay and bisexual men. Nevertheless, what is presented here has a wider application which we invite our colleagues to assess and debate. At the heart of the project's approach is a detailed analysis of the structure of sexual behaviour, which is notable for focusing attention not on the individual but concentrating on the process of sexual interaction, an approach which is invaluable in avoiding some of the pitfalls of the individualist fallacy.

### Sexual Acts

The logical primitives of any study of sexual behaviour are sexual acts, not identities, proclivities or preferences. From the specific point of view of HIV, this focus is crucial since each act carries a different probability of transmitting the virus. From the more general point of view, the formulation allows the complexity of sexual behaviour to be captured far more easily than approaches which begin with the individual. The project identifies a set of fourteen core sexual acts. These are: masturbation, fellatio, anal intercourse, anilingus, anodigital insertion, anobrachial intercourse, lindinism (urolagnia), coprophilia, enemas, frottage, inter-femoral intercourse, corporal punishment, massage, and deep kissing. A number of points need to be made at this juncture. First, although the list is long, it is not exhaustive. Other specific acts will be reported by individuals, whose range and the consequent length of the list of acts is limited only by inventiveness and physical ingenuity.

Second, and more specifically, there are some acts which will always, in our culture at least, be considered sexual. The insertion of the penis into the rectum, for example will always carry sexual connotations (as well as others). On the other hand, there are acts which become sexual only because they occur in an erotic, sexualized context. Massage, for example, can carry little or no erotic charge on some occasions, while on others it might be intensely erotic and sexually charged.

Third, by asserting the logical primacy of sexual acts, we are not engaged in a biological or behavioural reductionism. We are not seeking to confine these acts within sterile behavioural definitions. We are not, for example, saying that male masturbation is reducible to the stroking of an erect penis by the hand. Such an act becomes masturbation only when the actor so wills and understands it. The intention to masturbate gives the act meaning.

The above three points: infinity, contextuality and intentionality point to the fact that the exercise in which we are engaged in this chapter is a refinement of thought: an attempt to render coherent the actual use of these terms by individuals in our culture, not a confinement of behaviour within bounds formed by the inability to think clearly or in an imaginative manner about our sexual experiences.

Fourth, although it is in the nature of language to impose a logical framework on a fluid reality, it is not always possible to distinguish completely and absolutely the boundaries between acts. When does a massage of the genital area move to become a gentle masturbation? Does running the mouth and tongue along the shaft of the penis count as sucking? Just how much hand has to be inserted to count as fisting?

It is important to realise that these problems are neither unique to the study of sexual behaviour, nor do they vitiate any discussion of sexual matters in these terms. All language carries such ambiguity, yet we manage in everyday life and in scientific endeavour to cope with these problems. Such problems remain unanswerable in the abstract, but remain the stuff of scolasticism: how many angels were there on the point of the pin?

### Gendering of Acts

It is clear that sexual acts are asymmetric in the sense that doing $x$ to someone is not the same as having $x$ done to you. One way to capture this asymmetry is to consider acts from the point of view of an ego, the actor. It is then possible to modulate each of the acts above, so that it can be done either (i) by and to self, (ii) by ego to alter, (iii) by alter to ego or (iv) by ego to alter and by alter to ego simultaneously. In principle, therefore, $4 \times 14$ modulated acts are defined, but, as the alert reader will have noticed, some of these are physically impossible. Nevertheless, in the last seven years we have been surprised on a number of occasions when acts or combinations of acts that we had thought physically impossible were described by our respondents. Ingenuity and dexterity are great adjuncts to a healthy and varied sexual life.

Some of these modulated acts can be gendered, either physically or psychically. Some modulated acts are possible only between a man and a woman, such as penile penetration of the vagina. Other acts which are not so confined by biology are also gendered if, for example, they can be done 'by' a man 'to' a woman and by a man to a man, but not by a woman to a man.[2] In this latter case, we propose that the gender significance of the act remains when the act is performed in a homosexual context. Thus, a woman may suck a man's penis, but a man may not do this to a woman. We suggest that the gendering of the act is also present when a man sucks another man's penis, though, as we shall argue this does not necessarily mean that the suckee automatically becomes the feminine, only that this is a symbolic connotation that may be enhanced, subverted or transcended.

### Sexual Sessions

Sexual acts do not occur at random across space and time. We do not often meet a sexual act while walking around Marks and Spencer. The primary 'chunking' of sexual behaviour is into sexual sessions or sexual encounters. A session consists of an ordered set of sexual acts involving one or more people in a specific place over a relatively short period of time. It is worth considering each of the elements of this definition in some detail.

Definitionally, sessions consist of one or more sexual acts, ordered either sequentially or simultaneously. While there are some acts which are physically impossible, painful or difficult to perform simultaneously, there is no logical or a priori reason why acts should occur in particular sequences or groups. Yet there are clearly distinct patterns of acts and these are, we suggest, culturally informed.

Turner (1984) has described the ways in which the body is a prime site of social control and it would be perverse not to see in the agreed grammar of sexual interaction some form of cultural control. In the same way that it is not always possible to distinguish one act from another, so it is often not always easy to decide whether one or the other act follows, overlaps with or is simultaneous with another. This, though logically inconvenient, is not a major problem.

The timing of a session is sometimes difficult to determine. Whereas in some cases, the action begins, continues and comes to an end without interruption or pause, in many cases, sessions will have longeurs, while the participant(s) rest, have a spliff, get (un)dressed, answer the phone, feed the cat or do any of those things that had earlier been forgotten. How long a pause has to be before one extended session becomes two distinct ones is a matter of little practical import: a logical nicety, which the pedantic will delight in exploring at length. For men, a common marker of the end of a session is orgasm, but while this is common it is not universal: sessions may end without orgasm while others may continue after it. For women, such an obvious end-marker does not obtain. Other cues will inform the cessation of intimacies.

Though it may on first sight seem clear-cut, it turns out that the question of determining the number of participants in a sexual session is far from straightforward. Rather than consider the difference between a solo session and one involving two people as discrete entities, it is possible to think in terms of points on a continuum. This may seem odd, even perverse, but consider the following. A person alone in a room, wanking and doing whatever else turns them on will commonly fantasize, establishing in some cases, an imaginary or remembered other as the focus for erotic excitement. Otherwise, still photographs of individuals in states of undress or provocative dress might be employed as a concrete focus of erotic interest. Magazines which reproduce still photographs of sexual sessions, either of individuals or of two or moresomes, provide not only external focus, but also a sequence which the reader is invited to follow. Textual descriptions of sexual sessions, telephone lines which play pre-recorded verbal descriptions of sexual sessions, videos of people having sex, all provide not only a focus of erotic attention, but also guide it temporally, seeking to heighten arousal and interest over a period of time. The consumer will have differing degrees of control over the timing. In the telephone case, this is largely outside control, while videos and text allow choices to be made, boring bits skipped or particularly enjoyable sequences to be lingered over. All these modes of enjoyment involve only one participant directly but others are involved vicariously, either unknowingly, as in the fantasy built round the builder, the biker or the pizza boy casually encountered during the day, or more directly, as when people are filmed having sex together.

In any meaningful sense of the term, however, it is clear that these scenarios involve only one participant. It is from this only a small step, however, to consider an individual pleasuring him/herself in the presence of another(s). These others might indeed be the photographers, camera operators or spectators at a live sex show, in which case they themselves may or may not be sexually aroused and the main participant may seek to dismiss their presence from their minds, as do some strippers who report thinking about the shopping to distance themselves from the scenario. In other cases, the presence of the other can be a source of excitement. Having sex in public places carries an extra erotic charge because of the reactions of unwitting others. In specifically defined erotic spaces, however, the presence of another may also be a source of narcissistic pleasure. It turns me on that he is turned on by me, even though I find him physically unattractive. Otherwise it is the derived pleasure of the other which is itself reflexively exciting. He turns me on; seeing him getting turned on turns me on and great sex can happen without physical contact. In these cases, it makes sense to talk of two (or more) participants, even though it may be that no physical contact takes place, as on an interactive phone line.

It is useful, then, to make a distinction between participants and sexual partners. A participant becomes a partner when physical contact is made (but see below). Clearly, this criterion describes not a discrete class of events, but a continuum. Two men having sex in a cruising ground, for example, may be masturbating while watching each other. Physical contact might be non-existent, or confined to, say, the chest or the back and confined to friendly encouragement: a positive stroke. On the other hand, it might be specifically sexual and focused on particular areas, the nipples, the armpit, the toes, even the genitals, which give direct sexual charges. At this point participants become sexual partners and may engage in any or all of the acts mentioned above.

A similar continuum can be constructed between twosomes and threesomes, ranging from the couple constructing a fantasy scenario, through watching a video and tempering the action to the development of that session, or through the unwitting, witting, non-participation or involvement of another person. Further definitional complications arise in the case of threesomes if one person is excluded from the action for a period of time. The inimitable Victoria Wood described the end of an unsuccessful attempt at a sexual threesome: 'They got onto politics and I ended up watching "Take the High Road" with the sound down.'

The point to be made is that sex is not simple. A comprehensive study of sex and sexuality should include aspects of all of these. A study whose primary focus is HIV transmission can concentrate on partners and exclude from detailed consideration the complications of participation, erotic focus, intentionality and control that we have mentioned. Studies which seek to inform intervention must take these matters most seriously, however, since it is within this cultural matrix that both the hindrances to and the means to encourage safer sex are to be found.

It may come as a surprise given the examples that we have adduced so far, but it is only at the level of the session that the sex and the gender of the participants becomes relevant. The fact that the participants are, for example, both female will exclude the possibility of any act involving the penis. Two men will not be able to have vaginal intercourse. Certain combinations of acts will not be possible in specific circumstances. A man and a woman will not be able to fuck each other (if we take fuck to involve the penis). Each session therefore has a sexuality, derived from the sex of its participants.

The issue of gender is altogether more complicated. Sex is often subversive, in ways that are beyond the scope of this current discussion. The man who invites sexual domination from another man dressed as a woman is playing a subtle game, not only with sexuality but with gender. The widespread popularity of transsexual sex-workers in many countries points to a far less rigid set of gender roles than most commentators allow. This has important consequences for interventions, in that programs which have been successful in one cultural context will not necessarily translate into others where gender boundaries are differently drawn.

### Sexual Individuals

The sexual career of an individual can now be defined as the sum of the sessions in which she or he has participated. On this basis, it is possible, at least in principle (in practice, it is fraught with problems) to distinguish completely homosexual and completely heterosexual individuals and to describe also individuals with varying degrees of bisexual experience.

This is not to restrict the sexual to the physical. We recognize that sexual behaviour and sexual interest or preference are both logically and empirically distinct. A sexual identity does not predict absolutely sexual practice, nor does sexual behaviour predict identification. There are clearly degrees of deception. Married men have sex with other men in clandestine ways. Gay men covertly have sex with women and lesbians sleep with 'the enemy' for money or pleasure. Many more will have fantasies at odds with their chosen identification. The relationship between avowed identity and behaviour is at best probabilistic.

Although sexual individuals are logically third-order constructs, they are the primary focus of studies of sexual behaviour. This is mainly because it is not easy to think of practical methods of sampling directly sexual sessions in all but a few contexts. The best strategy to date is the method of recall, in which respondents are asked to recount relevant details of a recent sexual encounter (see, for example, Gold *et al.*, 1991). While this does not give, in the strict sense, a direct sample of encounters, such a method does, with heterogeneity in the group of individuals, at least focus attention on the session as the locus of decision-making.

## CODA

The history of AIDS is, among other things, the history of a search for simple solutions. There is a widespread and distressing tendency among many professionals, well-meaning and competent though they may be, to react with either incomprehension or ill-disguised animosity if their cherished, simple either incomprehension or ill-disguised animosity if their cherished, simple solutions are challenged. In the early days of the epidemic, there was a pressing need, in the face of ignorance about the causes and prognosis of AIDS, to do something quickly. Indeed, the early response in the gay communities of North America, for example, was remarkably effective in cutting annual incidence rates to extremely low levels. Many of the solutions were simple and effective and demonstrably appropriate. Ten years and more into the continuing pandemic, it should occasion neither surprise nor concern that those simple solutions become inadequate and increasingly inappropriate. There is no need to resort to the vocabulary of relapse to appreciate that living with the need for safer sex over a decade is a more difficult and complex process than adopting such practices in the face of an immediate and frightening new threat to life.

The role, even the duty, of social and behavioural scientists in the fight against AIDS is to describe and seek to understand the complexity of sexual decision-making in order to inform the next generation of health promotion initiatives. In so doing, we believe that a more sophisticated understanding of the relationship between individuals, preferences, partners, sessions and acts is vital if our understanding of sexual behaviour is to keep pace with the frightening expansion of the epidemic.

## Notes

1 Project SIGMA (Socio-sexual Investigations of Gay Men and AIDS) is a project funded jointly by the Medical Research Council and the Department of Health.
2 The gendering of sexual language and its rendition in terms of activity and passivity is pervasive. It does not seem to be possible, without absurdly long periphrases to avoid this. The terms are, therefore rendered in nonce marks.

## References

BANDURA, A. (1977) 'Self-efficacy: Toward a unifying theory of behavioural change', *Psychological Review*, 84, pp. 191–215.
BECKER, M.H. (ed.) (1974) *Health Education Monograph*, *2(4)*, special edition of the HBM, reprinted as *The Health Belief Model and Personal Health Behaviour*, NJ: Charles Black.
DAVIES, P. (1992) 'On relapse: Recidivism or rational response?', in AGGLETON, P., DAVIES, P. and HART, G. (Eds) *AIDS: Rights, Risk and Reason*, London: Falmer Press, pp. 133–41.
DAVIES, P.M., HICKSON, F.C.I., WEATHERBURN, P. and HUNT, A.J. (1993) *Sex, Gay Men and AIDS*, London: Falmer Press.
FITZPATRICK, R., BOULTON, M. and HART, G. (1989) 'Gay men's sexual behaviour in response to AIDS', in AGGLETON, P., DAVIES, P. and HART, G. (Eds), 1989: *AIDS: Social Representations, Social Practices*, London: Falmer Press., pp. 127–46.
GOLD, R.S., SKINNER, M.S., GRANT, P.J. and PLUMMER, D.C. (1991) 'Situational factors and thought processes associated with unprotected intercourse in gay men', *Psychology and Health*, 5, pp. 121–8.

KAHNEMAN, D. and TVERSKY, A. (1972) 'Subjective probability: A judgement of representatives', *Cognitive Psychology*, 3, pp. 430–54.

MCKUSICK, L., HARTMAN, W. and COATES, T.J. (1985) 'AIDS and sexual behaviour reported by gay men in San Francisco', *American Journal of Public Health*, 75, pp. 493–6.

ODETS, W.W. (1992) 'Unconscious motivations for the practice of unsafe sex among gay men in the United States' poster presented at the VIIIth International Conference on AIDS', *Amsterdam Abstract* No: PoD, 5191.

ROTTER, J.B. (1966) 'Generalised expectancies for internal versus external control of reinforcement', *Psychological Monographs*, 80(1).

TVERSKY, A. and KAHNEMAN, D. (1974) 'Judgement under uncertainty: Heuristics and biases', *Science*, 185, pp. 1124–31.

WEATHERBURN, P. (1990) *HIV, STDs and Perceived Risk: A Theoretical Overview and Two Pilot Studies*, Project SIGMA Working Paper no. 11, London.

Chapter 5

# Analysing Naturally-Occurring Data on AIDS Counselling: Some Methodological and Practical Issues

*David Silverman*

One of the least fruitful questions one can ask a sociologist is: 'to what school of social science do you belong?' For instance, although it would be easy to interpret this chapter as a defence of 'qualitative methodology', this would be misleading. As I will shortly explain, I reject the fashionable identification of qualitative method with an analysis of how people *see* things, preferring to focus instead on how people *do* things. Moreover, there are no principled grounds to be either qualitative or quantitative in approach. It all depends upon what you are trying to do. Indeed, often one will want to combine both approaches. For instance, I will shortly discuss how we have tested a hypothesis by using simple tabulations on fifty-odd examples of HIV counselling 'advice packages' whose form can readily be identified and counted.

Analytically, I follow in the tradition of many sociologists who have argued about the need to avoid reducing methodological issues to ones of technique (for instance, Mills, 1959 and Cicourel, 1964). I believe that analytical issues are central to methodological discussion. This means that I take to be the main question, at least in case-study research, the quality of the analysis rather than the recruitment of the sample or the format of the interview (see Mitchell, 1983).

My underlying theme is simple: the relevance to practice of rigorous micro work informed by analytical issues rather than by social problems. Practically, it is usually necessary to refuse to allow our research topics to be defined in terms of the conceptions of social problems as recognized by either professional or community groups. Ironically, by beginning from a clearly defined sociological perspective, I show how we can later address such social problems with, I believe, considerable force and persuasiveness.

Let me begin controversially by suggesting that there are two dangerous orthodoxies shared by many sociologists and by policy-makers who Commission social research. The first orthodoxy is that people are puppets of social structures.

According to this model, what people do is defined by society. In practice, this reduces to explaining people's behaviour as the outcome of certain 'face-sheet' variables (like social class, gender or ethnicity). Let me call this the *Explanatory Orthodoxy*. According to it, social scientists do research to provide explanations of given problems, such as why do individuals engage in unsafe sex? Inevitably, such research will find explanations based on one or more face-sheet variables.

The second orthodoxy is that people are 'dopes'. Interview respondents' knowledge is assumed to be imperfect, indeed they may even lie to us. In the same way, practitioners (like doctors or counsellors) are assumed always to depart from normative standards of good practice. This is the *Divine Orthodoxy*. It makes the social scientist into the philosopher king (or queen) who can always see through people's claims and know better than they do.

What is wrong with these two orthodoxies? The Explanatory Orthodoxy is so concerned to rush to an explanation that it fails to ask serious questions about what it is explaining. There is a parallel here with what we must now call a post-modern phenomenon. I gather that visitors to the Grand Canyon in Arizona are now freed from the messy business of exploring the Canyon itself. Instead, they can now spend an enlightening hour or so in a multi-media 'experience' which gives them all the thrills in a pre-digested way. Then they can be on their way, secure in the knowledge that they have 'done' the Grand Canyon.

This example is part of something far larger. In contemporary culture, the environment around phenomena has become more important than the phenomenon itself. So people are more interested in the lives of movie stars than in the movies themselves. Equally, on sporting occasions, pre- and post-match interviews become as exciting (or even more exciting) than the game itself. In my terms, in both cases, *the phenomenon escapes*. This is precisely what the explanatory orthodoxy encourages. Because we rush to offer explanations of all kinds of social phenomena, we rarely spend enough time trying to understand how the phenomenon works. So, for instance, we may simply impose an operational definition of unsafe sex or a normative version of good counselling, failing totally to examine how such activities come to have meaning in what people are actually doing in everyday (naturally-occurring) situations.

This directly leads to the folly of the Divine Orthodoxy. Its methods preclude seeing the good sense of what people are doing or understanding their skills in local contexts. It prefers interviews where people are forced to answer questions that never arise in their day-to-day life. Because it rarely looks at this life, it condemns people to fail without understanding that we are all cleverer than we can say in so many words. Even when it examines what people are actually doing, the divine orthodoxy measures their activities by some idealizied normative standards, like 'good communication'. So, once again, like ordinary people, practitioners are condemned to fail.

In what follows, I will outline how one can organize research in a way which seeks to satisfy three ends:

1   A focus on how a particular phenomenon is constituted, looking at what people are actually doing in real-life situations.
2   A search for explanations grounded in data drawn from these situations, so that we can address 'why?' because we have secure knowledge of 'how'.
3   An invitation to a dialogue with practitioners based on a sound knowledge of what they are doing *in situ*.

Given our common interest in social research on HIV and AIDS, I want to address these issues in the context of a continuing research programme, funded by the Health Education Authority and Glaxo Holdings plc, which, since 1988, has been assembling and analysing tape-recordings of counselling from nine HIV-testing centres in Britain, the USA and Trinidad. (More detailed discussions of this work are available in Perakyla, 1991a; Perakyla and Bor, 1990; Perakyla and Silverman, 1991a, 1991b; Silverman, 1989, 1990; Silverman and Bor, 1991; Silverman and Perakyla, 1990; Silverman, Bor and Perakyla, 1992, and Silverman, Bor, Miller and Goldman, 1992.)

Before I develop further the methodological implications of this research, it will be helpful to discuss some of our findings. In particular, what has our analysis of these tape-recordings revealed about how HIV counselling works? Let me relate these findings to what look like reasonable expectations about what goes on in counselling. Note that I am not, at this stage, assigning any empirical validity to these expectations, nor do I cite any supporting references. Let me simply propose that these are nothing more than reasonable expectations based upon conventional social science perspectives and upon common normative accounts of good counselling practice.

### Assumed Features of HIV Counselling

Although many kinds of counselling may deal with intimate matters, HIV counselling, with its presumed focus on such topics as sexuality and/or illegal drug use, seems to be concerned with particularly delicate issues. We might, therefore, predict that clients (and indeed some counsellors) may find it embarrassing to talk about delicate topics. However, social science teaches us to expect cultural and sub-cultural diversity. This suggests that we should expect to find cross-cultural variations in what constitutes a delicate matter and how people talk about it.

Given such variations, health promotion professionals usually assume that effective counselling works by eliciting the client's perspective rather than by imposing a body of information with an unknown relation to that perspective. Moreover, training programmes (whether for beginners or practitioners) may be presumed to work on the assumption that counsellors need to be taught the skills to practice effective counselling. These assumptions are summarized in Table 5.1 below:

---

1 Clients may find it embarrassing to talk about delicate topics.

2 We should expect cross-cultural variations in how people talk about their sexuality.

3 Eliciting the client's perspective is the basis of effective counselling.

4 Counselling skills can be learned through proper training.

---

*Table 5.1: Standard expectations about HIV counselling*

Our research has not invalidated any of these four assumptions. However, it has revealed that the situation has more nuances than we might expect. In turn, this has clear implications for counselling practice. Let me review each of the above assumptions in the light of our findings.

*Assumption 1: Clients may find it embarrassing to talk about delicate topics*

I have already noted (in Assumption 3 above) that it is usually assumed that effective counselling involves trying to elicit the client's perspective. This is reflected in a standard question asked by counsellors at an early stage at all our centres. This question is some variation of 'Why do you want an HIV test?' We find a version of this question in Extract 1 below (*C* is the counsellor and *P* is the patient; transcription symbols are given in an appendix to this chapter):

**Extract 1** (8A2)

```
1 C:   Can I just briefly ask why: you thought about having
2       an HIV test done:

3 P:   .hh We:ll I mean it's something that you have these
4       I mean that you have to think about these da:ys, and
5       I just uh:m felt (0.8) you- you have had sex with
6       several people and you just don't want to go on (.)
7       not knowing.
```

We might first note that P delays giving a response to C's question (via taking a breath and a preface 'We:ll I mean', line 3). Such delays are massively recurrent before patients answer this kind of question (see Silverman and Perakyla, 1990 and Silverman and Bor, 1991). It is tempting to see this as indicating potential embarrassment on P's part.

However, there are two reasons why we should avoid this temptation. First, we have no access to what *P* is thinking. So, any attempt to link her answer with her psychological state would be risky. Second, we do have access to what follows *P*'s turns. If we examine how these interviews proceed, on a line-by-line basis, we can find out what *follows* from the way *P* constructs her turn. This will give access to what she is doing (i.e., the function of her turn) rather than to the murky area of what she may be thinking.

Although not given here, after *P* has spoken, the counsellor, as in most other interviews, requests *P* to specify what she means by the descriptions she has offered. Such requests for specification typically occur in professional-client encounters where a professional requires more precision. By requesting specification, *C* thus makes *P*'s account into a 'gloss' or generalization which needs to be unpacked.

In the context of HIV pre-test counselling, how may *P*'s turn be heard as a generalization or gloss? First, *P* does not offer, straight off, any information about herself or about the presumably risky activities which have led her to want an HIV test. Instead, *P* opts for a 'business as usual' first reason for wanting an HIV test ('We:ll I mean it's something that you have these- I mean that you have to think about these da:ys'). This neatly locates having an HIV test within a range of ordinary activities that you engage in 'these days'. This allows her to delay information about her sense of her own exposure to risk until lines 5–7. Moreover, this information is delivered after multiple speech perturbations: a hesitation ('uh:m'), a 0.8 second pause and a repair ('you- you').

Second, *P* conveys the information about having 'had sex with many people' in the impersonal voice of 'you', thus linking it to what she has just said about what everyone does 'these days'. This functions to gloss over her own precise actions and their implications for her own life. For instance, one can 'have had sex with several people' in the context of serial monogamy without being unfaithful to any one partner.

We now see why *C* (data not given) might want to treat *P*'s answer as a 'gloss' and to request further specification. However, in Extract 1, the patient is a heterosexual woman. In Extract 2 below, *P* is a gay man being counselled at a Gay Mens' Health Clinic staffed by gay counsellors. If delay and lack of specification ('glossing') were consequences of 'embarrassment', we might predict that they would be less evident here.

Extract 2 is taken from a little way into the consultation. As in Extract 1, it begins with a very general question from the counsellor about why the patient wanted an HIV test.

**Extract 2** (56A WH)

```
1  C:   Would you tell me (0.3) what (0.2) what's happened you know
2       what [m- made you worry about [t this.
3  P:        [tch .hh                 [er: er:: Well I: (.) met
```

    4       this: (.) ma:n and we sort of like (.) (did) it for a while.
    5       (0.7) And he: knew my condition because (0.7) er it's very
    6       difficult for me to start you know up front you know boom you
    7       know. .hh Well this is what I am this is you know (.) so
    8       basically what I do is instead of like stating (0.8) I am
    9       negative and I expect (you to be negative) whatever I- I sort of
    10      like (0.2) go through a more: uh (0.7) er a roundabout way of
    11      saying it [P now talks about his nationality in regard to
            immigration]

Notice how P organizes the beginning of his answer in exactly the same way as
the patient in Extract 1. There are multiple delays and hesitations before a
partner is described, the description is given in very general terms (this: (.) ma:n)
and the risk activities are largely glossed (and we sort of like (.) (did) it for a
while). P only elaborates his answer when, shortly after, on line 24 below, C
requests specification:

### Extract 3 (56A WH continuation)

    24  C:  [(Well so [did you)- so did you =

    25  P:         [Which is-

    26  C:  = have [safe sex [(with him).

    27  P:         [.hhh    [Ye:s.

    28  P:  'Ye:s. But you know there were some parts that were rather:
    29      [risky:

    30  C:  [(                    ).

    31  P:  (When you're (.) in contact with [this you know.

    32  C:                                   [Ye:s.

    33  C:  Yeah.

    34  P:  Yeah. .hh There were certain times when I thought when I
    35      thought well maybe we shouldn't have crossed the line you
    36      know because we were sort of like borderli:ne [you know
    37
    38  C:              [Can you tell me: I mean I- it's not that I want to pry
    39                           [but I'm a little ] =

    40  P:                       [n- No no no] =

    41  C:  = [concerned about the validity.

```
42  P:    = [it's all right no of course of course [uhm

43  C:       [Could you tell me (              [    )

44

45  P:    [s-

46  P:    Well you know uhm (0.9) I understand that oral sex is the least

47        (0.5) er: risky.

48  C:    Ri:gh[t.

49  P:         [Another we did er: er oral sex (.) and when we did it we was

50        protected. .hhh U:hm (0.5) b- b-

51        But that [wa-

52  C:               [You each had a condom o:n when-

53               [when you- you do oral sex.

54  P:    [Right. Right yeah. But no- not necessarily at all ti:mes you

55        know and certainly not at the very beginning you know it was

56        sort of like (0.2) .hh

57                    (            )

58  C:    Mm hm

59  P:    a:nd (1.5) then I found out eventually that the guy was in fact

60        positive.
```

In Extract 3, notice how *P* responds to *C*'s request for specification with a straight 'yes', produced early and without hesitation. Immediately after, however, *P* qualifies his answer (But you know there were some parts that were rather: [risky:).[1] Notice how this is a very general answer, hearable by *C* as a gloss. Moreover, when *P* expands his answer, he uses formulae like 'crossing the line' and 'borderline' which again do not spell out the details. Only when *C* requests specification (line 38), thereby turning *P*'s 'borderline' into a gloss, does *P* produce a more specific description of the activity involved ('oral sex'). Notice once more how *P* initially offers the preferred answer (that a condom was used at all times) and only later qualifies this claim.

Extracts 1–3, therefore, show how people receiving HIV counselling skilfully manage their talk about delicate topics, as follows. First, through delays and hesitations, they mark out their understanding that certain matters are not ordinarily spoken about in general conversation. Thus, they prepare the way for an upcoming hearably delicate item. Second, they recognize the rules of 'preference organization', attending to what is hearable as the preferred answer to a question and producing it rapidly and without delay — only subsequently introducing qualifications (see Heritage, 1984: 265–80). Third, their answers initially are very general and hearable by counsellors as glosses requiring specification. Patients make it clear that, whatever their sexual orientation and the auspices of the counselling interview, they are not the kind of people who *straight off* will talk 'dirty' to a stranger. However, when the counsellor asks for specification, they indeed provide it because now they can produce intimate details as specifically demanded by the counsellor who is thus responsible for bringing them into the conversation.

In Extract 3, notice, however, that the counsellor also organizes his talk with reference to the delicate implications of the subject matter. C couches his request for specification within a question projection ('can you tell me', line 38). As Schegloff (1980) has noted, such formats mark an upcoming potentially delicate topic. This interpretation is supported by the fact that C does not immediately ask his question but adds another explanation for asking it ('it's not that I want to pry but I'm a little concerned about the validity', lines 38–41). It is only after *P* has shown that he accepts *C*'s version of the status of his inquiries (lines 40 and 42) and C repeats his request, that *P* tells more, using turbulent speech to mark oral sex as a delicate object.

Extracts 1–3 clearly indicate that our first assumption (Clients may find it embarrassing to talk about delicate topics) is severely limited. We may replace it with the following finding: the production and management of delicate topics is skilfully and co-operatively organized between professionals and clients.

*Assumption 2: We should expect cross-cultural variations in how people talk about their sexuality*

I have already noted the different genders and sexual orientations of the patients in Extracts 1 and 2–3. Despite this, we have found markedly *similar* features in how they organize their talk about their sexuality. This immediately casts doubt about assumed sub-cultural variations in this area. Moreover, Extract 1 is taken from an English sexually-transmitted diseases clinic open to all patients, whereas Extracts 2–3 come from a Gay Mens' Clinic in the United States. It now looks as though we are finding both sub-cultural and cross-cultural similarities rather than differences.

Let us vary the combination of factors. Extract 4 is taken from an English hospital setting. P is a gay man who is testing because his partner has just tested as positive.

### Extract 4 (SS-2-16.1A)

```
1  C:   Mm hm .hhh What sort of sexual relationship are you having
         at  ___
2        the moment with him.
```

3      (0.6)

4  *P*:   With X.

5  *C*:   Mm hm

6  *P*:   er::: (1.7) We:ll (0.6) hhh God how to go into this on camera:
7        I don't know. .hhhh er:: (2.6) Let me just say I'm on bottom
8        he's on to:p, (0.7) er:: There was a period at the very
9        beginni:ng (0.5) er:: (0.5)
10       where a condom was not- ((Clears throat))
11       excuse me was not used. (0.6)
12       er:[::
13 *C*:   [Are you using condoms now? = [Or er-
14 *P*:                                [uh We::ll (0.4)

15       yeah. Mm (1.0) er::: (.) There is: (.) still some oral se:x,
16       (0.6) er:: not passing any fluids alo:ng but they say: (0.4) that
17       yes you do pass fluid along. (0.4) So I'm still kind of nervous
18       about that. = However: .hhhh (0.2) er:uh::hhh (0.8) I:- I don't
19       know:: (0.5) what I don't know .hh is er:: (0.2) how: I would
20       have contracted it to him.

22 *C*:   Mm: =

23 *P*:   = er::: (0.7) I have not (1.1) er:: (1.0) had anal intercourse
24       with hi:m.

25       (0.8)

26 *C*:   Okay.

27 *P*:   er::: (0.5) He ha:s

28 *C*:   Mm

29 *P*:   er:: (0.5) performed oral sex on me:

30                        (.)

31 *C*:   M[m:

32 *P*:       [without a condo:m, (.) but I've not ejaculated
33       into his mouth

34 *C*:   Mm

Notice here how *P*, like his peers in Extracts 1–3, *delays* producing a detailed reply in response to *C*'s question. There is a 0.6 second delay (line 3). Then *P* asks *C* to confirm that it is *P*'s partner that he is asking about (line 4). Lines 6–7 consist of a series of hesitations, repairs and delays which make reference to the fact that, in this clinic, all interviews are video-recorded, with patients' consent, for training purposes. Finally, note how *P* prefaces his eventual answer with a projection format ('let me just say', lines 7–8) which, as we have already noted, serves to mark an upcoming delicate topic. Here, additionally, *P*'s use of 'just say' is hearable as inviting what follows to be heard as a gloss. It may thus be seen to constitute a tacit invitation to *C* to request that the gloss be unpacked. And indeed this is what now happens. *C* requests specification (line 13) and offers several response-tokens ('mm mm'), which serve to pass his turn during *P*'s elaboration. Having set up a context in which he may be required to tell more, *P* now does so.

Let us now switch continents once again. Extract 5 comes from a Trinidad hospital. This *P* has been given a positive test result but, even after a long information-delivery from *C*, has stated that he thinks this means that he has AIDS. We are interested in this extract because it is the first point in this interview where P's sexual orientation is mentioned.

### Extract 5 (91A)

```
1  C:   What is your your perception (1.0) of (0.7) this AIDS
2       business

3  P:   ((describes a social worker who had arranged to have his
4       blood taken by a doctor)) and and um his his approach was
5       different (.) and so (.) I gave my blood and that's how I
6       reached this stage (.) otherwise I wouldn't be proceeding
7       as you know (0.2) I'm not very sexually active and (.)
8       whenever I have sex (.) if the person wants to use a condom
9       I use it and if he doesn't or she doesn't (.) or if he
10      (0.3) because I'm homosexual (.) if he doesn't then I don't
```

Although *P* volunteers the self-description 'homosexual', note how it is prefaced by 'I'm not very sexually active' (line 7). This seems to work as a down-grade retrospectively (on *P*'s need for a test) and prospectively (on his sexual orientation). Immediately after this, *P* selects a term for a sexual partner ('person') which is neutral in terms of his own sexual orientation.

Only when *P* unpackages (what now becomes) his initial indefinite reference do we learn that he is gay. But note that his highly implicative use of 'he' to describe a sexual partner (line 9) is immediately repaired ('or she'), thus serving to keep the issue open. Only, finally, via a second repair, does *P* opt for 'he', together with a self-identification as 'homosexual'. So here expressive caution about what may be hearable as delicate matters is neatly set up in a step-by-step movement towards descriptions with more and more implications.

As already noted, this example is from Trinidad (in which it is difficult as a gay man to 'come out', and the sexual orientation of the counsellors is not apparent to the *P*). In the gay mens' clinic in the US, from which Extracts 2–3 derive, *C*s are also known to be gay. Therefore, we might not have predicted the same sort of expressive caution around describing one's sexual orientation or activities. In such a setting, presenting oneself as a patient at the clinic can be read as a category-bound activity which implicitly defines one's sexual orientation.[2]

Nonetheless, this prediction about cultural differences has not been upheld by our data. We are now in a position to offer a second finding: there is little evidence of either sub-cultural or cross-cultural variation in how people talk about their sexuality in counselling interviews; if anything, there is some suggestion of cross-cultural *uniformity*.

For reasons of space, let us now combine Assumptions 3 and 4 and see what our data reveals.

*Assumptions 3–4: Eliciting the client's perspective is the basis of effective counselling. Counselling skills can be learned through proper training*

We can review these assumptions most readily by examining our analysis of the delivery and reception of advice in HIV counselling which closely followed our remit from the Health Education Authority to investigate how safer sex was discussed in these interviews. Fortunately, an earlier study had paved the way for this part of our research.

Heritage and Sefi (1992) have analysed seventy instances of advice-giving sequences drawn from eight first visits to first time mothers by five different health visitors. They found that most advice was initiated by the professional, often prior to any clear indication that it was desired by the client. Health visitor (HV) initiated advice took four forms. First, stepwise entry in the sequence, such as an HV enquiry; a problem-indicative response by the client; a request for specification by HV ('a focusing enquiry'); a specification by the client, or advice-giving. The second form was the same sequence with no request for specification because the client volunteers how she dealt with the problem. The third form involved no client statement of how she dealt with the problem and no HV request for specification (thus stages c and d are omitted). In the fourth form the HV initiated advice without the client giving a problem-indicative response (i.e., the HV enquiry is followed by advice-giving).

The majority of advice initiations analysed were HV-initiated advice. Indeed, in many cases, even the HV's enquiry was not problem-oriented but was more concerned to topicalize the issue for which advice was subsequently delivered. The reception of advice by mothers took three forms. There were *marked acknowledgements* (MAs), such as 'oh right' or repeats of key components of the advice; Heritage and Sefi say such utterances acknowledge the informativeness and appropriateness of the advice. *Unmarked acknowledgements* (UAs), such as 'mm', 'yeah', 'right' — without an 'oh' — are minimal response tokens which, Heritage and Sefi argue, have a primarily continuative function; they do *not* acknowledge the advice-giving as newsworthy to the recipient, or constitute an undertaking to follow the advice, and can be heard as a form of resistance in themselves because, implicitly, such responses are refusing to treat the talk as advice. The third form is *assertion of knowledge* or competence by the mother. These indicate that the advice is redundant — hence may also be taken as resistance. This underlines Heritage and Sefi's argument about the advantages of stepwise entry into advice-giving. In this form of advice-giving, they find less resistance and more uptake displayed by mothers' use of marked acknowledgments. Here the HV's request for her client to specify a problem means that the advice can be recipient-designed, non-adversarial and not attribute blame.

Like Heritage and Sefi, we focused on the link between the form in which advice is delivered and its reception. Nearly all advice sequences were counsellor-initiated; some step-by-step sequences were identified, but the majority were truncated. As in Heritage and Sefi's study, step-by-step sequences were more likely to produce marked acknowledgements, truncated sequences usually produced unmarked acknowledgements. The data on uptake is shown in Table 5.2, which shows a very clear correlation between the way in which an advice sequence is set up and the response that it elicits from the patient. In the total of thirty-two cases where the counsellor delivers advice without attempting to generate a perceived problem from the patient, there are only three cases where the patient shows any sign of uptake. Conversely, in the other eighteen cases, where the advice emerges either at the request of the patient or in a step-by-step sequence, there are only four cases where the patient does *not* show uptake.

| Advice-format | Number | Type of Acknowledgement | |
|---|---|---|---|
| | | unmarked | marked |
| P-initiated | 2 | 0 | 2 |
| C-initiated: | | | |
| Step-by-step: | | | |
| full-sequence | 11 | 1 | 10 |
| shortened | 5 | 3 | 2 |
| Truncated: | | | |
| no P problem elicited | 32 | 29 | 3 |

*Table 5.2: Form of advice and degree of uptake\**

(based on 50 advice sequences)

\*'Unmarked' means only *unmarked* acknowledgements were given in the advice-sequence; 'marked' means that at least *one* marked acknowledgement was given.

So far, Assumption 3 — eliciting the patient's perspective is the basis of effective counselling — seems to be fully borne out. Heritage and Sefi's findings, and our own tabulations both suggest that uptake of advice is directly related to whether the professional attempts to elicit her client's own concerns. Moreover, a first look at an actual case where no such attempts are made may seem to imply that the counsellor concerned lacks the appropriate skills (Assumption 4). Take Extract 6 below:

**Extract 6** (SW2-A)

```
 1  C:    .hhhh Now when someo:ne er is tested (.) and they ha:ve a
 2         negative test result .hh it's obviously dealuh:m that (.) they
 3         then look after themselves to prevent [any further risk of =
 4
 5  P:                                           [Mm hm
 6  C:    = infection. .hhhh I mean obviously this is only possible up to
 7         a point because if .hhh you get into a sort of serious
 8         relationship with someone that's
 9         long ter:m .hh you can't obviously continue to use condoms
10         forever. .hh Uh:m and a point has to come where you make a
11         sort
12         of decision (0.4) uh:m if you are settling down about families
13         and things that you know (0.6) you'd- not to continue safer
           sex.
14         [.hhhh Uh:m but obviously: (1.0) you =
15  P:    [Mm:
16  C:    = nee:d to be (.) uh:m (.) take precautions uhm (0.3) and keep
17         to the safer practices .hhh if: obviously you want to prevent
18         infection in the future.
19  P:    [Mm hm
20  C:    [.hhhh The problem at the moment is we've got it here in
21         {names City} in particular (.) right across the bcar:d you know
22         from all walks of life.
23  P:    Mm hm
24  C:    Uh::m from you know (.) the sort of established high r- risk
25         groups (.) now we're getting heterosexual (.)
26         [transmission as well. .hh Uhm =
27  P:    [Mm hm
28  C:    = so obviously everyone really needs to careful. .hhh Now
           whe- when someone gets a positive test result
29         er: then obviously
30         they're going to ke- think very carefully about things. .hhhh
```

| 31 | | Being HIV positive doesn't necessarily mean that that person |
|---|---|---|
| 32 | | is going |
| 33 | | to develop ai:ds (.) later on. |
| 34 | | (.) |
| 35 | *P*: | Mm hm |

We can make three observations about this extract. First, *C* delivers advice without having elicited from *P* a perceived problem. Reasons of space do not allow us to include what immediately precedes this extract but it involves another topic (the meaning of a positive test result), and no attempt is made to question *P* about her possible response to this topic, i.e. how she might change her behaviour after a negative test result. Moreover, within this extract, *C* introduces fresh topics (what to do in a serious relationship on lines 6–13; the spread of HIV in the city on lines 20–22) without employing any step-by-step approach. Second, predictably, the *P* only produces UAs (variations on 'mm hmm'). While these may indicate that *P* is listening, they do not mark what *C* is saying as advice. Hence, at the very least, they do not show *P* uptake and may also be taken as a sign of passive resistance.

Third, *C* does not personalize her advice. Instead of using a personal pronoun or the patient's name, she refers to 'someone' and 'they' (lines 1–4) and 'everyone' (line 28).

Advice-sequences like these are very common at three out of the five centres examined here. So we have to ask ourselves why counsellors should use a format which is likely to generate so little patient uptake. However, since our preference is not to criticize professionals but to understand the logic of their work, we need to look at the *functions* as well as the dysfunctions of this way of proceeding.

The first thing we might note is that topic follows topic with a remarkable degree of smoothness and at great speed. This might indicate one function of this style of counselling. Moreover, there is no *active* resistance from P. Indeed, we might question Heritage and Sefi's assumption that there is any kind of resistance to advice here.

The reason is that the counsellor's depiction of the consequences of a negative test-result might be heard as information-delivery rather than as specific advice to this patient. For instance, *C* avoids referring directly to *P* but uses the non-specific term 'someone'. In such cases, then, we may be dealing with the uptake of what can be heard by the patient as *information* rather than advice. It follows that such uptake obviously need have no direct implication for what the patient does (as opposed to what he thinks) — unlike the uptake of advice.

Moreover, if this is hearable as information-delivery, unlike advice, patients are only interactionally required to give response-tokens (unmarked acknowledgements) (Perakyla and Silverman, 1991). This means that, in information-delivery, it is *optional* whether patients offer marked acknowledge-ments. When they do so, they do not implicate themselves in any future lines of action because they are only responding to what can be heard as information and not necessarily advice.

The optional character of the kind of patient uptake in information-delivery suggests that we need not interpret the occasional 'mms' of *P* in Extract 6 as resistance to advice — precisely because *P* need not hear what *C* is saying as advice at all. Rather it is hearable as information about the kind of advice she might give in certain circumstances. However, this does not explain why counsellors would want to package their advice in a way which makes patient uptake less likely. Are such counsellors necessarily lacking skills or poorly trained?

I would answer such questions in the negative. Instead, I would suggest that, by constructing advice-sequences that can be heard as information-delivery, counsellors manage to stabilize advice-giving. In Extract 6, we have seen an example of a counsellor constructing what we might call hypothetical advice sequences, concerned with the advice the counsellor *would give* if someone (i.e., not necessarily this patient) had a particular test result. A function of maintaining an ambiguous communication format is that the counsellor does not have to cope with the difficult interactional problems of the failure of patient-uptake, given the instability of advice-giving. Throughout our corpus of examples, counsellors exit quickly from personalized advice when patients offer only minimal response tokens or when they display overt resistance. A fascinating example of such resistance is found in two of our Trinidad extracts where patients overtly resist question-answer sequencs about safer sex by asserting that the counsellor should not be asking about their behaviour and knowledge but, as the expert, telling them directly.

Not only is advice-giving unstable but, if given in a step-by-step manner, it takes a long time. Clinics which use this method spend 30–45 minutes over their counselling interviews. This compares to the clinic from which Extract 6 is taken, where pre-test counselling interviews average been 10–15 minutes. Truncated, non-personalized advice sequences are usually far shorter — an important consideration for hard-pressed counsellors.

Another function of offering advice in this way is that it neatly handles many of the issues of delicacy that can arise in discussing sexual behaviour. First, the counsellor can be heard as making reference to what she tells 'anyone' so that this particular patient need not feel singled out for attention about his/her private life. Second, because there is no step-by-step method of questioning, patients are not required to expand on their sexual practices with the kinds of hesitations we saw in Extract 4. Third, setting up advice sequences that can be heard as information-delivery shields the counsellor from some of the interactional difficulties of appearing to tell strangers what they should be doing in the most intimate aspects of their behaviour.

Undoubtedly, then, there are gains for the counsellor in setting up advice-packages which are truncated and non-personalized. Obviously, however, there are concomitant losses of proceeding this way. As we have shown, such advice-packages produce far less patient-uptake and, therefore, their function in creating an environment in which people might re-examine their own sexual behaviour is distinctly problematic.

Two possible solutions suggest themselves from the data analysed by this study (see Silverman, Bor, Miller and Goldman, 1992). First, avoiding necessarily delicate and unstable advice sequences but encouraging patients to draw their own conclusions from a particular line of questioning. Second, since both this method and step-by-step advice-giving take considerable time, finding ways of making more time available for more effective counselling.

It should be noted that neither of these solutions fit Assumptions 3 and 4. The question of effective counselling and effective counsellors can only be addressed in the context of the management of the interactional and practical constraints on counselling practice. There are no simple normative solutions to these constraints — although my experience running workshops for such counsellors suggests the value of these kind of detailed transcripts in in-service training provision.

We may now present Finding 3: information-packages are functional for stable professional-client communication in the context of time limitations. The implication is that effective training begins from a close analysis of the skills of counsellors and their clients revealed in careful research rather than from normative standards of good practice.

To refer to careful research presupposes general agreement about what the characteristics of such research might be. In many respects the kind of research discussed here is very different from the mainstream of both quantitative *and* qualitative social research. To discuss why I have proceeded in this manner, I must discuss some basic methodological issues.

### Methodological Issues in Counselling Research

Our mandate from the Health Education Authority for England and Wales was to examine the health education consequences of counselling particularly from the point of view of safer sex. Given the nature of the problem, why study it via tape-recordings of counselling sessions?

There are at least two more obvious ways of evaluating counselling. First, using an experimental design where we might offer volunteers different forms of counselling and then interview them subsequently about their uptake of information (perhaps followed up, some months later, with a further interview about the effects, if any, on their behaviour compared to their reported behaviour prior to the experiment). Second, using a non-experimental design where existing counselling procedures are evaluated by a cohort of patients. Again, we might follow up a cohort some time later.

The advantage of such research designs is that they permit large-scale studies which generate apparently hard data, seemingly based on unequivocal measures. However, a number of difficulties present themselves.[3] These include how seriously are we to take patients' accounts of their behaviour? Furthermore, does not the first of these designs ignore the *organizational* context in which health-care is delivered, for example, relations between physicians and other staff, tacit theories of good counselling, resources available, staff turnover? Such contexts may shape the nature and effectiveness of counselling in non-laboratory situations. And is it not the case that both of these alternative designs treat subjects as 'an aggregation of disparate individuals' who have no social interaction with one another (Bryman, 1988: 39)? As such, they give us little hold on how counselling is organized as a local, step-by-step social process and, consequently, we may suspect that we are little wiser about how counselling works in practice.

The apparently unequivocal measures of information retention, attitude and behaviour that we obtain via laboratory or questionnaire methods have a tenuous basis in what people may be saying and doing in their everyday lives. Moreover, if our interest is in the relation of counselling to sexual practices, do such studies tell us how people actually talk about sex with professionals and with each other as opposed to responses to researchers' questions? Consequently, once more, the phenomenon escapes.

An example makes the point very well. At a recent meeting of social scientists working on AIDS, much concern was expressed about the difficulty of recruiting a sample of the population prepared to answer researchers questions about their sexual behaviour. As a result, it was suggested that a subsequent meeting should be convened at which we could exchange ideas about how to recruit such a sample. The irony of AIDS researchers meeting to discuss such a topic is evident. For, if we concede that our best chance of limiting the spread of HIV may be by encouraging people to discuss their sexual practices with their partners, then surely we cannot neglect naturally occurring talk about sexuality and reduce the whole issue to a technical problem of obtaining a sample?

To counter this problem, work is now being carried out on understanding how people ordinarily describe their own and others' sexual activities. Let me mention two forms of such work:

1   Asking respondents what they understand by a series of terms used by professionals to describe sexual activities — 'heterosexual', 'intercourse', etc. (Wellings *et al.*, 1990).
2   Asking people to keep diaries about their sexual encounters where they record, in their own terms, the number and nature of their sexual activities over many months. This method is currently being used by Coxon with a cohort of gay men in Britain (Coxon, Chapter 8, this volume).

Despite the apparent (and real) differences between experimental designs and qualitative subjectivist research like that described above, both share an unwillingness to examine how safe sex comes to be constituted as a topic in naturally occurring situations. Studies of the first type fail to recognize that, in everyday life, we are able to understand each other without ever having to define our terms. So the laughter that is usually generated by researchers' accounts of the apparently inept way in which laypersons misunderstand sexual terms is misplaced. Studies using the second approach are ingenious in that they avoid the need for researchers to suggest a vocabulary to respondents. However, keeping a diary about one's sexual activities is unlikely to be a routine situation for many people, and the descriptions present in it do not stand in any one-to-one relationship with the events depicted.[4]

Both kinds of research are fundamentally concerned with the environment around the phenomenon rather than the phenomenon itself. In quantitative studies of objective social structures and qualitative studies of people's subjective orientations, we may be deflected away from the phenomenon towards what follows and precedes it (causes and consequences in the objective approach) or to how people respond to it (the subjective approach). This can be illustrated diagrammatically in Figure 5.1.

---

**Objectivism**

causes⟩the phenomenon⟩consequences

**Subjectivism**

perceptions⟩the phenomenon⟩responses

---

*Figure 5.1: Objectivism and subjectivism.*

In both approaches, the phenomenon with which ostensibly we are concerned disappears. In Objectivism, it is defined out of existence (by fiat, as Cicourel, 1964 puts it). Equally, what I have called Subjectivism is so romantically attached to the authentic rush of human experience that it merely reproduces tales of a subjective world without bringing us any closer to the local organization of the phenomena concerned.

Both approaches derive their sense from a false polarity in social research. The social world is neither simply objective nor simply subjective but consists of a set of practices that researchers need to describe. One of those practices is distinguishing reality from illusion or thought from fact. This lay distinction is regularly seen as, say, policemen and stockbrokers try to discern underlying 'real' patterns in the 'facts' with which they deal. It is these activities and others like them which constitute a phenomenon that social researchers ignore at their peril. Another way or putting this is to say that, in social research, the objective/subjective distinction should be treated as a topic but not as a resource (see Garfinkel, 1967). Hence subjective approaches get us no closer to understanding the local organization of the phenomenon.

So much for critique. The reader may rightly now ask: what alternative is offered by the study of counselling that I have already described? I begin with the nature and advantages of the distinction between 'how' and 'why' questions.

## Institutional Contexts: Why? and How?

My argument will be that one's initial move should be to give close attention to how participants locally produce contexts for their interaction. By beginning with this question of 'how', we can then fruitfully move on to 'why' questions about institutional and cultural constraints. Such constraints reveal the functions of apparently irrational practices and help us to understand the possibilities and limits of attempts at social reform.

Schegloff (1991) has shown that a great deal depends on the pace at which we proceed.

> The study of talk should be allowed to proceed under its own imperatives, with the hope that its results will provide more effective tools for the analysis of distributional, institutional and social structural problems *later on* than would be the case if the analysis of talk had, from the outset, to be made answerable to problems extrinsic to it. (Schegloff, 1991: 64, my emphasis).

Quite properly, this will mean delaying what I have called 'why' questions until we have asked the appropriate 'how' questions. But how, eventually, are we to make the link between the two?

A solution is suggested in two recent accounts of institutional talk. Heritage and Greatbatch's (1992) study of news interviews begins by asking: how is a recognizable 'news interview' constructed? They demonstrate how both parties adopt what they call a 'news-interview footing', for example, the interviewee withholds a response until a question is asked, and the interviewer does not respond during the course of an answer. If this answers our 'how' question (about the local organization of a context), Heritage and Greatbatch show that we can then begin to move on to answer 'why' questions about the stability of the footing. They do so by looking at how this footing satisfies presumed cultural assumptions about such interviews — allowing the interviewer to maintain a neutral stance, while constituting the viewing audience as the primary addressee of the talk.

Similarly, Maynard's (1991) study of interviews between paediatricians and mothers begins by a close focus on how the parties locally produce patterns of communication. Maynard shows how paediatricians giving diagnostic information may use a 'perspective-display sequence' where they first invite the parents' views. He then moves on to the 'why?' question, relating the 'perspective-display sequence' to the functions of avoiding open conflict over unfavourable diagnoses. In this way, the device serves to preserve social solidarity.

Both these accounts end up by considering the functions of the forms they have discovered (for another example, see Perakyla and Silverman: 1991b). Ironically, the way forward in the macro-micro debate may be to reinstate a variant of the much criticised functionalist perspective in the context of much more sensitive sociology of work. The lesson is clear. We cannot do everything at the same time without muddying the water. For policy reasons, as well as from conventional sociological concerns, we may well want to ask the 'why' questions. There is no reason not to, providing that we have first closely described how the phenomenon at hand is locally produced. If not, we are limited to an explanation of something that we have simply defined by fiat.

So there is nothing wrong with the search for explanations, providing that this search is grounded in a close understanding of how the phenomena being explained are put together at an interactional level. This means that, wherever possible, one should seek to obtain naturally-occurring data in order to obtain adequate understanding, leading to soundly-based policy interventions.[5]

This close analysis of a few lines of data extracts may have over-extended the patience of readers more familiar with other research methods. If so, I beg their forgiveness. The aim has been to demonstrate a way of working with data which seeks to preserve the local production of social phenomena. However, a further methodological objection may be made to this kind of analysis. To what extent does it allow generalizable observations to be made?

## Reliability and Validity

I take it that few of us have any stomach for any remaining qualitative researchers who might maintain that our only methodological imperative is to 'hang out' and to return with authentic accounts of the field. Conversely, I would argue that issues of validity and reliability are relevant to any form of social research. I will deal first with the issue of reliability. Attempts to bypass this issue by appealing to the different ontological position of field research (see Marshall and Rossman, 1989) are unconvincing. As has been recently pointed out:

> Qualitative researchers can no longer afford to beg the issue of reliability. While the forte of field research will always lie in its capability to sort out the validity of propositions, its results will (reasonably) go ignored minus attention to reliability. For reliability to be calculated, it

is incumbent on the scientific investigator to document his or her procedure.

(Kirk and Miller, 1986: 72)

Kirk and Miller suggest that the conventionalization of methods for recording fieldnotes offers a useful method for addressing the issue of reliability. However, we need only depend upon fieldnotes in the absence of audio- or video-recordings. As I hope my data show, the availability of transcripts of such recordings, using standard conventions, satisfies Kirk and Miller's proper demand for the documentation of procedures.

Fortunately, there is no dispute that validity is a serious issue in field research. Although academic journals are still prepared to publish papers based on no more than a few carefully chosen examples, their authors need to demonstrate further the validity of their claims (see Bloor, 1978; Mitchell, 1983; Silverman, 1989b and Silverman, 1993). So my earlier close analysis of the co-production and management of potentially delicate issues has been developed by following the standard methods of case-study research, namely analytic induction based upon the constant comparative method and deviant-case analysis. The identification of deviant cases allows us to revise and strengthen the analysis.[6]

The method of analytic induction encourages us to generate and then to test hypotheses in the course of research. Note that this method, coupled with a close attention to the local organization of the phenomenon *in situ*, means that we can be more confident that deviant cases derive their status from a comparison with knowledge of participants' routine practices rather than with idealized concep-tions of those practices. The latter is a frequent concomitant of deploying hypo-theses, couched in 'operational definitions' of variables, prior to entry into the field.

The revised analysis can subsequently be applied to tapes of counsellor-patient consultations gathered at other centres, allowing for further revision. Indeed, as already noted, one of the fascinating upshots of our current research is the degree of invariance that we are discovering in the local management of delicacy, using settings as apparently diverse as Britain, the USA and Trinidad (see Silverman and Bor, 1991). This reveals that the comparative method has no less a place in the detailed analysis of naturally-occurring situations than in more conventional experimental, interview or life-history methods. So, contrary to the assumption of many social scientists, as well as funding bodies, validity need not be a problem in case-study research. Moreover, as I have already shown, simple tabulations are a useful way of testing hypotheses on field data (see also Silverman, 1985: Chapter 7).

### Conclusions

Despite some of the more polemica passages in this chapter, I share the belief that there is no right or wrong method in science. At some level, everything depends on what you are trying to do. Moreover, our findings, discussed earlier, arose because of the way that we have been working. I happen to be using methods drawn from conversation analysis (CA) in this study (see Heritage, 1984: especially Ch. 8). This explains my focus on the sequential organization of talk, the avoidance of appeals to what participants are thinking and, instead, the pursuit of what they are doing.

CA has been used for two reasons. First, because it is appropriate to an understanding of the complexity of my data — over 150 hours of audio-recordings of HIV counselling. Second, because CA has demonstrably established a fruitful dialogue with practitioners in a range of work settings (see Drew and Heritage, 1992). In this study, CA has encouraged me to look at the local functions of people's activities in a way which I believe has a direct bearing upon policy issues.

I began by arguing that one of the least fruitful questions one can ask a sociologist is, 'To what school of social science do you belong?' Too often we are seduced by false polarities which would have us believe that only objectivist, macro-studies based on hard data can provide satisfactory explanations of social phenomena which lead to successful policy interventions. As I have tried to show, there are good reasons to suspect the 'hardness' of such data. Moreover, the proposed alternative, subjectivist studies of meanings, works no better since it may reduce the sociologist to the role of the tourist or chat-show host, concerned with trapping decontextualised experiences.

Too much social theory and methodology sets up such artificial polarities (Silverman, 1985 and 1989b). These polarities stop us thinking through issues because they provide ready-made solutions. Instead, we need to develop a logic of thinking through and de-constructing these polarities in social theory and methodology.

Perhaps one consequence of such lateral thinking will be for sociology to make a more fruitful contribution to institutional change. In Britain, for instance, one is struck by the failure of both macro- and micro-sociology to give an adequate account of professional practice. By beginning with a fine-grained attention to the detail of naturally-occurring interactions and then broadening out into explanations which address structural constraints, one can succeed both analytically and practically.

## Notes

1   This agreement followed by a later qualification is typical of 'dispreferred' answers (Pomerantz, 1975). Preferred answers are produced rapidly and without qualification; dispreferred answers are delayed.
2   See Sacks (1992) on the crucial concept of 'category-bound' activities.
3   Of course, I recognize that these problems are recognized by researchers who use such research instruments. In turn, they have ingenious methods for dealing with them.
4   Once again, I would stress that such researchers do seek to address such issues.

Moreover, of course, the same argument could be made about our counselling tapes which are no more intrinsically life-like than diaries (except that counselling is a naturally-occurring event with routinized forms, whereas keeping a diary about one's sexual activities may, in members' terms, be regarded as an extraordinary activity). In both cases, however, the issue is not the quality of the data but whether we attempt to grasp the local production of description.

5  We often falsely assume that there is inherent difficulty in obtaining naturally-occurring data in many situations, such as family life or sexuality. However, this assumption trades off a commonsense perception that these are *unitary* phenomena whose meaning is constructed in a single site, for example, households, bedrooms. However, family life is going on all around us — in courtrooms and social security offices as well as households (see Gubrium, 1992). Equally, sexuality is hardly confined to the bedroom; discourses of sexuality are all around us (see Foucault, 1979).

6  For reasons of space, I have not included any deviant cases here. However, elsewhere, I have shown how deviant-case analysis can strengthen our explanations of advice-reception (see Silverman, Bor, Miller and Goldman, 1992).

## References

BLOOR, M. (1978) 'On the analysis of observational data: A discussion of the worth and uses of inductive techniques and respondent validation', *Sociology*, 12, 3, pp. 545–57.

BODEN, D. and ZIMMERMAN, D. (Eds) (1991) *Talk and Social Structure*, Cambridge: Polity Press.

BRYMAN, A. (1988) *Quantity and Quality in Social Research*, London: Unwin Hyman.

CICOUREL, A. (1964) *Method and Measurement in Sociology*, New York: Free Press.

DREW, P. and HERITAGE, J.C. (Eds) (1992) *Talk at Work*, Cambridge: Cambridge University Press.

FOUCAULT, M. (1979) *The History of Sexuality: Vol 1*, Harmondsworth: Penguin.

GARFINKEL, E. (1967) *Studies in Ethnomethodology*, Englewood Cliffs, NJ: Prentice-Hall.

GUBRIUM, J. (1992) *Out of Control: Family Therapy and Domestic Disorder*, London: Sage.

HERITAGE, J. (1984) *Garfinkel and Ethnomethodology*, Cambridge: Polity.

HERITAGE, J. and GREATBATCH, D. (1992) 'On the institutional character of institutional talk', In DREW, P. and HERITAGE, J.C. (Eds) *Talk at Work*, Cambridge: Cambridge University Press.

HERITAGE, J. and SEFI, S. (1992) 'Dilemmas of advice: Aspects of the delivery and reception of advice in interactions between health visitors and first time mothers', in DREW, P. and HERITAGE, J. (Eds) *Talk at Work*, Cambridge: Cambridge University Press.

KIRK, J. and MILLER, M. (1986) *Reliability and Validity in Qualitative Research*, Qualitative Research Methods Series, Vol. 1, London: Sage.

MARSHALL, C. and ROSSMAN, G. (1989) *Designing Qualitative Research*, London: Sage.

MAYNARD, D.W. (1991) 'Interaction and asymmetry in clinical discourse', *American Journal of Sociology*, 97, 2, pp. 448–95.

MILLS, C.W. (1959) *The Sociological Imagination*, New York: Oxford University Press.

MITCHELL, J.C. (1983) 'Case and situational analysis', *Sociological Review*, 31, 2, pp. 187–211.

PERAKYLA, A. and BOR, R. (1990) 'Interactional problems of addressing "dreaded issues" in HIV-counselling', *AIDS Care*, 2, 4, pp. 325–8.

PERAKYLA, A. and SILVERMAN, D. (1991a) 'Reinterpreting speech-exchange systems: Communication formats in AIDS counselling', *Sociology*, 25, 4, pp. 627–51.

PERAKYLA, A. and SILVERMAN, D. (1991b) 'Owning experience: describing the experience of other persons', *Text*, 11, 3, pp. 441–80.

POMERANTZ, A. (1975) *Second Assessments: a Study of some Features of Agreements/Disagreements*, unpublished PhD. thesis, Irvine, CA: University of California.

SACKS, H. (1992), JEFFERSON, G. (Ed.) *Lectures on Conversation* with an Introduction by SCHEGLOFF, E., Oxford: Blackwell, 2 volumes.

SCHEGLOFF, E.A. (1980) 'Preliminaries to preliminaries: "Can I ask you a question?" ', *Sociological Inquiry*, 50, 3/4, pp. 104–52.

SCHEGLOFF, E.A. (1991) *Reflections on Talk and Social Structure*. in BODEN, D. and ZIMMERMAN, D. (Eds) (1991) *Talk and Social Structure*, Cambridge, Polity Press.

SILVERMAN, D. (1985) *Qualitative Methodology and Sociology*, Aldershot: Gower.

SILVERMAN, D. (1989a) 'Making sense of a precipice: Constituting identity in an HIV clinic', in AGGLETON, P., HART, G. and DAVIES, P. (Eds) *AIDS: Social Representations, Social Practices*, London: Falmer Press.

SILVERMAN, D. (1989b) 'Telling convincing stories: A plea for cautious positivism in case-studies', in GLASSNER, B. and MORENO, J. (Eds), *The Qualitative-Quantitative Distinction in the Social Sciences*, Dordrecht: Kluwer.

SILVERMAN, D. (1990) 'The social organization of AIDS counselling', in AGGLETON, P., DAVIES, P. and HART, G. *AIDS: Individual, Cultural and Policy Dimensions*, London: Falmer Press.

SILVERMAN, D. (1993) *Interpreting Qualitative Data: Methods for Analysing Talk, Text and Interaction*, London: Sage.

SILVERMAN, D. and BOR, R. (1991) 'The delicacy of describing sexual partners in HIV-Test counselling: Implications for practice', *Counselling Psychology Quarterly*, 4, 2/3, pp. 177–190.

SILVERMAN, D. and PERAKYLA, A. (1990) 'AIDS counselling: the interactional organization of talk about "delicate" issues', *Sociology of Health and Illness*, 12, 3, pp. 293–318.

SILVERMAN, D., BOR, R., MILLER, R. and GOLDMAN, E. (1992) 'Advice-giving and Advice-reception in AIDS counselling', in AGGLETON, P., DAVIES, P. and HART, G. (Eds), *AIDS: Rights, Risk and Reason*, London: Falmer Press.

SILVERMAN, D., PERAKYLA, A. and BOR, R. (1992) 'Discussing safer sex in HIV counselling: Assessing three communication formats', *AIDS Care* 4, 1, pp. 69–82.

WELLINGS, K., FIELD, J., JOHNSON, A., WADSWORTH, J. and BRADSHAW, S., (1990) 'Notes on the design and construction of a national survey of sexual lifestyles', in HUBERT, M. (Ed.) *Sexual Behaviour and Risks of HIV Infection*, Bruxelles: Facultes Universitaires Saint-Louis.

### Appendix 1

#### Transcript Symbols

| | | |
|---|---|---|
| [ | C2: quite a [ while<br>Mo:　　　[ yea | Left brackets indicate the point at which a current speakers talk is overlapped by another's talk. |
| = | W: that I'm aware of=<br>C: = Yes. Would you confirm that? | Equal signs, one at the end of a line and one at the beginning, indicate no gap between the two lines. |
| (.4) | Yes (.2) yeah | Numbers in parentheses indicate elapsed time in silence in tenths of a second. |
| (.) | to get (.) treatment | A dot in parentheses indicates a tiny gap, probably no more than one-tenth of a second. |
| _ | What's up? | Underscoring indicates some form of stress, via pitch and/or amplitude. |
| :: | O:kay? | Colons indicate prolongation of the immediately prior sound. The length of the row of colons indicates the length of the prolongation. |
| WORD | I've got ENOUGH TO WORRY ABOUT | Capitals, except at the beginnings of lines, indicate especially loud sounds relative to the surrounding talk. |
| .hhhh | I feel that (.2) .hhh | A row of h's prefixed by a dot indicates an inbreath; without a dot, an outbreath. The length of the row of h's indicates the length of the in- or out-breath. |
| ( ) | future risks and<br>( ) and life<br>( ) | Empty parentheses indicate the transcribers inability to hear what was said. |
| (word) | Would you see (there) anything positive | Parenthesized words are possible hearings. |
| (( )) | confirm that<br>((continues)) | Double parentheses contain author's descriptions rather than transcriptions. |

*Samples and Populations*

## Chapter 6

# Some Methodological and Practical Implications of Employing Drug Users as Indigenous Fieldworkers

*Robert Power*

Illicit drug use is, by its very nature, a largely hidden activity. As Wiener (1970) rightly points out, drug using networks tend to be exclusive, functioning to prevent access and knowledge to non-users. As with any deviant or illegal activity, its participants are often wary of outsiders, particularly those who are inquisitive. However, it has become increasingly apparent, particularly over the last decade, that we need to collect research information on illicit drug users in the community. This has stemmed from a number of issues of concern: the realization that only a minority of problem drug users attend established services; the link between HIV infection and injecting drug use; the recognition that drug users not in touch with services are more likely to be involved in high-risk injecting practices; and the trend towards harm minimization policies and community-oriented interventions. Throughout the 1980s, the influential Advisory Council on the Misuse of Drugs (ACMD) highlighted the need to contact illicit drug users in the community who had minimal or no contact with the helping services and to gain an understanding of their patterns of behaviour (ACMD, 1982; ACMD, 1988; ACMD, 1989).

In the clinic or drug agency setting, where researchers can be vouched for by staff, research amongst drug users is relatively easy to accomplish. In the community context, where researchers do not have the safety, security and backing of an authoritative third party, much thought needs to be given to utilizing the most appropriate techniques for contacting relevant samples of drug users.

Since 1985 I have been involved, in one capacity or another, in conducting research amongst this 'hidden' population of drug users. The empirical and policy orientated questions have changed throughout this time, most crucially as a result of AIDS, but the methodological issues have remained. Central to the latter has been the drive towards developing and refining techniques and strategies that will elicit detailed, accurate and consistent data from a group of respondents that are often reluctant to come to public attention. In this chapter I examine a number of methodological and research issues that arise from the social behaviourial study of illicit drug users, particularly regarding the employment of current or recovering drug users as research workers.

## Participant Observation and Illicit Drug Use

Social researchers have always been interested in accessing difficult to reach subgroups, and participant observation (a method often used to gain an understanding of deviant populations) has a rich tradition in drugs research (see, for example, Becker, 1963; Preble and Casey, 1969; Feldman, 1974; Plant and Reeves, 1976; William 1989). Such a methodology aims to provide an insider's view of the social network or milieu being studied. This is often only achieved after many hours of careful observation and informal conversation. Although participant observation can be conducted without forming relationships with the subjects (for example, by observing drug dealing locations), it does facilitate access to information hidden from most observers. Once the researcher gains the trust and respect of the subjects, then he or she becomes accepted by the group and can engage in detailed participant observation. In my earlier work on drug users patterns of 'help-seeking', many hours and days were spent in nurturing relationships with individual and networks of drug users in order to gain access to their secret worlds (Power, 1989).

Yet the potential exists for drug users themselves to become more than just the subject in the study. We need only to be reminded of the role of 'Doc' in Whyte's (1955) study of street gangs, or 'Tally' in Liebow's (1967) work, to recognize the importance of the 'key informant' or 'gatekeeper'. Such individuals can be used to great effect to guide the researcher through the world of illicit drug use, in terms of its spatial aspects and its subcultural mores and norms. This is especially the case when the key informant is a well-respected or high status member of the drug-using fraternity. In the company of such individuals the researcher accrues a certain status, indicating to other members of the population that he or she is worthy of respect. In my own experience, this was best exemplified by the relationship I developed with a well-known heroin dealer in London's Soho area. In part due to the strength of my relationship with him I was accepted into one of the main heroin dealing sites in London. This 'copping site', ostensibly a pool-room situated above a striptease club, was accessed through an unmarked door. Heroin was purchased and consumed twelve hours a day and many of those who patronized the venue were chaotic street-drug users who were not in touch with the helping services (Power, 1987). Such key informants are not only invaluable in facilitating entry to difficult to access arenas, but they also act as ambassadors for the research project. This is especially the case amongst illicit drug users where word-of-mouth communication and recommendations play an important role in everyday life.

## Drug Users as Research Workers

Whereas participant observation and the role of the key informant are now an established part of social behaviourial research into illicit drug use, the use of recovering or active drug users as research workers is a relatively recent phenomenon, particularly in Britain. Although Hughes (1977) employed drug users as research staff (in this case, methadone-maintained opiate users) on his prevalence study of heroin use in Chicago, it was not until AIDS became an issue that this strategy was widely adopted. Since the mid-1980s, action research projects, combining both epidemiology and AIDS prevention interventions that employ indigenous drug users as researchers and outreach workers, have been funded with great success throughout the USA (see Wiebel, 1988; Broadhead and Fox, 1990).

My first experience of using indigenous research staff dates back to 1986, where a user-dealer was employed on a piecemeal basis to conduct interviews amongst his own social network of regular heroin users. Subsequently, using nomination and snowballing techniques, the study on which I was working began to identify key contacts that could be used as part-time temporary interviewers to access hitherto difficult to reach networks such as cabaret artistes and the punk sub-culture (Power *et al.*, 1992). Shortly after this time, Stimson *et al.*, (1988) adopted similar strategies in the evaluation of syringe exchange schemes.

Since its inception in January 1990, the Centre for Research on Drugs and Health Behaviour, in London, has used what we now term indigenous fieldworkers as an important element of many social behaviourial studies. This methodology has been especially efficacious in studies targeting drug users outside of the treatment context. Indigenous fieldworkers (both current and recovering drug users), selected for their knowledge of particular milieus, have been employed on a range of research projects. These include a World Health Organization study of HIV seroprevalence amongst injecting drug users; research into the HIV risk behaviour of ex-prisoners; the evaluation of a district health authority community drug team; an examination of drug users' experiences of methadone prescribing regimes; and a Department of Health study into the informal coping strategies adopted by drug users to control their substance misuse and injecting practices.

Once recruited under the generic term of indigenous fieldworkers, such individuals can be employed in a variety of roles according to the aims and objectives of the research project. Primarily, we have used them as indigenous interviewers, to contact appropriate respondents and conduct relevant research interviews. Indeed, the main concerns of this chapter focus on indigenous interviewers. But ex- and current- drug-users can also be used in a number of other contexts. 'Contact tracers' are used to provide research subjects from targeted networks that can then be interviewed by full-time research staff. 'Community guides', who have an intimate knowledge of a particular drug-using location that has been selected for research, are valuable in orientating researchers and explaining the functions and locations of specific drug using milieus. They are especially useful in the context of a research site that is little known to the research team.

Future developments for indigenous fieldworkers would be as indigenous observers (regularly reporting on drug-using patterns and trends in the areas with which they are familiar), and as indigenous advocates (taking on a peer education and health advocacy role). For further discussion on the nuances of these tasks see Power and Jones (1993).

Employing recovering or current drug users as research workers, in whatever capacity, raises a plethora of issues. Some of these concerns are methodological: How can we verify the data? How reliable and standardized can we hope the data to be? Others touch on matters of ethics: are we placing these individuals in potentially damaging situations, especially if they are striving towards abstinence? What responsibilities should we have in terms of career development for such workers? Additionally, there are a host of practical issues: How do we recruit them? What level of training and supervision should be provided? How do we arrange payment for these workers, many of whom are involved in the 'grey' economy? How do we co-ordinate a group of often transient workers spread over a wide geographical area?

## Reliability and Validity

Questions around reliability and validity are a common concern to social scientists. This is especially the case regarding self-reported data on illicit behaviours, such as drug use. Using ex- and current drug users as indigenous fieldworkers adds an extra dimension to the methodological and practical issues involved. Although there is a large area of overlap, it is worth making a semantic distinction between our understanding of validity and reliability. Questions of validity concern the extent to which a true and accurate impression is obtained of the phenomenon being studied. Those around reliability address issues relating to the research process itself, such as the extent to which the research tools employed and the methodologies adopted facilitate observations that are replicable.

Before addressing the specific problems of validating the research produced by indigenous fieldworkers, we first need to look briefly at the general question of the validity of self-reported data collected from illicit drug users. As Stephens (1972) rightly points out (despite a slight tendency towards stereotyping) part of the 'addict role' is to deceive and mislead. Much of the daily round of the drug user is concerned with striving or 'hustling' for money and drugs, and many activities centre on cheating or defrauding others. Becker (1963) comments that deviant groups involved in illegal behaviour have a vested interest in concealing the precise nature of their proscribed behaviour. Stephens (1972) adds that this may spill over into interactions with others, such as in the therapeutic setting, and researchers need to be aware of this problem, especially in the context of self-reports.

However, Ball (1967) flips the coin and notes that deviant subjects will faithfully report their actions under appropriate research procedures. His study of the validity and reliability of data derived from fifty-nine Puerto Rican drug users confirms this contention. These drug users were followed up after an initial interview, requestioned on a number of matters, and the data was checked against existing source material, including hospital records. There was considerable agreement on the main items addressed: age (83 per cent); age at first drug use (66 per cent); type and place of first arrest (54 per cent, with a further 26 per cent reporting an earlier arrest); and total number of arrests and criminal history (71 per cent). In addition, urine analysis showed a 92 per cent concurrence with self-reported current drug use.

Similarly, Stephens (1972) followed-up 100 drug users discharged into an aftercare phase of a treatment programme. A questionnaire was constructed to look at various aspects of the drug user's life and to examine the level of agreement between the aftercare counsellor, the client and a relative of the client. The questions covered issues such as drug use, work-related problems and criminal history. High levels of agreement were found when comparing accounts from patients and relatives (82 per cent agreement) and patient and counsellors (89 per cent). More recently, Amsell *et al.* (1976) attempted to validate the self-reported criminal and drug-taking activity of 1500 drug users. The authors, concluding that overall they were confident that 829 responses (55 per cent) were fully reliable, added the caveat that unreliable police records and urinalysis reports hindered their work.

Clearly, the more sensitive and potentially threatening the questioning, the more likely respondents will be resistant to providing valid answers. Nevertheless, as Stephens comments, 'Researchers need not concern themselves with the veracity of addict informants any more than they would with a less deviant sample. Letting addict informants know that their responses may be checked with independent sources possibly might assure more truthful responses' (1972: 57). Where feasible, non-reactive measures, such as physical examinations and independent records, should be used to validate self-reported data.

In order to safeguard the veracity of a study, validity and reliability checks need to be carried out on interviews completed by indigenous fieldworkers. In our own studies a number of controls were incorporated into the research designs. Intraquestionnaire safeguards are routinely included in questionnaire design and can take a number of forms. The essential purpose is to check for consistency between questions and within the overall context of the respondent's replies. Thus, the same question, or subtly different aspects of a theme, can be asked in different forms within a single questionnaire. For instance, this could be around drug-use patterns, economic activity and revenue raising. Amsell *et al.* (1976) found that 13 per cent of questionnaires contained at least one inconsistency between frequency of illegal activity and amount of income derived from illegal sources. Additionally, inconsistencies were reported in 7 per cent of responses around cost of drug habit and weekly income and 7 per cent around cost of habit and frequency of drug use.

When using indigenous interviewers it is often difficult to determine if a discrepancy within a completed questionnaire arises from inaccuracies in recording information or inconsistencies in the respondent's account. Thus, we have instituted a further check of the re-interview procedure. This entails re-interviewing a random selection of respondents. Often, the mere threat of implementing such a procedure is sufficient to encourage valid information. In practice, it is often problematic to enforce this procedure with indigenous interviewers. This is because, by the very nature of their task, they frequently interview other drug-using acquaintances who are not prepared to be met by a third party. At the very least we insist on meeting one or two selected respondents from each indigenous interviewer so that baseline data (such as socio-demographics and drug-use history) can be validated against the research interview. In the Amsell *et al.* (1976) study, spot-checks on three questions were carried out to test for comparability. Interestingly, this study found a high level of congruence: drug use (97 per cent); illegal activities (97 per cent); and alcohol 'highs' (69 per cent). Less directly, socio-demographic and behaviourial profiles can be checked against secondary sources, such as relevant datasets, official statistics, and, through triangulation, by confirmatory interviews with significant and knowledgeable others. Where possible, researchers should observe indigenous interviewers as they interview a sample of respondents, and should be involved in participant observation and ethnographic work concerning the social networks and milieus being studied. In a recent study where indigenous interviewers were used at three separate field sites, full-time research staff conducted ongoing ethnography amongst the same networks, and at the same locations from which interviewees were recruited (Power and Jones, 1993).

Whereas no single validation check is foolproof, a combination of those outlined above will go a long way to maintaining the integrity of the project. We also need to limit sampling bias. One method is to restrict each interviewer to a quota of interviews. This strategy is important as interviewers are often selected to access distinct networks of drug users. Unless quotas are applied, the data is liable to be skewed by over-sampling particular networks and friendship groups who have similar characteristics.

Notwithstanding the need for careful scrutiny of the research process, evidence suggests that the use of indigenous fieldworkers does produce particularly reliable and valid data. In their study of crack cocaine use in New York, Dunlap *et al.* commented that the use of ex-drug users as interviewers 'was frequently the key to obtaining . . . accurate personal information about topics without reluctance or suspicion' (1988: 129). In Britain, a similar observation has been made by Davies and Baker (1987). Their work showed that respondents interviewed by ex-users were more likely to provide personal details of drug use that matched independently recorded information than those who were interviewed by researchers with no personal experience of drug use. In fact, when interviewed by the latter, respondents consistently presented themselves as heavier users and as more dependent. As Ball (1967) notes, the interviewer's knowledge of, and familiarity with, the target group and milieu is an important consideration in ensuring the validity of data. Feedback from a study of twenty-one indigenous interviewers confirms this point (Power and Harkinson, 1993). Many pointed to the importance of their own drug-using past as an asset. This was not only in terms of contacting and being accepted by the respondent, but also in reducing the likelihood of false information being provided and in understanding the vernacular of drug users.

Commentators have noted the positive role of indigenous fieldworkers in terms of data validity. Gallmeier (1991) makes the important point that the validity of qualitative data is often impeded by the reactive effect of the observer upon the observed. Webb *et al.* (1981) suggest that the subjects will behave in an atypical manner, strive to make a good impression, and emphasize aspects of their character which they deem most appropriate to the observer's presence. Whereas any observer is liable to influence the actions or those around them, this will be limited when that individual is an accepted member of the social group and is familiar and at ease in the environment. One disadvantage that the indigenous worker has in this context is the potential to fail to record that which is deemed commonplace to them. In this context, rigorous and routine debriefing, as we note below, is an essential part of the research process.

### A Question of Ethics

A number of ethical issues arise from the employment of indigenous interviewers, both in terms of the role itself and their relationship to respondents. Regarding the latter, they become party to sensitive personal information and need to observe rules of confidentiality common to all researchers involved in work with illicit drug users. This is even more pertinent when interviewers are working with contacts and networks known to them, where information divulged might have multiple repercussions.

Other ethical considerations arise out of employing indigenous fieldworkers with drug-using backgrounds. We have a responsibility to safeguard them from either compounding their current drug use or else breaking their abstinence. The problems of 'going native' have long been recognized in the sociological literature concerned with ethnography (see Hughes, 1957), yet expecting an ex-drug user to return to former venues and mix with old acquaintances in a drug-using context throws up a different set of ethical issues. It is here that the value of careful recruitment and appropriate training, supervision and debriefing become apparent.

The temptation to use drugs is an issue that must be faced by all ex- or current drug users employed as research workers. One way of addressing this is to provide clear guidelines that not only raise the issue, but also state unequivocally that no illicit drugs are to be used during the course of fieldwork. This does not mean that we abdicate responsibility for any indigenous fieldworker who develops a drug problem. Indeed, it is our ethical responsibility to be proactive in this respect and offer sensitive and practical support. Interestingly, many of the ex-drug users interviewed in our feedback study commented that the work had furthered their resolve to remain drug free (Power and Harkinson, 1993). As one individual stated: 'Meeting people who are still using has positively reinforced my determination to keep living a drug free life.'

The temptation to use drugs was noted by a number of indigenous interviewers, but none stated that it had led to an increase in their personal use or to a breaking of abstinence. Nevertheless, comments were made concerning increases in the use of tobacco and alcohol, particularly as social lubricants:

'I have started smoking again after twenty years. This is very serious; I must stop.'

'My brandy consumption goes up sometimes when I need to deal with post-interview blues.'

Interestingly, a number commented on the positive impact of the work in relation to their own drug use:

'At first I felt dreadful because I wanted to use when interviewing people who did. This job has helped me to get off and stay off drugs and I feel a deep gratitude.'

We clearly have a particular responsibility for this group of workers, however casual their employment may be. Due to their backgrounds of substance misuse they may be vulnerable to the specific stresses of conducting fieldwork amongst populations for which they feel special empathy. This will be compounded for those working within networks already known to them. Many commented on the strain of working with acquaintances who were still using drugs and who were experiencing serious personal and social problems: 'Meeting old friends after years and nothing's changed. Still saying the same old things, like "I'm coming off" or "I'm reducing". I found this quite depressing.'

From their experiences of employing ex-drug users as researchers and outreach workers in Chicago, Schick and Wiebel (1991) recognize the stresses endemic to this type of employment: over-identification with subjects, temptation to return to drug use, feelings of helplessness in the face of HIV disease, and frustration at being unable to effect change. This latter point is a recurring issue with indigenous fieldworkers, many of whom find it difficult to accept the boundaries imposed upon them by the parameters of the research role. Many of these issues can be addressed and monitored in the context of appropriate recruitment, training and supervision.

## Some Practical Considerations

*Recruitment*

A crucial initial issue to be addressed is that of recruitment. Experience has shown that it is not only important to consider the personal qualities of potential indigenous fieldworkers, but also attention needs to be paid to the venues from which they are recruited. Both these factors will be influenced by the particular requirements and nature of any given study. However, as with any form of recruitment, it is important at the outset to assess the individual's personal qualities and suitability.

Importantly, we must gauge the extent to which the person's knowledge and access to particular networks of drug users matches the aims and objectives of the study in question. It is also important to gain some appreciation of their role and status in drug-user networks, as this will influence their ability to penetrate any given drug scene.

The question concerning the source of recruitment of indigenous fieldworkers is a complex one and is again linked to the aims of specific studies. If the research issue concerns injecting practices then we might turn to syringe exchange schemes for prospective workers. More generally, they can be sought from all manner of venues: clubs, pubs, and the range of arenas where drug users congregate; through other drug user contacts and existing indigenous fieldworkers; from drug agencies. Respecting the latter, it is of great importance that agencies are informed and, where applicable, involved in this process. Staff members may well be in a position to recommend suitable candidates. If staff are not informed of the demands on their clients then the potential for conflict arises, as in the case where staff judge a prospective indigenous fieldworker to be too vulnerable for such work. In all aspects of research it is critical that due concern is given to sensitive and respectful agency liaison. In this case such an imperative has both practical and ethical implications.

*Training and Supervision*

Personal experience of drug use and drug-using milieus does not automatically equip an individual with the necessary skills to undertake research tasks. Our experience has shown that such a background normally ensures that the individuals will feel at ease in the fieldwork context and that they will be accepted by respondents in the drug using community. However, it is essential that indigenous fieldworkers receive sufficient initial basic training to ensure both personal competence and standardized practice. Where practical, group training sessions should be conducted at the beginning of a new study, with any additionally recruited fieldworkers being inducted on an individual basis.

Any training has cost implications, particularly where the study is spread geographically, with fieldworkers emanating from different regions of the country. The cost of any centralized training session needs to be carefully accounted for in any new research budget. Issues covered by initial training of indigenous interviewers should include: aims and objectives of the study, review of fieldwork guidelines, criteria for sample recruitment, basic interview techniques, the need for objectivity and methods for recording qualitative data. It is during this basic training that administrative and payment issues can be discussed, along with any other personal or substantive issues. It also enables the indigenous interviewers to meet their colleagues, be introduced to the research centre and its staff, and generally feel a broader sense of involvement in the project.

If feasible, discussion or focus groups should be conducted with these indigenous fieldworkers. This is particularly useful at the beginning of a study, when issues and ideas can be explored and knowledge and experience of such groups can be used to full advantage. When combined with a training session, such focus groups are a particularly good use of scarce resources.

Although all aspects of induction and basic training are necessary to the successful adoption of this research methodology, it is particularly important that clear fieldwork guidelines are produced and disseminated. Individual projects might produce specific guidelines (such as the procedure for administering anonymous HIV saliva testing), but there needs to be core guidelines to cover issues such as personal safety, lines of communication and assistance, alcohol policy, professional conduct and relations with the police. The guidelines should also state the terms and conditions of employment and clearly outline the nature of payment.

Given the stressful nature of the work and the non-academic backgrounds of the majority of these interviewers, debriefing and close supervision is essential. Where practical, and certainly during the early stages of fieldwork, debriefing sessions should take place after each completed interview. This has a number of important functions. First, any problems with the research instrument can be discussed and clarified and any difficulties the interviewer is having in the field can be aired. Second, the details of the interview can be reviewed and examined and the interviewer can be questioned about individual respondents. This is a useful and practical validity check and often produces additional data, especially of a qualitative and contextual nature. Third, quality assurance and standardization can be monitored and sampling issues, such as quotas, overseen. Fourth, the debriefing session functions as a safe forum for the indigenous fieldworker to offload any issues that may be concerning them respecting fieldwork.

Further to this, each indigenous fieldworker should be assigned to a fulltime member of research staff to act as supervisor on a day-to-day basis. Even where fieldworkers are spread throughout the country and frequent face-to-face contact is not always possible, regular telephone contact should be maintained.

*Payment*

A recurring practical problem with employing ex- and current drug users as research workers concerns method of payment. The majority of these individuals favour cash payment. Many are involved in the 'grey economy' and are reluctant for their names to be entered on to any computerized payroll. Others claim social security and are concerned that their benefits will be jeopardized by a relatively minor source of income.

Payment may be on an hourly basis, but for specific interviewing work, the most satisfactory system is for piecemeal payment per completed interview, plus an agreed maximum sum for expenses. To arrive at this figure it is important to pilot the interview (or whatever research instrument is being used) and then gauge the average time taken to make contact with the potential interviewee, conduct the interview and write it up. It is also important that the indigenous fieldworker is aware of what else is expected within the package, such as the safe delivery of the interview to the research centre and time for debriefing.

Rarely have we been able to offer indigenous fieldworkers sufficient regular work to justify their relinquishing their claim on state benefit. In most instances cash payment is impractical, particularly when the research institute is part of a larger bureaucratic organization where stringent accounting systems are in place. We are therefore only able to employ fieldworkers willing to provide a national insurance number and who are prepared to have their names entered on the payroll. This limits the range of individuals that can be formally employed as indigenous fieldworkers, highlighting the need for more secure and regular work for these types of people.

Due to the nature of contract research, the work is spasmodic. Yet over the past two years we have compiled a register of indigenous fieldworkers, listing personal identifiers, contact addresses, knowledge of specific drug scenes and areas, hours available for work and other relevant information. Thus, as new projects come on stream we can match the profiles of indigenous fieldworkers to appropriate studies. Although it is difficult at this stage to envisage how a formal career structure can be constructed for such casual work, it is pleasing to note that at least two of our former interviewers have used the experience to gain fulltime posts in the drugs field.

## Final Remarks

It can be argued that the use of indigenous fieldworkers detaches the fulltime researcher from the subject of study. It is important, as noted above, that the fulltime researchers involved in projects using this resource maintain firsthand experience of fieldwork. This can be through a combination of ethnographic work at the sites where the research is taking place and by conducting a sample of the interviews.

Yet, in spite of the practical and ethical issues that need to be addressed and overcome, there are many advantages to using ex- and current- drug-users in social research. This is especially the case in terms of contacting elusive networks of drug users that would be extremely difficult for the uninitiated to access. In this context it should become an established component of social behaviourial research in the drugs field.

Although the bulk of the discussion above has emphasized the value of using indigenous fieldworkers in a research context, we should look at ways in which this role can be expanded. In the USA, indigenous workers have been employed on community-based outreach prevention programmes in both research and outreach capacities, particularly in the context of reducing the spread of HIV infection amongst injecting drug users. By adopting this dual role their depth of experience of local drug scenes is used to its full benefit, thereby highlighting the importance and value of this largely untapped resource. Outreach services in Britain would greatly benefit from examining the potential and applicability of these models. With suitable training and supervision, ex- and current- drug-users could be used alongside existing outreach teams as indigenous advocates, working as peer educators amongst networks and at venues with which they are familiar. Thus, we may realise the greater potential of indigenous workers in the field of drug abuse, expanding their activities, not only in research, but also in the context of community-based interventions aimed at particular groups and networks of drug users.

## References

ADVISORY COUNCIL ON THE MISUSE OF DRUGS (ACMD) (1982) *Treatment and Rehabilitation*, London: HMSO.

ADVISORY COUNCIL ON THE MISUSE OF DRUGS (ACMD) (1988) *AIDS and Drug Misuse Part I*, London: HMSO.

ADVISORY COUNCIL ON THE MISUSE OF DRUGS (ACMD) (1989) *AIDS and Drug Misuse Part II*, London: HMSO.

AMSELL, Z., MANDELL, W., MATTHIAS, L., MASON, B. and HOCHERMEN, I. (1976) 'Reliability and validity of self-reported illegal activities and drug use collected from narcotic addicts', *International Journal of Addictions*, 11, 2, pp. 325–36.

BALL, J. (1967) 'The reliability and validity of interview data obtained from fifty-nine narcotic drug addicts', *American Journal of Sociology*, 72, pp. 650–4.

BECKER, H. (1963) *Outsiders: Studies in the Sociology of Deviance*, New York: Free Press.

BROADHEAD, R. and FOX, K. (1990) 'Takin' it to the streets: AIDS outreach as ethnography', *Journal of Contemporary Ethnography*, 19, pp. 322–48.

DUNLAP, E., JOHNSON, B., SANABRIA, H., HOLLIDAY, E. (1990) 'Studying crack users and their criminal careers', *Contemporary Drug Problems*, Spring, pp. 121–43.

FELDMAN, H. (1974) *Street Status and the Drug Researcher: Issues in Participant-observation*, Washington, DC: Drug Abuse Council.

GALLMEIER, C. (1991) 'Leaving, revisiting, and staying in touch: neglected issues in field research', in SHAFFIR, W. and STEBBINS, R. (Eds) *Experiencing Fieldwork*, London: Sage.

HUGHES, E. (1957) 'The relation of industrial to general sociology', *Sociology and Social Research*, 41, pp. 25–6.

HUGHES, P. (1977) *Behind the Wall of Respect: Community Experiments in Heroin Addiction Control*, Chicago, IL: University of Chicago Press.

LIEBOW, E. (1967) *Tally's Corner*, Boston, MA: Little Brown.

PLANT, M. and REEVES, C. (1976) 'Participant observation as a method of collecting information about drug taking: Conclusions from two English studies', *British Journal of Addiction*, 71, pp. 155–9.

POWER, R. (1989) 'Participant observation and its place in the study of illicit drug abuse', *British Journal of Addiction*, 84, pp. 43–52.

POWER, R. and HARKINSON, S. (1993) 'Accessing hidden populations: a survey of indigenous interviewers', in AGGLETON, P., DAVIES, P. and HART, G. (Eds) *AIDS: Facing the Second Decade*, London: Falmer Press.

POWER, R. and JONES, S. (1993) *Lifestyles* (Part Two): *Coping Strategies of Illicit Drug Users*, Final report to the Department of Health, Monograph.

POWER, R., HARTNOLL, R. and CHALMERS, C. (1992) 'Help-seeking amongst illicit drug users: Some differences between a treatment and nontreatment sample', *International Journal of Addictions*, 27, pp. 889–906.

PREBBLE, E. and CASEY, J. (1969) 'Taking care of business: The heroin user's life on the streets', *International Journal of Addictions*, 4, pp. 1–24.

SHICK, J. and WIEBEL, W. (1991) 'Sources of stress and stress reduction needs among indigenous AIDS outreach workers', AIDS Outreach Intervention Program, Chicago, IL: Chicago School of Public Health, University of Illinois. Mimeo.

STEPHENS, R. (1972) 'The truthfulness of addict respondents in research projects', *The International Journal of Addictions*, 7, 3, pp. 549–58.

STIMSON, G., ALDRITT, L., DOLAN, K. and DONOGHOE, M. (1988) Injecting Equipment Exchange Schemes — final report, Monitoring Research Group, London: Goldsmiths' College, University of London, Monograph.

WEBB, E., CAMPBELL, D., SCHWARTZ, R., SECHREST, L. (1981) *Nonreactive Measures in the Social Science*, (2nd ed.) Boston, MA: Houghton Mifflin.

WHYTE, W. (1955) *Street Corner Society*, Chicago, IL: University of Chicago Press.

WIEBEL, W. (1988) 'Combining ethnographic and epidemiologic methods in targeted AIDS interventions: the Chicago Model', in BATTJES, R. and PICKENS, R., *Needle Sharing Among Intravenous Drug Abusers: National International Perspectives*, NIDA Research Monograph 80, Rockville, MD: NIDA pp. 4–12.

WIENER, R. (1970) *Drugs and Schoolchildren*, London: Longman.

WILLIAMS, T. (1989) *The Cocaine Kids*. New York: Addison-Wesley.

# How Many Prostitutes? Epidemiology out of Ethnography

*Neil McKeganey, Marina Barnard and Michael Bloor*

The language of AIDS is a discourse overflowing with statistics. We have statistics on those who are HIV-positive, those who have AIDS, those who have died, and those who are at risk. We have statistics by age, by transmission category, by gender, by geographical place of residence, and — in the case of prostitutes, by occupation. Statistics, of course, can be strangely comforting in a context where so much is uncertain. To quote an HIV prevalence figure for a particular group gives us the impression of a minor victory against the disease — we may not be able to control it, or cure it, but we can at least measure it. And that, in the context of these other failures, is no small victory.

The comfort of measurement depends to a large extent on the accuracy of our measurement tools; yet in many areas related to AIDS and HIV we are working at the very limit of what it is possible to measure or estimate. In this chapter we will describe recent work that we have been undertaking in our aim to estimate the number of women working as prostitutes on the streets in Glasgow and the proportion who are HIV positive. We will describe some of the practical as well as some of the ethical difficulties that we have encountered in this research which involves the surveillance of a hidden population.

## Prostitutes and HIV Infection

Studies into the prevalence of HIV among prostitutes in Europe have shown much lower rates of infection than has been found among prostitutes in certain Sub-saharan African countries and some parts of Asia (Nkya *et al.*, 1992; Bhave *et al.*, 1992). Research in the United Kingdom has shown that about 1 to 3 per cent of female prostitutes might be HIV-positive (Ward *et al.*, 1992; McKeganey *et al.*,

1992). In an Israeli study 180 female prostitutes were HIV tested, of these 1.1 per cent had a positive test result (Modan *et al.*, 1992). A recent study in Spain tested 1665 prostitutes for antibodies to HIV, 12.5 per cent of this sample were found to be antibody positive (Estébanez *et al.*, 1992). A 1988 study of female prostitutes in The Netherlands reported an HIV prevalence of 28 per cent amongst female prostitutes (van den Hoek *et al.*, 1988). Within a number of these studies the link between prostitution and drug injecting has been shown to be crucial. In the Glasgow study reported by McKeganey and colleagues, all of the prostitute women testing HIV-positive were drug injectors; similarly, in the Spanish study reported by Estébanez and her colleagues, the overall HIV prevalence figure of 12.5 per cent masked an important difference depending upon whether the women were injecting drugs. Amongst those women who were prostituting and injecting drugs, the HIV figure was 50.9 per cent, amongst those prostitutes who were not injecting drugs the seroprevalence of HIV was 3.4 per cent. Such results have underlined the importance of looking at HIV amongst both drug injecting and non-drug injecting prostitute women, and of trying to estimate the proportion of prostitute women injecting drugs.

Although it is clearly of importance to be able to identify the percentage of prostitute women (or for that matter clients) who are HIV-positive, such figures can appear to tell us more than they are able to do. A major difficulty in interpreting these figures is one of not knowing the size of the referent population. It makes a good deal of difference, for example, depending whether one is talking about 50 per cent of 100 prostitutes being HIV-positive or 50 per cent of 2000 women being HIV-positive. In planning health services we need to know not only the percentage of people who may be HIV-positive but also the actual number of individuals involved. To estimate the number of female prostitutes who may be HIV-positive you need to estimate the number of women who may be working within an area. But how do you estimate the number of people involved in a hidden and stigmatized activity? Recent research we have been carrying out in Glasgow has suggested that one way round this problem may be to customize methods that field ecologists have used to estimate the size of bird and wild animal populations.

### Mark/Recapture Studies

The typical approach used by field ecologists involves capturing a sample of birds or animals, tagging them mechanically or electronically, releasing them into the wild, capturing a second sample and estimating the size of the overall population on the basis of the proportion of tagged birds in the second sample. Basically, the bigger the overlap in the second sample the smaller the estimate of the population size. We have tried to apply a modified version of this technique in estimating the number of women working as prostitutes on the streets in Glasgow.

### The Glasgow Prostitute Study

The Glasgow research has involved carrying out extensive fieldwork within the city's red-light area (McKeganey and Barnard, 1992). In the first year of our study we conducted fieldwork on fifty-three nights within Glasgow's main red-light area over a seven-month period, totalling more than 156 hours of observation. This fieldwork was structured in accordance with strict time sampling covering every night of the week between the hours 8.00 pm to 1.00 am.

Practically, this work involved the two main researchers, McKeganey and Barnard, walking around the entire set of streets comprising the red-light area. A detailed record was kept of the total number of women seen working and the proportion of women directly contacted by the researchers. All of the women contacted were asked to provide an unnamed saliva sample which was then tested for antibodies to HIV. In total 80 per cent of the women asked to provide a saliva sample agreed to do so.

To facilitate our fieldwork in the red-light area we combined a research role with that of an outreach service provision role. All of the women contacted were provided with condoms, information on HIV risk reduction and if they required it, sterile injecting equipment. In return, all of the women were asked to provide us with a unique identifier — in this case their initials and the day and the month of their date of birth. It is this latter information which is critical in estimating the number of women working on the streets.

At the outset all of the women contacted were new to us; this was reflected in the list of unique identifiers following our first night of fieldwork. As our work within the red-light area progressed, however, a growing proportion of the unique identifiers recorded each night were ones that we had recorded on a previous night. By recording this information we were able to build up a 'capture history' for each of the woman contacted over the duration of our fieldwork. In effect, each night of fieldwork represented a mini-capture/recapture study with the sequence of nights representing a series of such studies of women socially tagged through their initials and date of birth data.

To estimate the number of women working on the streets we have analysed the capture history data on the women using statistical modelling techniques. Basically, the question one is asking is what is the most likely size of the prostitute population to have produced the particular combination of new and repeat identifier details recorded over the period of fieldwork? The statistical methods underlying this research have been detailed elsewhere (Leyland et al., 1993). Using this approach we have estimated that there may be something in the region of 1150 women working on the streets in Glasgow over a twelve-month period, approximately twenty-nine of whom are likely to be HIV positive (McKeganey et al., 1992).

Recording the identifier information on the women following each night of fieldwork has also enabled us to look at the working patterns of different women. For example, we have been able to identify two distinct groups of women, namely a small group of women who work very frequently and a much larger group of women who work on only an occasional and infrequent basis. This distribution can clearly be seen in Figure 7.1.

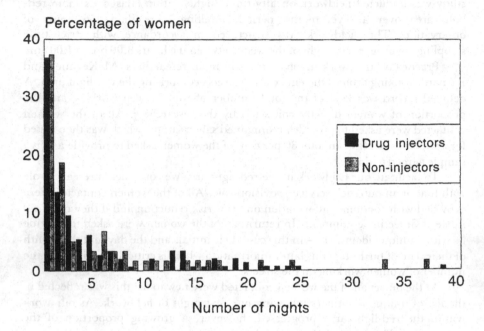

Observations made over 53 nights

*Figure 7.1: Working habits of female prostitutes.*

At the right hand side of the chart are those women who were contacted on virtually every night of fieldwork. At the left hand side by contrast are those women who were seen working on only one or two nights.

In the remainder of this chapter we look at some of the methodological and ethical difficulties encountered in this work.

### Methodological Considerations

*Heterogeneity*

One of the fundamental assumptions underlying early mark/recapture studies is that individual birds or animals within one's study population have an equal likelihood of being contacted. In fact, this is rarely the case. We know some of the reasons why certain birds may be more or less contactable at different times, for example migratory or reproductive habits. We know much less about those factors which might influence the contactability of members of a human population. One of the factors influencing contactability in our own research is the nature of the relationship which we have established with the women. Some of the women with whom we have been able to establish good working relationships actively engage us in conversation during fieldwork. Other women, with whom we have a much more distant relationship, are less likely to be contacted by us, and some women actively avoid contact with us. This difference in our field relationships is very evident in the extracts below:

> The first woman we saw this evening was Trisha. Although we have met her on only three or four previous occasions she greets us warmly, she remembers Marina's name and not mine though previously it had been the reverse. Trisha chats about her family in Birmingham and about her working in London. She said that she had been arrested a few nights previously by a policeman who thought she was an injector. Trisha also chatted about having worked previously in one of the Glasgow saunas and having left when business became really slack. Once having worked on the streets, she said, it would be really difficult for her to go back into the sauna scene since all of the sauna owners thought that women on the streets were using drugs. Trisha also chatted about sexual services saying that an increasing number of men were requesting oral sex, often without a condom, which she said she would never do.

> We met up with Eileen who was standing with another woman who we had not met before. As we approached the two of them, Eileen, who is always a bit stand-offish, moved to one side and answered all of Marina's questions about recent drug deaths with a body language that said, 'Why don't you piss off.' I've noticed that Eileen often does this although on the nights that the drop-in clinic is closed she'll come up and ask for condoms and needles in a more affable manner.

The quality of the relationships we have established with different women is only one of the factors influencing the likelihood of their being contacted. In addition, women differ significantly in the amount of time they spend standing on the streets waiting for clients. Women who are particularly attractive, or younger, or who provide particularly desired sexual services spend less time on the streets between clients and are less likely to be contacted by us as a result. Other women, by contrast, spend a great deal of time between clients and are much more likely to be contacted by researchers.

We have sought to minimize the effects of such heterogeneity by keeping a record of the number of women who are seen only fleetingly, but who are never actually contacted by us. The fact that such heterogeneity exists, however, introduces an unavoidable 'guesstimate' into any calculation we make. The nature of the relationships we have established and the physical attractiveness of different women are only two of the possible dimensions of heterogeneity which may be influencing our work.

### False Identifiers

The identifier information the women provide is clearly a crucial component in our population estimate. Nevertheless, it has to be recognized that some women will have provided different identifiers on different occasions. One of the reasons why this might occur is contained in the extract below:

> We met up with one young woman who greeted us really warmly. We had not seen her for ages and had thought that she must have stopped working altogether. She explained that she had stopped working because at the time she was only 15. I remembered her telling us ages ago that she could not go into the drop-in though she had not explained why. She added that she was now 17. She also said that when she met us before she had given us a false identifier and that now she was older she could give us her correct details.

Where one is dealing with a population which for very good reasons is very wary of official agencies requesting personal information there is always the likelihood that the information provided will be false. We have tried to reduce the likelihood of such inaccuracies in our work in a number of ways. First, we reassure all of the women that the identifier information they provide is collected only in order to maintain a record of the number of different women contacted and that this information will not be passed to any third party. Second, we maintain a list of identifying nicknames (either assigned by ourselves or suggested by the women) which is then linked in our own records to a note of the women's identifier details. This enables us to maintain a regular check on the accuracy of the details some women provide and to amend our records accordingly. Third, in addition to noting the identifier for each woman we also record whether the individual is a new contact or a woman whom we have contacted on a previous occasion. This allows us to check whether a new identifier is being given by a woman whom we have previously contacted and alerts us to the need to pay particular attention to the individual and the identifier she provides on subsequent occasions. We have found it invaluable to carry a hand-held electronic notebook which allows us to record and access identifier details on a continuous basis during fieldwork.

### Women Working Who Are Not Contacted

Any surveillance system of a hidden or covert population will always be less than 100 per cent accurate. In our own work we continually walked around the entire set of streets comprising the red light area. While this widened the range of women contacted it also increased the likelihood of missing those women entering streets we were leaving.

By carrying out fieldwork over an extended period we hope to have minimized the number of women who remained invisible to us. In this research we have consistently been able to contact or identify around 90 per cent of the women seen working during each period of fieldwork. By repeatedly returning to the red-light area those women missed on one night should still be contacted on a subsequent night.

## Working Patterns

By recording the identifier information on each woman following each occasion she is contacted it is possible to look for differences in the working patterns of different women. We have already shown how this approach has enabled us to identify a small number of women who work very frequently and a much larger group of occasional workers. We have also been able to look at the frequency with which drug-injecting and non drug-injecting women work. As a result of carrying out this research over a lengthy period (the second year of data collection has recently been completed) it has also been possible to identify a common pattern of temporary migration from prostitution which many women adopt. This latter information is important since it allows us to characterize the prostitute population not only in terms of estimates of overall numbers, but also in the frequency with which the population changes.

Women who cease selling sex during the course of fieldwork represent a particular problem for our method. Our population estimate is based upon contacts established with the women. An individual who stops prostituting ceases to be contactable by us and is therefore lost to our study. It is very difficult to distinguish between those women who have stopped working temporarily and those women who have stopped working altogether. When we re-contact a woman after a period of non-contact it is possible to ask about the reason for her absence:

> We met up with a woman whom we used to see a lot of last year. She remembered us and said she'd been living in Southampton with her boyfriend for the last year. They had both been off drugs while there. She said she had prostituted there, 'Y'know just to get money, no' for drugs though.' She and her boyfriend made the decision to come back to Glasgow. 'We said, "we'll no' take drugs we'll just live there", What a joke! The first day we were right back into it, so that was us and now I'm back down here again.'

Those women who we cease to contact over an extended period are assumed to have stopped street prostitution in our study area. It is entirely possible that they may have moved to work in another city or have begun working from a non-street venue.

### The Risks of Research on the Streets

Violence is an integral feature of street prostitution. Much of that violence arises from clients and is directed at prostituting women. In the course of this research hardly any of the 300 or so streetworking women contacted by us have avoided being physically threatened or attacked at some time by clients. Two women have been brutally murdered and numerous others have had their life put at risk:

> Last night I went with a punter in a motor. We parked and I did business with him for £20. Then this other bloke gets out the boot of the motor. They stole ma leather jacket, ma money and they raped me and they didnae wear a condom either, so I'll have to go and get that AIDS test done.

Not all the violence though is perpetrated by clients; there were occasions when violence flared between the women themselves:

> We were standing talking with one of the women when we heard May shouting out to Andrea who was standing on the other side of the road to us. When she caught up with her she immediately punched her in the face. The woman standing with us commented how she was sick of it, that May was stealing Andrea's money, taking £10 off her every night because she knows that Andrea earns a fair bit of money. By this time May had landed another blow to Andrea's head with her handbag and was verbally threatening her. Andrea broke away and crossed the road to where we stood. She was obviously pretty shaken up but defiant and showed us a mark on her breast where May had stubbed out a cigarette.

The atmosphere on the streets at night is one in which the potential for violent assault is ever present. Although we have never been threatened ourselves there have been occasions where a night's work has been prematurely concluded to avoid potentially threatening situations developing.

The use of a mixed-sex pairing in work of this kind is very important. A single male researcher is liable to have his intentions misread by the women, similarly a lone female researcher, or two women working together, may be approached by clients requesting sex or be perceived by working women as competitors. A mixed-sex pairing avoids many such problems and offers some greater security to the researchers.

In the remainder of this chapter we will look at some of the ethical issues raised in our work.

### Ethical Considerations

We would like to draw attention to three ethical issues involved in this work. First, there is the issue of providing sterile injecting equipment, second, the question of informed consent, and third, the ethics of carrying out surveillance of a hidden population.

#### *Providing Sterile Injecting Equipment*

Earlier we noted the advantages of combining a service provider role with that of a research role. There is little doubt in our minds that the success we have enjoyed in building close links with working women has been achieved as a result of providing a useful function for them. Elsewhere we have estimated that as many as 70 per cent of street prostitutes in Glasgow are injecting drugs (McKeganey *et al.*, 1992). In the light of this figure the importance of being able to provide sterile injecting equipment to the women is very obvious.

It might be said of our providing the women with condoms and sterile injecting equipment that it is entirely appropriate for researchers to do what they can to reduce HIV-related risk behaviour. Accepting this view at a general level does not necessarily resolve some of the practical dilemmas that can surface in connection with such work (Barnard, 1992). We can illustrate one area of difficulty by taking a concrete example from fieldwork:

> There's a young girl who during the time that we've been coming down here seems to have become more and more involved in the life of the area. First time we encountered her she was completely drunk, running around shouting and screaming through the town. Last night she asked for condoms and needles. She asked me about needles asking whether I had anything 'stronger' than a 2 ml syringe. This made me suspicious because the size of the syringe is not really about anything other than what type of drug is being injected. I gave her needles all the same but felt a bit ambivalent about doing so. When Neil asked her for her identifier she let slip the last bit of her date of birth which makes her no more than 14-years-old. On the basis of this we have decided that we cannot supply her with needles and will advise her in future that she has to get them from the drop-in clinic operating in the area. We are not sure if she is injecting or even if she is prostituting.

By continuing to provide injecting equipment to this 14-year-old girl we might have been guilty of actively encouraging her initiation into drug injecting. However, the decision to stop such provision might have increased her chances of borrowing someone else's injecting equipment and possibly contracting HIV. This dilemma was not helped by the absence of any guidelines covering the researchers activity in this respect.

*Informed Consent*

The requirement that individuals should know and understand the nature of the research in which they are being invited to participate is fundamental to research with human subjects. Muddying the distinction between research and service provision, however, can have important implications to do with the clarity with which informed consent may be elicited.

For many of the women we contact the most salient aspect of our work is the fact that we provide them with condoms and injecting equipment. This is likely to be the case even though we carry and show personal identification cards noting our attachment to the university. To an extent this is probably inevitable. The role of service provider is a good deal more familiar to many of the women than that of a university researcher. The process of data collection for qualitative researchers most often consists in encouraging the free flow of conversation which is then recorded in a fieldwork diary by the researcher, most often when she or he has left the immediate situation. The very informality implied in this process can serve to further mask the research role.

The fact that the role of service provider somewhat eclipses our identity as university researchers places us under an additional obligation to avoid publishing our findings in a form that might increase the stigma and discrimination faced by women who work as prostitutes. We have purposefully avoided publishing our results within any of the tabloid press who from time to time have contacted one or other of the authors of this chapter. We are certainly fortunate in this research in having identified only very few women who are HIV-positive. The relative lack of HIV infection among prostitute women is not as powerful a headline as a high level of infection would undoubtedly have been. Nevertheless, had we identified a high level of infection we would then have faced the dilemna of where to draw the balance between concerns for one's research subjects and the concern to publicize a possible public health threat.

## Surveillance of Hidden Populations

Finally, there is the issue of the ethics of surveillance. Because of the perceived public health threat associated with AIDS and HIV it is now deemed acceptable to carry out research on some of the most intimate and hitherto hidden aspects of people's sexual and drug using behaviour. For some this is an acceptable price to pay in the face of the AIDS pandemic.

For others, however, studies such as our own conveniently gloss over the fact that female prostitutes are only one-half of the commercial sex equation. Men who buy sex are rarely the targets either of police attention or that of researchers. We know very little about the sexual behaviours of prostitute's clients. There is a need then to extend work of the kind that we have described to include male clients. And yet would such an extension overcome the ethics of surveillance? Is such surveillance made acceptable by being more inclusive? If we are able to show that prostitution is not associated with HIV spread should we cease trying to include prostitutes in research? Should we re-focus our research more broadly to include aspects other than HIV of prostitute/client encounters? In addition to our work on estimating the prevalence of HIV infection amongst street prostitutes we have also looked at violence as a feature of prostitute client encounters (Barnard, 1993), the sexual services purchased by male clients (Barnard *et al.*, 1993) and the motivations of male clients (McKeganey, 1994).

## Conclusions

The use of capture/recapture methodology for estimating the size of the street prostitute population in Glasgow clearly has its advantages. Not the least of these is that it is based on direct contact rather than being dependent on partial sampling from different agencies. It is evident, however, that the method raises many issues, some of which we have addressed here. It is true that in this area, as in many others related to AIDS, we are working at the very margins of what is possible. We are developing methods of data collection and analysis in relation to questions that are still relatively new.

This method of population estimate may have applications beyond a concern with HIV. For example, it may be possible to use a similar approach to estimate the number of homeless people within a given area. It is likely though that any such extensions of the approach will raise other problems of both a practical and an ethical nature.

## Acknowledgements

The research described in this chapter is funded by the Medical Research Council. We are grateful to Alastair Leyland for providing statistical support to our project. The Public Health Research Unit is funded by the Chief Scientist Office of the Scottish Home and Health Department and the Greater Glasgow Health Board. The opinions expressed in this paper are not necessarily those of the Scottish Home and Health Department.

## References

BARNARD, M.A. (1992) 'Working in the dark: Researching streetworking prostitutes, in ROBERTS, H. (Ed.) *Women's Health Matters*, London: Routledge, pp. 141-56.
BARNARD, M.A. (1993) 'Violence and vulnerability: Conditions of work for streetworking prostitutes, *Sociology of Health and Illness*, 15, 5, pp. 683-705.

BARNARD, M.A., MCKEGANEY, N.P., LEYLAND, A., COOTE, I. and FOLLET, E. (1993) 'HIV-related risk behaviours among male clients of female prostitutes', *British Medical Journal*, 307, pp. 361–2.

BHAVE, G., WAGLE, U., DESAI, S., MANDEL, J., HEARST, N. and SETH, G. (1992) 'HIV-II prevalence in prostitutes of Bombay', VIII International Conference on AIDS, Amsterdam, PoC 4623.

ESTÉBANEZ, P., RUA-FIGUEROA, M., AGUILAR, M.D., FITCH, K., PALACIOS, V., PÉLEZ, L. and NAJERA, R. (1992) 'HIV prevalence and risk factors in Spanish prostitutes', VIII International Conference on AIDS, Amsterdam, PoC 4189.

LEYLAND, A., BARNARD, M. and MCKEGANEY, N. (1993) 'The use of capture-recapture methodology to estimate and describe covert populations: An application to female street-working prostitution in Glasgow', *Bulletin de Méthodologie Sociologique*, 38, pp. 52–73.

MCKEGANEY, N. (1994) 'Why do men buy sex and what are their assessments of the HIV-related risks when they do?' *AIDS Care*, (in press).

MCKEGANEY, N.P. and BARNARD, M.A. (1992) *AIDS, Drugs and Sexual Risk: Lives in the Balance*, Buckingham, Open University Press.

MCKEGANEY, N.P. and BARNARD, M.A. (1992) 'Selling sex: Female prostitution and HIV-risk behaviour in Glasgow', *AIDS Care*.

MCKEGANEY, N.P., BARNARD, M.A., LEYLAND, A.H., COOTE, I. and FOLLET, E. (1992) 'Female streetworking prostitution and HIV infection in Glasgow', *British Medical Journal*, 305, pp. 801–4.

MODAN, B., GOLDSCHMIDT, R., RUBENSTEIN, E., VONSOVER, A. and ZINN, M. (1992) 'Prevalence of HIV antibodies in transsexual and female prostitutes', *American Journal of Public Health*, 82, pp. 590–2.

NKYA, W., HOWLETT, W., KLEPP, K., NYOMBI, B. and ASSENGA, C. (1992) 'HIV-cohort study of self-proclaimed prostitutes in Moshi and Arusha Towns, Northern Tanzania', VIII International Conference on AIDS, Amsterdam, PoC 5645.

VAN DEN HOEK, J., COUTINHO, R., VAN HAASTRECHT, J., VAN ZADELHOFF, A., and GOUDSMIT, J. (1988) 'Prevalence and risk factors of HIV infections among drug users and drug using prostitutes in Amsterdam', *AIDS*, 2, pp. 55–60.

WARD, H., DAY, S., DUNLOP, L., DONEGAN, C., WHITAKER, L. and DE LA COURT, A. (1992) 'Commercial sex and HIV risk: A six-year study of female sex workers', VIII International Conference on AIDS, Amsterdam, PoC 4186.

*Methods of Data Collection*

*Chapter 8*

# Diaries and Sexual Behaviour: The Use of Sexual Diaries as Method and Substance in Researching Gay Men's Response to HIV/AIDS

*Anthony P.M. Coxon*

The Human Immunodeficiency Virus (HIV) is transmitted primarily in sexual activity; hence detailed information is needed about the sexual context in which that transmission occurs if accurate epidemiological estimates are to be made and the spread of the pandemic to be understood and contained. How such information may be obtained, and how its reliability and validity may be assessed form the basis of the research reported in this chapter. Very little can be taken for granted in such research and the methodological problems are considerable. From the outset we know that sexual behaviour such as vaginal and anal intercourse are particularly implicated in transmission, but the evidence is much less clear for oral sex and other sexual activities and it is therefore necessary to investigate the whole range of activities which could *possibly* lead to transmission.

The individual is at the centre of that investigation and is normally the source of such data, so it makes sense to collect data from his or her (ego's) perspective. But since any implicated sexual activity involves at least one other person, the real unit of investigation is the dyad (couple), and the behaviour and characteristics of the other person (alter) are also crucial.

Information of a particularly intrusive kind is needed for analysing HIV transmission. Since the mechanism involves the 'exchange of bodily fluids' — especially semen, blood and saliva — they too must be tracked and reported and details of whether and how ejaculation of semen occurs is an integral part of the analysis. Our research focus does not, however, cover all types of sexual behaviour, it is restricted to the sexual and social lifestyles of *men who have sex with men*[1] (and possibly with women).

If we were interested primarily in the actual mechanisms of sexual transmission of HIV, then direct observation might well be the appropriate method for obtaining information, as in Masters and Johnson's (1966) work. But such a method is likely to lead to highly biased estimates, since only a highly atypical sub-population is likely to consent, and the presence of an observer would itself be highly reactive. Observation as a method is therefore far from unobtrusive and would involve major problems of consent and organization (and cost). It would also be illegal, at least in England and Wales (but not in Scotland).[2]

In order to obtain relevant information, we have to rely on subjects' own reports or accounts of sexual activity have to be obtained, and the interview setting provides the most usual context of data-collection. In Project SIGMA[3] the yearly Core Question Schedule includes as a central element the Inventory of Sexual Behaviour (ISB) (Coxon *et al.*, 1992b), asking respondents a systematic set of questions about whether (and if so, how often) they had engaged in these detailed activities (for prevalence) and within a given period of time (for incidence). But how accurate are such subjects' estimates likely to be? From the outset of our enquiries the data gave good grounds for scepticism: the numbers given in answers were often suspiciously vague, rounded or approximate (Coxon, 1988b), suggesting problems of accurate recall. Moreover, when questions (identical or implied) were repeated later in the interview, the number given was rarely the same, suggesting problems of reliability. When cross-checks were made with estimates given by their partners the numbers were (to varying degrees) often at variance with the respondent's, suggesting problems of validity.

Much information obtained about sexual activity is also atomistic and out of context — we learn whether or how often something was done, but rarely the context in which it took place, the sequence in which it occurred, or the person with whom it occurred. Such factors make a big difference to the meaning of sexual behaviour, but they are also important, we believe, in attempting to understand sexual risk. That sexually risky behaviour takes place is important, but if people are to be encouraged to lessen or avoid risk then we need to know the significance of such behaviour to the person, and we also need to identify its context in order to find out whether risk-taking varies systematically by situation, rather than simply by individual. Again, the number of sexual partners a person has is an important variable epidemiologically, but it is even more important to know whether they are one-off or regular partners, whether sex with such partners involves penetrative or unprotected (risky) sex, whether alcohol or drugs such as nitrites have been used (possibly as disinhibitors) . . . and so on. In the normal way such questions are asked separately, and even if recall is excellent we can know nothing about how they co-occur with sexual behaviour and combine in a particular sexual situation to increase or decrease risk. Finally, the order in which sexual activity occurs (and the position in a sequence in which an act occurs) can have quite different effects. An example is the differing risks of hepatitis infection when oral sex follows anal intercourse as opposed to preceding it. Similarly, the probabilities of transmission are very different according to whether a person is anally receptive or insertive, and we knew little indeed about the prevalence and possible mixture of sexual role playing in male-with-male sex (Coxon and Coxon, 1993a).

The interaction of these issues is highly complex, and answers to them cannot be obtained by simple questionnaire methods. But they are pressing issues, whose answers could have radically different consequences for understanding and predicting the spread of the pandemic and for health education and interventions. It is not just that recalling complex behaviour is more difficult than recalling simple behaviour but that many people are unaware of how these factors combine in their own case, or simply cannot give a verbal account of it. A rather different method is therefore called for which can provide information in a manageable and a systematic way: we developed the diary method for this purpose.

Diary-keeping is a very natural way to elicit data of the sort we require. Almost everyone has kept a diary at some point and it is often the chosen way to confide and record one's thoughts and actions. It is, as Plummer (1983) rightly dubs it, a 'document of life'. Used as a social science method, it can be a valuable non-reactive method (when previously written, uncommissioned diaries are used as a resource), or it can be a specially elicited record, typically focused on one domain such as purchases or alcohol consumption or, as here, on sexual activity. Like its natural variant, it suffers similar problems of motivation; many start diaries but fewer finish them.

How does the diary method compare with other methods? As in *Content Analysis*, diaries are usually written in natural language format, and are subject to the same forms of analysis including syntactic, semantic and thematic analysis. But in diaries, the focus and domain of interest is usually narrower than in most naturally-occurring prose. Like the similar methods of *Life- Case- or Event-history*, the diary method is time-structured and sequential, but it is usually more detailed and discursive in content and has a much smaller time-span than a history. There are even some similarities with the *questionnaire*. The questionnaire can differ in how structured it is and whether it is self-completed or administered in an interview situation, and so can the diary method. The main difference is that diary data are not elicited in a pre-ordained, conditional branching sequence of questions, as in the case of the questionnaire.

### The Sexual Diary

The diary method has been developed within Project SIGMA (Coxon, 1988a; Davies and Coxon, 1990; Coxon *et al.*, 1992b; Coxon and Coxon, 1993b) as a parallel to the Project's more conventional methods, and has now become the preferred (indeed, the unique) method for obtaining certain sorts of information about the detail of gay men's sexual activity. It is important to enter a series of provisos at this point:

(i) We are restricting attention here to sexual *behaviour*; other methods are used to establish the meaning and context of that behaviour and other forms of data collection are useful in relation to other research questions.

(ii) The need to concentrate on sexual behaviour capable of leading to HIV transmission means that considerable (perhaps undue) attention is paid to ejaculation and its *sequelae*. This aspect can, of course, be ignored and omitted.

(iii) Although the sexual diary method has been developed in the context of studying homosexual behaviour there is nothing to restrict it to this orientation. Indeed, sexual activity between homosexual men and their female partners forms a natural part of this study.

Project SIGMA has developed a theory (or schema) for the representation and analysis of sexual activity (Coxon *et al.*, 1992b), which forms the basis for obtaining systematic information about the prevalence and incidence of sexual behaviour in both the Interview/Questionnaire context and that of the sexual diary (See Davies, Chapter 4, this volume). This makes aggregation and comparability of data from these different data sources a straightforward matter, and it also gives SIGMA's use of the diary method a very distinctive flavour. The theory itself arose both as a way of systematizing and inter-relating the components of sexual behaviour relevant to HIV transmission and as an attempt to connect the structure of sexual behaviour to Talcott Parsons' account of the Unit Act in the structure of social action, and to communication processes. At an early stage we had realized that the structure of sexual behaviour has a striking resemblance to linguistic structure, and that to interpret it in this way gives added insight to the analysis and meaning of sexual behaviour. In this interpretation, the self-contained unit of communication analogous to the sentence is the sexual session; the constituent words corresponded to the sexual acts, and the inflections of the word could encode the activity, the modality and the outcome. The information transmitted in a sexual session is basically a predication of the form:

WHO *does* WHAT, TO WHOM *and with* WHAT OUTCOME

which encodes the agent (who), the sexual behaviour (what), the other sexual recipient (to whom) and whether and how ejaculation occurred (what outcome).

This same structure can then be used to define question-formats for questionnaires (such as the ISB) and for diary instructions and makes it possible to compare data having many different formats.

### Advantages and Disadvantages

Before proceeding with a specification of how the method of diaries is applied to sexual behaviour, it is worth pausing to summarize the advantages and disadvantages of the sexual diary method. The sexual diary method is a more 'natural' method than most, both in the sense that it exists as a common social practice and that it is written in natural language. The diary makes it possible to obtain information in far greater detail than other methods, since it is designed to minimize recall and memory errors and cognitive strain. It is especially adapted to gathering reliable information on the time-sequence of events, so that change is easily charted. The information can be obtained in a contextually-specific manner, without relying on recall; thus variation due to such things as particular partners or particular settings can be directly studied. Quantitative information is derived directly from the data, without recourse to the errorful estimating procedures used by survey questioning or respondent recall. The sexual diary can be augmented to obtain other concurrent information such as alcohol and drug use in sex (see Weatherburn *et al.*, 1993), and the data obtained are, on present evidence, more reliable than those obtained from retrospective recall in surveys (see Janson, 1990). These advantages are impressive, but need to be balanced against the undoubted disadvantages, some of which can be ameliorated.

The main disadvantages of the sexual diary method have to do with bias in recruitment of respondents rather than with the method of data collection *per se*. But there is undoubted selection bias with respect to those who do and those who do not agree to be diary respondents or return information. In the case of hidden populations like gay men (SIGMA, 1990, Coxon and Joyce, 1993) selection bias in the recruitment of those prepared to keep a diary exists in addition to that in the initial sampling procedure of Project sample members. The sources of bias are very similar to those in other studies relying on volunteer subjects (Rosenthal and Rosnow, 1975:225) who tend to be educated, of higher social class, intelligent, approval-motivated and sociable; (the last characteristic takes the form of being more likely to be 'out' as gay men). Those volunteering tend to be more sexually active (in the sense of having more sexual sessions and more partners) than those who do not volunteer.[4] For longitudinal studies there is undoubted 'step-wise attrition' — it is far easier to persuade men to keep a diary for consecutive months than regularly on a yearly basis. The type of data generated cannot readily by analysed by conventional packages, and rely on an intermediate stage of string-manipulation software (see section entitled 'Sexual diary data' below).

### Implementation of the sexual diary

Keeping a sexual diary is not a novelty to many gay men (Joe Orton is a notorious instance; Lahr, 1986); some have been keeping one intermittently all their life. Sometimes this is instrumental (in case of infection with a sexually transmitted disease, so that partners can be informed), but more often it is intrinsically interesting, especially to those with a full and/or complex sex life, or who wish to note their adventures for later enjoyment or as an aide-memoire to masturbation.

At each wave of the Project, the SIGMA respondent is taken through the last week of his[5] sexual activity by the interviewer according to a specified format. Originally this was done to ensure that the respondent understood the instructions for keeping the diary. The interviewer often assisted in its recall and wrote the actual transcript. Subsequently, this procedure also provided useful information on autobiographical memory: how far back could he recall the detail of sexual activity?[6] At the end of the interview, a month-long diary and set of instructions (see SIGMA, 1993) were given to the respondent for completion and return (an example of a completed week of such a diary is contained in Appendix One).

Respondents are told that accounts of sexual activity should be written down as soon as possible, and if possible on the same day they occurred; only to complete a diary if they are prepared to be completely honest, and not to invent or 'shade' what they do; that the basic unit of their account should be the 'session' ('one or more sexual acts by yourself or with the same person/s at one time'). The format of each session, derived from the 'structure of sexual action' (see Coxon, *et al.*, 1992b) is then explained. The components are:

- *Time, place and antecedents*: Day, hour; location (for example, in whose accommodation or external sites, such as parks, toilets, the activity took place), together with antecedents such as the use of alcohol, drugs and nitrites;
- *the participants*: (if any); description of the sexual partner/s[7] involved in this session;
- *the sexual activity*: for each constituent sexual act in a session — the behaviour; the modality (who did it to whom) and the outcome (whether and how ejaculation occurred);
- *accompaniments*: especially use of condoms, lubricants, 'toys', etc.

The relevance of the participants and sexual activity components has already been explained above, but the inclusion of the others needs a brief explanation. *Time* is necessary for sequencing sessions during a day (what one does sexually in the morning often differs dramatically from what happens in the evening). *Place* or location allows us to separate out home-based from casual or out-of-doors activity. *Antecedents* are part of the scene-setting which makes it possible to inspect the effect of precursor activities (poppers or alcohol before, as opposed to within sexual activity); together they define the situation and hence reduce problems of indexicality. *Accompaniments*, by contrast are part of the scene and sexual activity which do not usually have a direct effect of the probability of transmission.[8]

*The Sexual Act*

The sexual act forms the basic building block — the word of the session's sentence — and the structure here is crucial for later analysis. In SIGMA's schema, all description is ego-centric, i.e., viewed from the respondent's (ego's) position in the proceedings, and the question of which sexual actor is doing a given act to the other is dealt with by the relational modality[9] of the act. Thus, Active always means that ego does *x* to alter, and Passive always means that alter does behaviour *x* to ego. A simplified[10] form of the specification of the sexual act is as follows:

| ⟨ACT⟩:: = | {⟨MODE⟩⟨BEHAVIOUR⟩⟨EGO'S ORGASM[11]⟩⟨ALTER'S ORGASM⟩⟨MODIFIER⟩} |
|---|---|
| ⟨MODE⟩:: = | {S\|A\|P\|M} |
| ⟨BEHAVIOUR⟩:: = | {W\|S\|F\|Ri\|Fg\|Dk\|Fi...} |
| ⟨EGO's | |
| = ALTER'S ORGASM⟩:: = | {N\|I\|X\|O\|H\|M\|C} |
| ⟨MODIFIER⟩:: = | {null\|/ ⟨associated object list⟩⟨modifier⟩} |
| ⟨OBJECT⟩:: = | {P,L,D,T,...} |

The symbol :: = may be read as 'can be replaced by' or 'consists of'; it links the basic term (*definiendum*) on its left hand side and its specification on the right. The symbol | may be read as 'or' or 'such that'. The most fundamental units (behaviours, modes, orgasm/ejaculation, conjugators and objects or 'accompaniments') are specified as a list of letters denoting the contents in the code. In brief:

a *sexual act* consists of:
        a *behaviour* [masturbation,[12] fellatio . . .], where
        the *mode* is [self, active, passive, mutual . . .] and
        *ego's ejaculation* and *alter's ejaculation* can occur in a specified manner
        [in him, on me, in a condom . . . to be explained later],

together with
        *modifier/s* such as [poppers, lubricants . . .].

When the respondent is asked to specify these details (in natural language) for each act he will write, for example:
    'I fucked him; I came in him; he didn't come.'

which is interpreted as:

> *behaviour* anal intercourse; *modality* active;
> *ego's orgasm* in alter; *alter's orgasm* no
> (*modifier/s* none).

The specification of the sexual act is open; the list of behaviours can be extended as new activities, such as inter-femoral intercourse, are encountered and such is the imaginativeness of human sexual behaviour that even modality is not closed.[13]


### The Sexual Code

The structure of the sexual session can readily, simply and efficiently be represented in an encoded form as a string, which greatly simplifies storage and facilitates data analytic operations like comparing the structure of two sessions. The details of the coding system in this context would be rebarbative and need not detain us; suffice it to say that the coded form is isomorphic with the structure of the act, and has an easily remembered mnemonic form. Earlier and simpler versions of the code were used by respondents themselves as an encrypting device and some of these are still used to save unnecessary repetition.[14]


### Sexual Diary Data

The problems of representation and analysis which arise in the case of sexual diaries are similar to those encountered in content analysis, where one is faced by a large amount of natural language material subdivided in various ways (sources, chapters, sentences and words) each with their own syntax and semantics. The same is true for sexual diary information, although coding is fortunately an easier prospect because the structure of sexual behaviour is (by design) much more tightly defined than ordinary language, and much complexity has been reduced by the preliminary coding.

To illustrate the high degree of structure and redundancy in a typical set of sexual diary data consider this coded version of a week of a respondent's sexual activity (each session is a sentence ended by a period):[15]

---

PF,NM/1.AS AS&PS PRI ARI ATF AF,HN/1 PF/1 HW,NI. (*PS AS PS ACP PRI ARI AF,HN&HW*)/*p*. PRI PF,NM/1 PW. AW PW. AS. PF/1. HW PW,XN&HW,NX/1. PF/1. PS AF,HN/1,p,t. PW PRI PF,NM/1 (PS ACP AF,HN/1)/p. PW AFG HW,NX AF/1.

---

### Context and Acts: Data record and string

The original diary version of third sentence/session above was:

[...when we got home after the club I stripped him and, kneeling before me] he sucked me. After moving to the bed, I sucked him. Then I lay back and he started again sucking me. Lying face down I then took the belt to him and began using it on him and after a while he then moved round and began rimming me. I did exactly the same to him, preparing him. Then, with him lying on his back, I then fucked him using KY whilst he wanked himself. I came in him; he didn't come. We used poppers throughout.

Clearly, the purely sexual information has been abstracted and some incidentals (such as stripping and positional information) have been removed. Each session is a separate data base record[16] as follows:

---

NO: cf****/1 | TYPE: vi | STATUS: Neg | DAY: tues | DATE: ******
TIME: 0100 | PLACE: home, after the club
PERSON: P2 Regular, 31, sex 4 yrs, Neg
ACT: (*PS AS PS ACP PRI ARI AF, HN&HW*)/p
POPPERS: tnt | CONDOMS: no          | LUBS: ky
OTHER: leather belt       | DRUGS: alcohol beforehand.

---

Each field of the record is in upper case (FIELD:) and the entries are in lower-case. Identifying information is denoted by asterisks. The contextual information makes it possible to select out subsets of data with particular characteristics of descriptive or explanatory relevance. Some of the more important ones evident from the above fields of the record include:

- *Home area and ID* (cf denotes Cardiff; **** is ID number and /1 refers to Wave 1).
- *Age-group and Relationship type* of Ego (type vi signifies 'Over 39 and in an open relationship').
- *Time:* day (to see whether sexual activity is different on Wednesdays as opposed to Saturdays); hour (to allow sequencing within a day but also to enable contrast between morning, afternoon, evening and early morning sex).
- *Place:* Most men are not co-habiting with a sexual partner, so location of sexual activity is interesting. This field also allows for outside sex, for example, parks or toilets to be selected.
- *Person:* each current sexual partner is allocated a sequential number and

described in terms of his (or her) characteristics (but not named) at the beginning of the diary form, and if other sexual contacts occur during the month they are added to the list, to form a *dramatis personae* of partners. The Project's ethical code promised that identifying information and names of partners (if known) would not appear on any records, thus precluding sexual network tracing — or almost so.[17]

- *Accompaniments:* Nitrites (poppers) are a commonly-used accompaniment to gay sex, and drugs sometimes are. The use of prophylactics (chiefly condoms but occasionally and more recently dental dams) are a major focus of safer sex.

### The Sexual Diary Database

Project SIGMA has been collecting sexual diary data systematically since 1986. As well as the monthly diaries (and week-long retrospective interview diaries), there have been several one-off appeals for volunteers via the gay press, especially in the *Gay Times* in 1986 and 1987, and in *Boyz* in 1992. In toto, there are probably close to 1000 diaries, but the maintained data-base keeps a subset of these:

---

| | |
|---|---|
| 852 | diaries in up to 5 Waves containing: |
| 17,664 | sessions involving: |
| 39,011 | acts for: |
| 569 | individuals from 10 SIGMA sites and 4 other sources |

---

These data exist as data-base records and in more efficient internal format and are accessible[18] with the specially-written package for the PC: SDA/pc (Sexual Diary Analysis) SIGMASOFT.™

### Reliability and Validity

The validity and reliability of the diary method has not been much studied, but there is a common assumption that it is less reliable and probably less valid than questionnaire methods. Although the validity of diaries as a method for collecting sexual behaviour has been questioned by McLaws *et al.* (1990). James *et al.* (1991) find a good fit between interviews and a self-administered questionnaire and Conrath *et al.* (1983) show the greater reliability of diary recording techniques (applied to sociometric data in this instance).

The reliability and validity of diary methods compared to interview methods are currently under systematic investigation in Project SIGMA,[19] and any results must therefore be tentative. In these investigations various methods are used. For a balanced subset of SIGMA panel members, comparison is made of the number of sexual acts per month given in the current interviews, and the estimates derived from their sexual diary (these refer to adjacent months, of course). A specially recruited national sample completed a month diary and returned it. After its return they were sent a form asking them to estimate the number of times they had done a set of sexual acts during that month (and given an incentive to do so).[20] Comparison was thus possible for the same month period between a diarist's counts derived from his sexual diary and the numbers estimated directly by him. Studies were made of the encoding process (both in the cognitive and the technical sense). In the former sense, the focus is upon how people differentially perceive and 'chunk' visual or verbal stimuli (of sexual behaviour); in the latter sense the focus is upon how Project coders turn subjects' accounts into their coded version.

Even at a preliminary stage the results of this research radically undermine the common assumption that data derived from questionnaire/interview data are more reliable and valid than diary data.

*Reliability*

Reliability refers to stability and internal coherence. Internal reliability in the psychometric sense of alternative forms or split-half reliability are not feasible proposals for diary entries; test-retest methods are virtually impossible to implement and can generate understandable and counter-productive hostility among diarists. Moreover, any attempt to implement independent or repeated entries fast run up against problems of memory recall for detailed data (Linton, 1986) and hence confound any reliability estimation. In SIGMA studies we have therefore concentrated on inter-coder reliability (how far do different coders encode natural language diary entries in the same way) and direct coding (from visual stimuli). Coders are presented first with a spoken or written account from a given diary, and asked to encode it (separately and without collaboration) according to the rules of representation.[21] The coded versions are then compared; inter-coder agreement is assessed by comparing the codings (which are strings) and measuring how similar they are to each other by using a Levenshtein distance (Sankoff and Kruskal, 1983). Distance (dissimilarity) values are generally excellent, averaging better than 0.10.

The visual experiments consist of showing two three-minute sections from a gay porn video collection called *Gay Weekend II*, produced in the United States but brought into Britain from the Netherlands. Experiments have so far been restricted to project staff and coders. The main purpose is to see how, given a specific visual stimulus of homosexual behaviour (a sequence taken from the video), experienced coders 'chunk' this continuous and sometimes ambiguous material in terms of the Project coding schema (which works in terms of a sequence of discrete events) and go on to ask how similar these accounts are. A major problem that emerges is how to reconcile codings which differ primarily in 'fine-ness' or detail, where, for instance, one coder will report that nipple fingering was followed by anal fingering, whilst another will interpose active masturbation between these two acts because the hand went over (and possibly lingered) over the penis. It is still too early fully to assess these visual experiments, but acts which resulted in ejaculation are always recorded, and in the correct sequence, which is reassuring.

### Validity

Short of observing sexual behaviour directly, it is not immediately obvious what forms validation can or should take. Since SIGMA diarists filled out their diaries in the months following their yearly interview it is possible to identify each diarist's interview data and compare the two sources. The most cited text treating validity (Campbell and Stanley, 1963) properly distinguishes internal and external validity (or, confounding and generalizability problems). Where there are two or more forms of instrument or method, each with its uniqueness component, they have also stressed the role of triangulation to deal with convergent validity.

### Comparing interview and diary estimates of the same behaviour

Several forms of investigating validity are currently being used (see 'Reliability and Validity'). These concentrate primarily on the extent of agreement between accounts — derived from different methods (interview estimates vs. derived diary counts) and from different individuals involved in the same sexual session. Internal threats such as instrumentation and selection biases are particularly liable to occur in these contexts, and selection bias in particular undoubtedly occurs among volunteers who agree to do sexual diaries. However, since the SIGMA diarists are a subset of the main panel, demographic and other factors (such as higher rates of sexual activity) which differentiate the two groups can be used to estimate the degree and sources of selection bias.

The main focus in the SIGMA studies is on comparing the similarity between accounts and finding out if (and how) different estimates of the same sexual activity vary. At the aggregate level (i.e. incidence figures over all individuals) agreement is excellent and gives an important clue about the likely relationship between interview estimates diary counts (calculated from the daily-completed diaries; see Coxon and Coxon, 1993b). In particular, rank-order correlation between the aggregate diary counts and the aggregate interview estimates is modest ($\tau = 0.77$), but the linear correlation is considerably higher (r = 0.93). The regression of the diary counts on the interview estimates gives a regression coefficient close to unity (b = 0.94) and an intercept of 15.5. Taken together this suggests that, overall, respondents consistently over-estimate the frequency of their sexual activity in their retrospective recall in the interview situation by a constant addition (intercept). The aggregate data are presented in Figure 8.1.

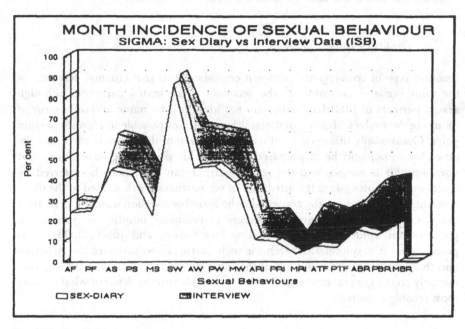

Sexual Behaviour Codes:

MODALITY (1st letter):  Active Passive Mutual/Simultaneous

BEHAVIOUR (Subsequent letter/s:)

| Code | 'Street Term' | Behaviour |
|------|---------------|-----------|
| F | Fuck | Anal Intercourse |
| S | Suck | Fellatio |
| W | Wank | Masturbation |
| RI | Rim | Oral-Anal |
| TF | Thigh Fuck | Inter-femoral |
| BR | Body Rub | Body Rub |

*Figure 8.1: Aggregate diary vs. interview estimates of sexual behaviour*

Until recently, the main alternative explanation for any observed differences between interview and diary counts was that the two months were not the same; the interview questions referred to the month *past*, whilst the diary was not started until after the interview, and the data hence referred to the *subsequent* month. In the most recent experiment, however, this has been overcome; on return of their diary, diarists were sent a new (and unannounced) sheet asking them to estimate the number of times in the last month (i.e. of the diary) they had done various acts, and how sure they were of each estimate. In this way the retrospection involved in answering the interview question is simulated, whilst a separate estimate is available by counting frequencies the diary.

### Comparing partners' accounts

Another type of convergent validation consists of two participants' accounts of the same event — in this case, the accounts of the sexual partners. Although sexual partners of SIGMA diarists are not identified by name and only some of them are themselves SIGMA diarists, it is sometimes possible to identify partner pairs. Occasionally this occurs naturally where one of the partners mentions the other by name, and he is prepared to solicit his partner's co-operation. But normally this is not so, and the sexual partner can sometimes be inferred by matching attributes (since the attributes of sex partners are described in the diary account) or by matching the contents of the actual sex session itself. This method has been used with a degree of success to estimate 'number of partners of partners' for epidemiological modelling (see Coxon and Joyce, 1993). It is proposed to do a systematic search for such partners and compare the structure and 'fine-ness' of the two codings of the same events, and thus gain information not only on the general convergent validity, but also on the detail of what acts are most reliably reported.

## An Example: Risk Behaviour in Anal Intercourse

We proceed now to an example of how the diary procedures are used in a specific research problem, namely that of anal intercourse and risk. The primary source of risk in sexual transmission of HIV among gay males is anal intercourse. Safer sex messages advise that risk should be minimized by the use of a condom, in conjunction with a water-based lubricant. If risk is to be monitored it is crucial to ensure that information about involvement in anal intercourse and the use of condoms is accurate, reliable and valid. The usual way of investigating this central issue is by the interview or questionnaire method, with the interviewer defining levels of sexual risk for the respondent and then asking whether or not he has engaged in any of the risky behaviours, and if so, how often.

There are good reasons for expecting that such data will underestimate the actual incidence of risk as respondents will tend to deny or underestimate such infractions of safer sex, and prevalence figures from interview or questionnaire data are best taken as lower estimates. Diary data offer definite advantages for investigating such issues. First, the estimates are obtained by the researcher *post factum* from the diary accounts, and there is no need to involve the respondent in identifying risk occurrences at all, since these, too, are identified *post factum* by the researcher. Interviewer and social desirability effects can thus be avoided.

In monitoring the incidence of anal intercourse and use of the condom, most studies (including SIGMA) usually rely upon the respondent to report upon his condom use, and often content themselves with a graded scale of frequency of condom use.[22] But, again, respondents' reports and estimates from interview contexts are liable to be defective and subject to systematic distortion.[23] Indeed, few can reliably give accurate estimates of their condom use, and yet fewer can remember which occasions involved their use.

### Characteristics of anal intercourse

As a preparation for the risk analysis let us turn first to some general findings about anal intercourse derived from analysis of the diaries.

- If anal intercourse occurs, it is typically an end-marker to a sexual session. This is especially so when it culminates in ejaculation on the part of one or more of the partners. Once ejaculation has happened it is unlikely that any significant sexual activity follows, and if it does, it often simply establishes a reciprocation.
- Anal intercourse plays a crucial role in determining the power aspect of a session; Davies and Coxon (1990) show that a sexual session tends consistently to be either reciprocal (symmetric) or dominant (asymmetric).[24] In the reciprocal session the pattern of events follows an A,P alternation ('I do it to you, and you then do it to me', or vice versa), in the dominant session power positions are established: one partner becomes the active partner and remains so throughout the session. Fucking is often the lynch-pin of such sessions.
- The pattern of acts which immediately precede anal intercourse has a clear structure: In an earlier paper we have been able to show that the rule is, 'If I fuck a guy, sucking is most likely to precede it (rather than wanking) and I'm most likely to be sucked by him first' (Coxon and Coxon, 1993b). Correlatively, passive (receptive) anal intercourse is typically preceded by fellatio, and usually by *active* fellatio.

### Ejaculation and Risk

Since many sexual acts carry the potential of orgasm, ejaculation is allowed for in the schema and in the coding. Initially, the only distinction noted was whether or not orgasm occurred, since the question of which partner did so was normally clear from the context of the behaviour and its modality. Next, the outcome suffix was made two-place — the first for ego, the second for alter — making the detail of mutual orgasm easy to code and clearing up residual ambiguity. Finally, the two-place form was further differentiated to specify the actual destination of the ejaculate (semen), so that even potentially risky behaviours (such as alter masturbating himself and ejaculating on ego's body, which might have lesions . . .) could be explicitly identified. To do this we have developed the form shown in Figure 8.2.

| CODE | EJACULATION DESTINATION |
|------|-------------------------|
| 1. N | No ejaculation |
| 2. X | Elsewhere (e.g. on floor, or unspecified) |
| 3. O | On him (alter), i.e. skin or body surface |
| 4. I | On me (ego) |
| 5. C | into a Condom |
| 6. H | In him (alter), either anally or orally |
| 7. M | In me (ego), either anally or orally |

*Figure 8.2: Alternatives for destination of ejaculation.*

The seven outcomes are arrayed as a weak order of risk of HIV transmission: no ejaculation (1) — ejaculate elsewhere (2) — ejaculate *on* a partner (3, 4) — ejaculate *in* a condom (5) — ejaculate *in* a partner (6, 7). This order differentiates the 'On rather than In' safer sex message and the full form also specifies which partner receives the semen. The fifth alternative (the condom) might at first sight seem anomalous, but belongs there as perhaps the most important 'destination', being the main form of prophylaxis. These ejaculation (outcome) codes will now be used to examine risk behaviour involving anal intercourse.

### 'Volume' Analysis of Risk and Anal Intercourse

The basic data used for the risk analysis are all the 2107 acts of anal intercourse in the data base and the unit of analysis will be the act rather than the individual (so-called volume or outlet analysis; Coxon and Coxon, 1993b).

Anal intercourse accounts for 5.6 per cent of all sexual acts of gay men in the database (13.4 per cent of all acts excluding masturbation), almost exactly evenly divided between the active/insertive and the passive/insertee modalities. (This percentage markedly differs from the usually reported incidence *per man* during a month; about a third of gay men engage in either active or passive anal intercourse a median number of two times a month according to SIGMA studies (SIGMA, 1990)).

To investigate levels of risk in anal intercourse we need first to examine the frequency with which the various forms of ejaculation occur. The percentage distribution is given in Table 8.1. The information in this Table reveals several interesting points. One is that coming *on* a partner is actually a very uncommon activity; ejaculation elsewhere (basically, avoiding the partner's body) is a much more likely eventuality.

| Code | Outcome | Per cent | Risk level |
|------|---------|----------|------------|
| N | No ejaculation | 30.5 | 0 |
| X | Elsewhere | 12.4 | 1 |
| O | On him (alter) | 1.9 | 2 |
| I | On me (ego) | 1.7 | 2 |
| C | into a Condom | 16.6 | 3 |
| H | in Him | 23.5 | 4 |
| M | in Me | 13.4 | 4 |
| | | 100.0 | |
| | | (N Acts = 2107) | |

*Table 8.1: Destination of ejaculate in anal intercourse.*

Putting the information hierarchically — out of 100 acts of anal intercourse, 70 involve ejaculation of semen. Of these ejaculations: 17 are into a condom, 53 are unprotected, 12 go elsewhere, 4 go on the partner's body and 37 go into the partner's anus. The actual level of high-risk behaviour revealed is disturbingly high since over one-third of the acts of anal intercourse are in the highest risk category of all. High-risk sexual behaviour thus appears in this analysis to be much more prevalent than normally reported in studies of gay men, possibly because high-risk behaviour is concentrated in particular individuals. In the next section we shall therefore enquire whether there is significant variation among particular *types* of gay man.

*Condom-use* also presents a disturbing picture. It is well-known that condom use is far from universal among gay men who practice anal intercourse. But the figures in Table 8.1 derived here from their diary accounts shows that if ejaculation occurs in anal intercourse, a condom is used in *less than a quarter of the instances*. Moreover, protected ejaculation (into a condom) occurs only half as frequently as the most high-risk behaviour of unprotected ejaculation.

Have these fractions changed over the four annual waves represented here? Table 8.2 presents the relevant information. The percentage of protected acts of

| Anal Intercourse Ejaculate: | WAVE 1 | WAVE 2 | WAVE 3 | WAVE 4 |
|------------------------------|--------|--------|--------|--------|
| Condom [C] | 20 | 13 | 18 | 21 |
| Unprotected [H,M] | 33 | 33 | 36 | 37 |
| Ratio: [C]/[H,M] | 0.61 | 0.39 | 0.50 | 0.56 |

*Table 8.2: Percentage of acts where anal intercourse involves a condom [C] or is unprotected [H and M] by wave.*

anal intercourse (i.e., where a condom is used) actually drops by a third in the second wave (a phenomenon noticed elsewhere), and only climbs back up again over the next two; the fraction of unprotected acts of anal intercourse[25] actually increases over this period. The ratio of protected to unprotected acts was highest in the initial wave (1987), fell dramatically in the second wave and although increasing subsequently has not yet reached the initial level.

### *The Effect of Age and Relationship on the Volume of High-Risk Activity*

Having found this variation, how is it to be explained? Power and sex-role almost certainly have a part to play (Coxon and Coxon, 1993a), and knowing that receptive anal intercourse is the more risky would normally lead us to differentiating active and passive modalities of anal intercourse in the analysis before going any further. But instead, in the space available, it may be more profitable to see how unprotected anal intercourse varies by the two factors that we have found to be repeatedly the most potent in explaining variation in gay men's sexual behaviour — age and relationship-type (Coxon, 1987). Because these factors are themselves associated, it will be best to take their combined effect on the unprotected anal intercourse.

The nine-fold SIGMA typology of three age-groups by three relationship types is now used to look at the percentage of acts of unprotected anal intercourse within the nine cells. This is presented graphically in Figure 8.2 with Table 8.3.

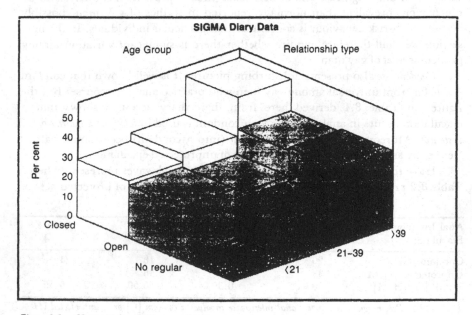

*Figure 8.3: Unprotected anal intercourse by type.*

| Relation↓ Age→ | Less than 21 | 21–39 | Over 39 |
|---|---|---|---|
| Closed Relation | 30.1 | 34.7 | 55.1 |
| Open | 27.8 | 24.5 | 38.2 |
| No Regular | 0.5 | 22.0 | 40.0 |

*Table 8.3: Percentage of unprotected acts of anal intercourse, by age and relationship type.*

There is clearly a very substantial amount of variation in these rates of unprotected anal intercourse. High-risk activity is positively related to age (the older groups have increasingly higher rates). Relationship also has a systematic effect: highest-risk anal intercourse is highest in closed relationships, slightly lower in open relationships, but considerably lower among those who have no regular relationship. This conforms well to findings from the panel-based data of the project (Weatherburn *et al.*, 1991; Hunt *et al.*, 1993), where issues of intimacy and trust rather than recidivism or relapse (Davies, 1992, 1993) are shown to explain such differences. Nonetheless, it is important to have some idea of whether age or relationship is the greater influence, and where the most important combinations occur. From the start of diary analysis (Coxon, 1987) we have used a resistant method of analysis to answer this question: means analysis with a median polish (Mosteller and Tukey, 1977: 165–202).

The analysis is a simple additive model: the table entries are the sum of the overall average (typical value TYP, here 27.8 per cent) plus the row (relationship) effect, plus the column (age-group) effect plus the combination/interaction/residual effect. In terms of main effects, age-group has a greater effect than relationship type, but this is primarily due to the older group (having an effect almost two-thirds the size of the overall effect). Being in closed relationships have the highest and positive effect. The most striking thing about the combination-effects is that the youngest age group who are not in a regular relationship have a remarkably lower rate — again, almost two-thirds the size of the overall effect. In brief, there are major variations in the rates of unprotected sex among these types of gay men; being older men (40 and over) and (to a lesser extent) in a closed relationship increases the rate of high-risk sex, and having no regular relationship and being young (under 21) serves to decrease the rate. Over and above this, young men with no regular relationship have a considerably lower rate than would be expected.

| Relation↓ Age→ | Under 21 | 21–39 | Over 39 | Row Effects |
|---|---|---|---|---|
| Closed Relation | 0 | 0 | 2.4 | 6.9 |
| Open | 7.9 | 0 | – 4.3 | – 3.3 |
| No Regular | – 16.9 | 0 | 0 | – 5.8 |
| Column effects: | – 4.6 | 0 | 18 | TYP = 27.8 |
| | | | | Per cent |

*Table 8.4: Median polish of percentage of unprotected acts of anal intercourse, by age and relationship.*

On this analysis of the sexual diary data, then, the youngest age group who are in no regular relationship have a very markedly lower rate of unprotected high-risk sex than any other. This is an encouraging (if not entirely unproblematic[26]) finding, and accords with other trends documented by SIGMA (Davies *et al*, 1992): young gay men conform far more to safer sex guidelines than any other group.

## Conclusions

The diary method provides an excellent tool for the study of sexual behaviour, yielding fascinating detailed and often unique information. If combined with an explicit theory or schema of sexual behaviour, comparison with other methods is straightforward. However, it is undoubtedly a demanding method (on both respondents and analysts) even if analysis is aided by recently-available software. Validity studies suggest that while aggregate data correlate extremely well with those derived from other methods there is an undoubted selection bias in those who agree to keep such diaries.

The most striking substantive conclusion is that there is a remarkable amount of highest-risk activity (unprotected anal intercourse to ejaculation) among gay men — far more than would be suspected from individual-based analyses. This highest-risk activity is concentrated in older gay men and is markedly under-represented in young gay men who have no regular relationship. It would have been impossible or totally unfeasible to use questionnaire or interview methods to obtain this striking result.

### Notes

1   This rather ugly clause is more accurate than homosexual or gay, which imply restriction to this orientation, or identification with it. In the rest of the chapter gay will be used to denote behaviourally homosexual males.

2   The presence of a third person (here the social scientist) would render homosexual activity illegal under the 1967 Sexual Offences Act as being no longer a private activity. Scottish law does not contain this restriction.

3   Project SIGMA (*Socio-sexual Investigations of Gay Men and Aids*). The research in this article was funded by the Medical Research Council and by the Department of Health (UK). Work on Sexual Diary software and on the validity and reliability of the sexual diary method reported here is funded under a series of grants from the Department of Health. The views expressed in this article are those of the author and not necessarily those of the Council or of the Department.

4   We have been able to show that it is selection bias toward those with busier sex lives rather than exaggeration of activity that is primarily producing bias.

5   The male pronoun is used descriptively throughout this chapter as we are referring exclusively to gay men.

6   As a rule of thumb, this is usually less than a three-day period for detailed accounts

of sexually active men. Particular, rare or risky behaviour can often be recalled for a longer time, but even here the contextual information and surrounding sexual activity is poorly recalled (see Brewer, 1988; Neisser and Winograd, 1988).

7    The ethical undertaking given by the Project was that the name of someone identified in an interview would not be part of a Project record. This was undoubtedly important in maximizing response and trust initially, but prevented any record linkage and severely limited network analysis. The ethical issue is discussed in Coxon *et al.*, 1993c, and the practical network issues in Coxon and Joyce, 1993.

8    But also because they could have such an effect: condoms can act as a barrier (and are anyway encoded into the outcome information), lubricants can increase the probability if not water-based and may decrease it if containing Nonoxynol-9; toys such as dildoes, if shared may potentially transmit the HI virus.

9    This distinction is in common use in the gay community. It is not to be confused with the inserter/ee distinction often used in this context. Many (indeed most) sexual acts are not penetrative.

10    See Coxon *et al.*, 1992b for a fuller specification and treatment.

11    Orgasm and Ejaculation are used interchangeably, though it is recognized that they are not necessarily equivalent.

12    The entries in square brackets are instances taken from the appropriate list. The letters in the behaviour list are the first letter of the street term of the behaviour, e.g., *Wanking, Sucking . . .*

13    We had to include a new modality 'H' to deal with situations where alter did something sexual by himself, which could still have relevance to HIV transmission. An example is where he masturbates himself but ejaculates on his partner.

14    The most common activity is solitary masturbation to ejaculation/orgasm. This is now well-known in the gay community by its SIGMA code of 'SWO'.

15    Everything but the sexual session data has been removed — time, place, partner, etc.

16    Using either dBase or CARDBOX-Plus software. Selection using boolean operators is done within the database and then exported as ASCII or Basic (comma-delimited) format to specially designed or commercial software.

17    In order to derive information on partner mixing for the Imperial College group of epidemiological modellers (Anderson, 1986) an estimate of the number of partners of partners was needed. The network procedures used to do this on a Diary dataset are described in Coxon and Joyce, 1993.

18    The Programs and data are available at cost from the author.

19    This sub-project on reliability and validity is funded by the Department of Health.

20    The incentive consisted of donating £2 to the Terrence Higgins Trust on their behalf on return of a completed estimate sheet.

21    The same rules are presented in the instructions to diary keepers (SIGMA, 1993). Originally respondents were invited to encode some or all of their data but this is now discouraged except for very common events such as solo masturbation.

22    SIGMA uses the 7-point gradation: Always / Almost always / More than half the time / Half the time / Less than half the time / Very seldom / Never.

23    The direction of distortion can be upwards or downwards, though it is more likely to be downwards. Upward distortion is a kind of Don Juan effect: boasting about one's sexual prowess, and downward distortion usually arises because anal intercourse is known to be most risky and subject to disapproval by health education authorities.

24    It is important to stress that this is a contextual and *not* an individual property. Some individuals will always engage in one of the two types of session or always adopt an active or passive role, but these are in a minority. Most gay men shift modality in different settings or with different partners or even within the same session.

25  Throughout this and following sections of the chapter the phrase 'unprotected anal intercourse' means unprotected anal intercourse *to ejaculation*.
26  This group is relatively small in size (51/569); spread across 4 waves it is difficult to see a stable trend. Selection bias could account for some of the unexpected very low value, but not the relative amount.

## References

ANDERSON, R.M., MEDLEY, G.F., MAY, R.M. and JOHNSON, A.M. (1986) 'A preliminary study of the transmission dynamics of the human immuno-deficiency virus (HIV), the causative agent of Aids', IMA *Journal of Mathematics Applied in Medicine and Biology*, 3, pp. 229–63.

BREWER, W.F. (1988) 'Memory for randomly sampled autobiographical events', in NEISSER, U. and WINOGRAD, E., pp. 21–90.

CAMPBELL, D.T., and STANLEY, J.C. (1963) *Experimental and Quasi-Experimental Designs for Research*, Chicago, IL: Rand McNally.

CONRATH, D.W., HIGGINS, C.A. MCLEAN, R.J. (1983) 'A comparison of the reliability of questionnaire versus diary data', *Social Networks* 5, 3, pp. 315–21.

COXON, A.P.M. (1987) 'The effect of age and relationship on gay men's sexual behaviour: A preliminary analysis of sexual diary data', Cardiff: SRU Working Paper (ISBN 0 948 935 06 5); reproduced in amended form in SIGMA (1990).

COXON, A.P.M. (1988a) 'Something sensational . . .' The sexual diary as a tool for mapping detailed sexual behaviour', *Sociological Review*, 36, 2, pp. 353–67.

COXON, A.P.M. (1988b) 'The numbers game: Gay lifestyles, epidemiology of AIDS and social science. In AGGLETON, P. and HOMANS, H. (Eds), *Social Aspects of AIDS*, Lewes: Falmer Press.

COXON, A.P.M. and COXON, N.H., WEATHERBURN, P., HUNT, A.J., HICKSON, F.C.I., DAVIES, P.M. and MCMANUS, T.J. (1993a) 'Sex role separation in sexual diaries of homosexual men', *Aids*, 7, 6, pp. 877–82.

COXON, A.P.M. and COXON, N.H. (1993b) 'Risk in context: The use of sexual diary data to analyse sequences of homosexual risk behaviour', in TEM BRUMMELHUIS, H. and HERDT, G. (Eds) *Culture and Sexual Risk: Anthropological Perspectives on Aids*, New York: Gordon Breach (Preliminary version: SIGMA WP38 Working Paper 38).

COXON, A.P.M. and JOYCE, C. (1994) 'Networks and nemesis: Social networks as method and substance in researching gay men's response to HIV/Aids, to appear in PARKER, R. and GAGNON, J. (Ed.) *Conceiving Sexuality: Approaches to Sex Research in a Post-Modern World*, London: Routledge. (Preliminary version: SIGMA Working Paper 37).

COXON, A.P.M., WEATHERBURN, P., HUNT, A.J. and DAVIES, P.M. (1992b) 'The structure of sexual behaviour', *Journal of Sexual Research*, 29, 1, pp. 61–83.

COXON, A.P.M., DAVIES, P.M., HICKSON, F.C.I., HUNT, A., MCMANUS, T.J., REES, C.M. and WEATHERBURN, P. (1993c) 'Strategies in eliciting sensitive sexual information: The case of gay men', *Sociological Review*, 41, 3, pp. 537–55.

DAVIES, P.M. and COXON, A.P.M. (1990) 'Patterns in homosexual behaviour: Use of the diary method, in HUBERT, M. (Ed.) *Sexual Behaviour and Risks of HIV Infection*, Brussels: Facultés Universitaires Saint Louis.

DAVIES, P.M., WEATHERBURN, P., HUNT, A.J., HICKSON, F.C.I., MCMANUS, T.J. and COXON, A.P.M. (1992) 'Young gay men in England and Wales: Sexual behaviour and implications for the spread of HIV', *AIDS Care*, 4, 3, pp. 259–72.

DAVIES, P.M. (1993) 'Safer sex maintenance among gay men: Are we moving in the right direction?', *AIDS*, 7, pp. 279–80.

HUNT, A., WEATHERBURN, P., HICKSON, F.C.I., DAVIES, P.M., McMANUS, T.J. and COXON, A.P.M. (1993) 'Changes in condom use by gay men', *AIDS Care* (in press).

JAMES, N.J., BIGNELL, C.J. and GILLIES, P.A. (1991) 'The reliability of self-reported sexual behaviour', *AIDS*, 5, 3, pp. 333–5.

JANSON, C.G. (1990) 'Retrospective data, undesirable behaviour and the longitudinal perspective', in MAGNUSSON, D. and BERGMAN, L.R. (Eds) *Data Quality in Longitudinal Research*, Cambridge: University Press.

LAHR, J. (Ed.) (1986) *The Orton Diaries*, London: Methuen.

LINTON, M. (1986) 'Ways of searching and the contents of memory', in RUBIN, (Ed.) *Autobiographical Memory*, Cambridge: University Press, pp. 50–67.

McLAWS, M.L., OLDENBURG, B., ROSS, M.W. and COOPER, D.A. (1990) 'Sexual behaviour in AIDS related research: Reliability and validity of recall and diary measures', *Journal of Sex Research*, 27, 2, pp. 265–81.

MASTERS, W. and JOHNSON, V. (1966) *Human Sexual Response*, Boston: Little Brown.

MOSTELLER, F. and TUKEY, J.W. (1977) *Data Analysis and Regression*, Reading, MA: Addison-Wesley.

NEISSER, U. and WINOGRAD, E. (Eds) (1988) *Remembering Reconsidered: Ecological and Traditional Approaches to the Study of Memory*, Cambridge: University Press.

PLUMMER, K. (1983) *Documents of Life*, London: Allen and Unwin.

ROSENTHAL, R. and ROSNOW, R.L. (1975) *The Volunteer Subject*, New York: Wiley.

RUBIN, D.C. (Ed.) (1986) *Autobiographical Memory*, Cambridge: University Press.

SANKOFF, D. and KRUSKAL, J.B. (Eds) (1983) *Time Warps, String Edits and Macromolecules: The Theory and Practice of Sequence Comparison*, Reading, MA: Addison-Wesley.

SIGMA (1990) *Longitudinal Study of the Sexual Behaviour of Homosexual Males under the Impact of AIDS*, Final Report to Department of Health, Project SIGMA.

SIGMA (1993) 'Notes on keeping a sexual diary', Colchester, Project SIGMA.

WEATHERBURN, P., DAVIES, P.M., HICKSON, F.C., HUNT, A.J., COXON, A.P.M. and McMANUS, T.J. (1993) 'No connection between alcohol use and unsafe sex among gay and bisexual men', *AIDS*, 7, 1, pp. 115–19.

## Appendix 1: Example: sigma sexual diary form

ID Number: _____ /_____ /5
WEEK BEGINNING: _____ 3/MAY _____ /1992 ____
                           (day)      (month)            (year)

*Remember, each session should include:*

- The Time, the Place, the Partners (from partner list).
- Then, the session in your own words.
- If you 'come' (ejaculate) in the session, remember to be explicit about where it goes and *always* to record the use of condoms.
- List any accompaniments you use (poppers, lubricants, drugs, sex toys...)

| | |
|---|---|
| Sunday<br><br>_____DAY | 9am. My flat, P1.<br>We deep kissed, and moved into a '69'. Whilst doing it I began to finger him. Then he wanked me (both using poppers) and I came. Following that I wanked him till he came. |
| Monday<br>_____DAY<br>4th | 12.30pm. Lunch-time wank at work; I didn't come. |
| Tuesday<br>_____DAY<br>5th | |
| Wednesday<br>_____DAY<br>6th | 11.30pm. Hampstead Heath, P2.<br>We wanked each other off; both came.<br><br>12.15am. (Thurs), P3.<br>I sucked him, then he put on a condom and fucked me; he came. |
| Thursday<br>_____DAY<br>7th | (see above: Wed). |
| Friday<br>_____DAY<br>8th | 8.30. Reading porn: quick wank to orgasm.<br><br>11.00pm. P1's flat.<br>After eve at The Bell (4 pints), I sucked P2, then he fucked me and came (no condom). |
| Saturday<br>_____DAY<br>9th | 7.30am.<br>I woke up to find P1 wanking me. Then he sucked me off, and I came in his mouth. We began using poppers and I sucked him, carrying on to fuck him (with condom), whilst he wanked himself. He came, I didn't. |

Chapter 9

# Social Science Methods used in a Study of Prostitutes in the Gambia

*Helen Pickering*

The need for field techniques to provide rapid and detailed data on complex social and behavioural phenomena has been given considerable impetus with the advent of HIV/AIDS. It has highlighted the contrasting approaches of epidemiology and the social sciences. Traditionally, epidemiologists study a limited number of variables in large samples to provide statistical evidence of relationships. The parameters of the study are firmly established before data collection begins. But interest has grown in aspects of the relationship between health and behaviour not amenable to so strict a format of scientific investigation. Anthropologists, in particular, have cultivated the opposite end of the methodological spectrum, looking in great detail at small groups over long periods of time. The anthropologist might start work with no hypothesis as such — only an area of interest and the theoretical constructs of anthropological theory. A study of a group's cultural concepts of sickness and health, for instance, could well provide descriptive knowledge of great depth and detail, highly relevant to the health issues of that particular people. Such findings are likely to be of limited generalizability, however, and to rely on data-gathering skills irreducible to repetitive structured techniques. The social and demographic characteristics and the mortality an morbidity of large populations, typically the concern of epidemiology, are beyond the scope of classic anthropological work.

The objectives of the study of prostitution in The Gambia discussed in this chapter were broadly epidemiological, but in the course of reviewing some of the problems that arose I aim to show that social research into HIV/AIDS and other health problems most usefully steers a course between the two methodological extremes. I hope to illustrate in particular the danger of relying, as many epidemiological studies do, almost entirely on findings from questionnaire-based survey data.

### Context

The Gambian AIDS and Prostitution study looked at the social backgrounds, working patterns and economic activities of female prostitutes within the context of broader clinical and epidemiological investigations of the spread and natural history of HIV-2 infection conducted by the Medical Research Council (MRC) unit in The Gambia, West Africa. It had earlier been established that prostitutes showed a much higher rate of infection with both HIV-1 and HIV-2 than the population as a whole (30.7 per cent against 1.7 per cent) and therefore almost certainly held the potential to contribute disproportionately to the further transmission of these viruses (Pepin *et al.*, 1991; Wilkins *et al.*, 1991).

The original research design envisaged a detailed study of four bars in two urban locations in The Gambia over a fourteen-month period. All individuals living and working in the bars and as many customers as was feasible would be included, and their interactions studied. It quickly became apparent that few women stayed in any one bar for more than a few days or weeks at any one time. An earlier notion that the bars could be treated as 'villages', each with a fairly stable population, had to be dropped. The investigation was broadened to include other locations and bars, and to focus on the individual women, recruited in the bars under study, their mobility and social networks.

The broadened scope of the study inevitably increased demands on fieldworkers. The anthropologist traditionally draws assistance from the population he or she studies. The epidemiologist sends out a team of fieldworkers with questionnaires to administer. The former cultivates relationships with informants from within the group being studied, but the latter relies on intermediaries. The two local fieldworkers employed full-time in the present study were both experienced data collectors, one of whom knew something of the world of bars and prostitutes. As the study progressed, both became closely involved with the study participants and soon functioned as 'brokers', interpreting and discussing what they observed and heard with the principal investigator, who had limited knowledge of the local languages.

Quantitative data was gathered first by means of a questionnaire administered to each of the 248 women who worked in the main bars studied at any time during the investigation, and second by daily records kept by fieldworkers in a prepared format of each woman's sexual activity and her movements around the region. Data on incomes and expenditure was obtained from sixteen of the less mobile prostitutes. Questionnaire data was also obtained from 795 men immediately after their contact with a prostitute. This provided basic demographic data on clients, and enabled some assessment of the accuracy of prostitutes' diaries to be made by asking the men details of the sexual contact they had just completed.

Both the diary and client data were collected almost daily in the bars, providing the research team with a context in which to sit around observing behaviour, to hold in-depth interviews and to challenge statements obviously at odds with what had been observed. This continual contact allowed the research team to get to know the women well and to be invited to accompany them on visits home and other expeditions. Both fieldworkers and the principal investigator developed a good rapport with the prostitutes and the men who worked or hung around the bars. Regular observation gave the researchers confidence in the accuracy of the diary data, as well as providing qualitative information that proved crucial to the development of the study.

The Gambia is a predominantly Islamic country in which few people drink alcohol. Prostitution is associated with a low-life scene centred on bars. This made it relatively easy to identify prostitutes and to study their behaviour in different parts of the country. The use of the term 'prostitute' in an African context has been challenged. It has been argued that many non-marital sexual relationships in Africa have an element of commercial exchange, and that a term such as 'free woman' would be more appropriate. But the women enrolled in the Gambian study formed a group with distinct sexual practices conforming in every respect to the customary model of prostitution. They described themselves as 'prostitutée' (most spoke some French). They did not discriminate among potential clients; they accepted any man willing to pay an agreed price, and confined the relationship to a brief sexual encounter. The majority practised from the generally recognized 'red-light' bars. They worked independently, with virtually no pimping or other exploitation beyond high rental charges for rooms in the bars. Many came from Senegal where prostitutes were required at the time to register with the police and undergo medical inspections every two weeks. Condoms are available from Senegalese clinics and nearly all women working in The Gambia were familiar with their use. A detailed description of the women participating in the study is available elsewhere (Pickering *et al.*, 1992).

Prostitution is illegal in The Gambia itself but that did not prove a significant problem in the research process. The Medical Research Council has been conducting research and providing medical facilities at a number of sites in The Gambia for over forty years. The reputation it enjoys gives MRC researchers easy access even to marginalized groups such as prostitutes. The women enrolled in the study valued both the medical services offered, and the prestige of being involved in an MRC study. Many aspects of this study would not have been feasible without the very considerable advantages of the MRC's unique long-term position in The Gambia.

### Prostitute questionnaires

On her first appearance in one of the bars being monitored, and on agreeing to join the study, each prostitute was interviewed using a prepared questionnaire covering basic demographic variables, family history, marriage history, future ambitions and information on sexual behaviour with clients and boyfriends. Subsequent information largely confirmed the demographic data thus obtained but threw a good deal of doubt on answers to other questions. The questionnaires, basic demography aside, turned out to be more useful in showing how prostitutes wished to be seen, what stories they wanted to tell of their lives, than in providing raw material for statistical analysis.

The questions to which women later proved, usually on their own admission, to have given inaccurate answers included matters such as their experience of abortion and use of drugs. Other questions, such as the use of sexual stimulants and lubricants, caused fieldworkers embarrassment and were often left blank. Local stimulants could have been abrasive, causing scratches or areas of inflammation which might have facilitated HIV transmission. Information on stimulants was obtained through discussion, as well as through visits to local markets with key informants, who would point out the different substances available and describe their effects.

A number of other questions, concerning regular but variable activities, proved difficult for respondents to answer accurately. They included one quite crucial question, asked in almost every study of HIV transmission and prostitution, 'How many clients per day?' This is rather like asking, 'How many cups of tea do you drink a day?' Only a respondent with a relatively fixed routine, would be in a position to offer a dependable reply. The women frequently guessed, or gave the number they happened to have had last night. They did not take into account days on which they did not work, which made a great difference to the average figure. According to the questionnaires, prostitutes had an average of 3.8 clients per night, with a range from 1 to 12. Data from the sexual activity diaries, however, showed the figure to be 1.6, with a range from 0 to 25. The diaries also showed that prostitutes might get a lot of work at one bar for a while, then move somewhere else and get very little, or vice versa. Such variations were not reflected in the questionnaire replies.

Similarly, questionnaire responses to the prices prostitutes charged were unlikely to have been accurate. In their replies many women gave the price they would like to charge, usually a figure slightly above the more or less generally agreed price at the bar in which they were currently working. The results were distorted not only by the difficulty of remembering but by the status the prostitutes attached to the ability to attract high prices. Overall, the sexual contact diaries recorded lower prices. Furthermore, each woman charged less or more according to her present location. She might halve her price when she moved away from the Gambian coastal area to a rural market town, or double it when working in Senegal or at an international hotel. Questionnaire data on prices failed to record the variations that emerged when the same women were asked similar questions in different locations (Pickering *et al.*, 1993).

The difficulties with the questionnaire data on number of clients and prices charged were picked up by the sexual contact diaries and client surveys, discussed below. The misleading responses of the women to questions concerning their personal circumstances and their reasons for starting prostitution would probably have gone unchallenged without the research team's prolonged acquaintance with the prostitutes. Many of the women became true informants rather than the subjects of a social survey. On first being enrolled in the study, the vast majority gave sad stories. They were orphans, or had old, blind or crippled parents to support and dependent siblings. Older women related histories of divorce or the sudden death of husbands leaving them with no support and young children to care for. With few exceptions these accounts were subsequently discovered to be untrue. One middle-aged woman told a particularly moving, tragic tale that on further enquiry was found to have no relation at all to her own life; it had been lifted straight from a film recently shown in the vicinity. Another girl told of being desperately poor, with her father dead and her mother crippled. Yet she wore quite expensive clothes and jewellery; a few weeks later she happened to mention that her father drove a Mercedes. A subsequent trip with her to her home in Senegal confirmed that she came from a comparatively wealthy family, that was unaware of her occupation. Such examples demonstrate the danger of relying on data from questionnaires not followed up by observation and acquaintance with the subjects concerned.

### Sexual contact diaries

After enrolment in the study, each woman was contacted four or five times a week while she remained at the bar and again whenever she reappeared there or at another location being studied. A prepared form was used to record on a daily basis her place of work and details of every sexual contact, including the price charged, whether a condom was used, the type of relationship (a boyfriend, casual or regular client), whether the man stayed all night and how many contacts he had during the night. This data collection was done mainly by the two local fieldworkers. Few of the prostitutes were sufficiently literate to complete the forms themselves. The very high mobility of prostitutes in The Gambia meant that there were, on average, only 87 women working in the study bars at any one time.

The sexual contact diaries produced a substantial database, covering nearly 15,000 woman-days and over 26,000 sexual contacts, from which variables such as rates of condom use, numbers of clients and prices could be calculated. Some of this data overlapped with that derived from the questionnaires first administered to the women. Diary data was preferred on several grounds. Deliberate daily falsification of diary reports would have been difficult to sustain, particularly when the person collecting the data had opportunities for observing behaviour and querying answers which appear to be untrue. The number of clients women reported was generally confirmed both by observation, and by peer agreement. Only events of the night before had to be remembered, and the women were not asked for their impression of what an average figure might be. Sometimes women who had been drunk forgot how many clients they had had the previous night, but they were often prompted by their co-workers, and usually at least remembered how much money they had made. In most bars a standard price per contact was agreed among the women; a minimum number of contacts could usually be worked out (some clients may have paid a lower price and boyfriends would not have paid at all, but relatively few clients paid more than the agreed price). Whether the man was a client or boyfriend and the length of the man's stay (possibly all night, involving more than one contact) did not appear to lead to discrepancies.

Interviews with clients, as we shall see below, provided a check on two areas of diary data — condom use and prices charged. It was ethically required of the research team that they simultaneously distribute and encourage the use of condoms. A sense among the prostitutes that they ought always to have been using them may have led to some over-reporting of condom use, but reported variations in use by individual women, over festivals, in different locations and when there were shortages in the country, together with the client surveys, suggested the contact diary data was reasonably accurate. Condoms were always in demand and not seen to be disposed of in other circumstances than immediately after a sexual contact. Observation suggested that almost all women normally made some attempt to use a condom with most of their clients, though perhaps not many insisted on a condom every time. When challenged on observed instances of a discrepancy between her report and that of a client on condom use, some women stated they were able to put a condom on clients without their knowledge. Women who were often drunk appeared to be least diligent in condom use.

Diary data was less reliable in the case of prices charged, a subject on which it emerged that for peer group reasons prostitutes could be highly defensive. In most bars a minimum price was agreed; women were free to charge higher prices but not to undercut each other. Women who were discovered to have been accepting lower prices were ostracized or even driven out of the bar. No prostitute working in a bar ever admitted accepting a lower price than the agreed standard. A third of the clients, however, reported that they paid up to 50 per cent less than the standard price. Local men with whom this matter was discussed disagreed with the research team's interpretation of the discrepancies, believing that while a client would not mind people knowing he had visited a prostitute, he might well be embarrassed by how much of the family budget he had just spent, and therefore tended to understate the price paid.

The diaries provided useful data on prostitutes' patterns of work. They showed that on average women worked only two days out of three and that there was a certain amount of seasonal variation. The number of clients increased significantly over festivals and during the dry season, when many men are away from home trading. The detailed information from the diaries combined with observation showed that over festivals when the numbers of contacts increased condom use decreased. At the same time alcohol consumption rose, fights sometimes broke out and the atmosphere in the bars became rather tense.

### Economic Monitoring

Sixteen prostitutes who were relatively stable or regular in their patterns of movement and thirty-one age-matched non-prostitute divorced or widowed women were asked to participate in daily monitoring of all their monetary transactions over a four-week period. Thus each day all income (from whatever source) was recorded together with details of every expenditure.

This part of the study was useful in building up a picture of the lives and economic standing of some of the women and of the choices they made. Eighty-eight per cent of prostitutes' income came from prostitution, 11 per cent from other work and the remainder from loans or theft. The other work included hairdressing, petty trading and drug dealing. Many were earning considerably higher sums than middle-rank civil servants and could easily have satisfied their commonly expressed ambition of setting themselves up in some kind of business if they had truly wished to do so. Most of the non-prostitute divorced and married women were supporting themselves by trading, cooking and selling food, sewing, or other of the many earning opportunities open to women in the informal sector (Pickering *et al.*, 1993).

Economic monitoring cast further doubt on another claim — that the women had turned to prostitution only as a last resort in order to support their families. Most of the prostitutes had children, but contributed on average no more than one per cent of their income to their support. Almost all children over the age of two were being cared for by the prostitute's family. Their comparatively high earnings went on high rents in the bars, travel, clothes, cosmetics, alcohol and cigarettes. Very few women ever admitted to having any money available. This appeared to be true in many cases; when cash was plentiful it was spent or given away very liberally; when it was scarce most women knew that they could earn sufficient in a night to cover whatever needs they had.

### Client Surveys

We obtained basic information on the clients of prostitutes, a group at high risk of HIV infection. Clients were approached immediately after their contact with a prostitute, asked to answer a very short questionnaire and to supply a saliva sample for HIV testing.

Interviewing clients meant sitting outside the prostitutes' rooms at night waiting for their customers to emerge, a difficult, labour-intensive exercise. At various times in the course of the study four additional fieldworkers were employed to help with the collection of this data. The areas by the rooms were dark and often full of rubble; clients were rarely talkative and sometimes drunk. All the fieldworkers, but in particular the males, were reluctant to approach clients under these circumstances and would only do so when the principal investigator was present. Sexual contact between clients and prostitutes was always straightforwardly vaginal and conducted in a perfunctory manner with the minimum of conversation. Most encounters lasted less than ten minutes from negotiation to departure.

For a while it proved difficult at some of the bars to persuade any of the men to talk to us. It quickly emerged that the prostitutes were telling their clients not to co-operate. They did not like us asking the men how much they had paid; they were afraid that instances of undercharging would become known. The problem was overcome, partly by asking the prostitutes to participate in this survey by collecting saliva samples from their clients and partly by prostitutes becoming confident of our discretion.

A number of men were suspicious of the salivettes used for collecting saliva; some were afraid there was a drug in the cotton wool, others feared they could be identified through the test. We collected saliva samples from a smaller number of men than we did answers to the client questionnaire.

The questionnaires administered to clients were anonymous. We were unable to check the accuracy of the answers. The demographic questions covered only basic factors such as age, occupation and place of residence; replies are not likely to have been deliberately falsified. It was noticed when the questionnaire was being piloted that questions on history of sexually-transmitted diseases and on number of sexual partners in the last four weeks were sometimes resented. It was felt that responses were unlikely to be accurate and the questions were dropped. The second half of the questionnaire, concerning details of the sexual encounter they had just had, could be compared with the prostitute's report in her daily diary. Discrepancies between prostitutes' and clients' reports on the price charged were more frequent than on the use of condoms.

## Discussion

The prostitute and client questionnaires, the sexual contact diaries and economic monitoring produced a great deal of data amenable to statistical analysis — a social and demographic profile of prostitutes and clients, patterns of work, rest and mobility, numbers of clients, earnings and expenditure, rates of condom use and contacts with boyfriends (a group of particular importance in the transmission of the HIV viruses). We have seen that these sources of data served to check and qualify each other. The diaries, for instance, showed data from the initial questionnaire survey of prostitutes to be inadequate in many respects. Diaries corrected misleading questionnaire replies on the number of clients, a vital epidemiological factor, and recorded wide variations in individual sexual activity over time and the high mobility of prostitutes, significant points that would have been missed in a questionnaire survey alone. In turn, the client survey questioned prostitutes' diary claims, to some extent, regarding condom use and prices charged. Economic monitoring cast new and interesting light on prostitutes' responses to questions concerning their financial situation and motives.

But these broadly epidemiological methods were themselves called into question at several crucial points and modified by information accumulated in the course of prolonged day-by-day observation and discussion with prostitutes, bar owners, boyfriends and clients. Anthropological looking and asking did more than merely provide additional, non-quantifiable impressions: it proved crucial to the success of the epidemiology. The prostitutes themselves later treated as a great joke our initial acceptance of their tragic accounts of the circumstances that had driven them to prostitution. Yet many studies of prostitution take such replies to questionnaires at face value. It was joining prostitutes on visits home and observing the relatively easy circumstances of many of their families that suggested the value of economic monitoring. Comparing prostitutes and non-prostitute single women showed clearly that women continued in prostitution not by necessity but as a choice among several possible ways of maintaining their freedom of movement and independence. Prostitutes generally present the opposite picture; questionnaire surveys too often merely report their replies as fact. Policy implications follow: a programme to offer prostitutes alternative livelihood strategies would need to look at why they do not avail themselves of those already available.

Observation of the prostitutes and their milieu allowed other significant developments in the course of the research work. If the study parameters had been fixed in advance and data collection carried out in a standardized manner by largely unsupervised field staff, the unexpectedly high mobility of prostitutes, while not perhaps going unnoticed, would certainly have reduced the usefulness of the data obtained. Discovering that prostitutes were doing the rounds of weekly village markets opened an entirely unsuspected area of investigation and potential intervention.

No hard and fast rules on the integration of epidemiological and anthropological methods can be laid down, though one rule of thumb may be suggested. When fieldworkers operate at the end of a chain of command and merely hand in results, report a few superficial problems, and reserve their impressions and gossip for each others' ears, the investigator has lost control. The same goes for social surveys delegated, for instance, to clinic staff. The investigator must be a constant presence at the point of investigation. He or she should be in a position to detect factors which may be distorting respondents' replies to questionnaires. In the present study the prostitutes had motives that sometimes helped, sometimes hindered the research. They feared the client survey would show they had been undercutting an agreed price and tried to stop the men talking to us. They were very willing, on the other hand, to have us visit their homes — they could then explain to their families that their high incomes came from working for an expatriate. It is always said that questionnaires dealing with sensitive subjects need to be carefully prepared and administered. We should be ready at every stage to be surprised by the pattern of interests and assumptions that unfold in the course of a respondent's replies.

### References

PEPIN, J., MORGAN, G., DUNN, D., GEVAO, S., MENDY, M., GAYE, I., SCOLLEN, N., TEDDER, R. and WHITTLE, H. (1991) 'HIV-induced immunosuppression among asymptomatic West African prostitutes: Evidence that HIV-2 is pathogenic, but less so than HIV-1', *AIDS*, 5, pp. 1165-72.

PICKERING, H., TODD, J., DUNN, D., PEPIN, J. and WILKINS A. (1992) 'Prostitutes and their Clients: a Gambian Survey', *Social Science and Medicine*, 34, 1, pp. 75-88.

PICKERING, H. and WILKINS, A. (1993) 'Do unmarried women in African towns have to sell sex, or is it a matter of choice?' (1993) *Health Transition Review* 3, supplementary issue on sexual networking and HIV/AIDS in West Africa, pp. 17-28.

PICKERING, H., QUIGLEY, M., HAYES, R., TODD, R. and WILKINS, A. (1993) 'Determinants of condom use in 24,000 prostitute/client contacts in The Gambia', *AIDS*, 7, pp. 1093-8.

WILKINS, A., HAYES, R., ALONSON, P., BALDEH, S., BERRY, N., CHAM, K., HUGHES JAITEH, K., OELMAN, B., TEDDER, R. and WHITTLE, H. (1991) 'Risk factors for HIV-2 infection in The Gambia', *AIDS*, 5, pp. 1127-32.

*Chapter 10*

---

# Focus Groups: Method or Madness?

---

*Jenny Kitzinger*

Focus groups: — method or madness?[1] I chose that sub-title because it reflected some of my feelings when faced with analysing transcripts of 52 group discussions. Here was a record of over 300 people's conversations about AIDS, almost 2000 pages of people arguing, brain-storming, making faces at each other, sharing jokes, telling stories, and deviating from the point.

It is not the kind of data that are easy to quantify or even to classify. Statements are often incomplete: people's sentences tail off into silence or their friends finish what they are saying on their behalf; some points of view are drowned out by ridicule and people contradict themselves and change their minds. The data are messy and sometimes incoherent. However, these are precisely the sorts of problems that, I believe, make focus groups a useful method for exploring people's understandings and experiences. The technique enables the researcher to examine people's different perspectives as they operate within a social network and to explore how accounts are constructed, expressed, censured, opposed and changed through social interaction.

This chapter introduces the focus group method and compares it to the two more popular data collection techniques of questionnaires and interviews. It concludes that focus groups can make a unique contribution to data collection: providing insights into how and why people think as they do, locating their sources of information, identifying their explanatory frameworks and highlighting different forms and levels of 'knowing'.

### The Focus Group: What is it, where did it come from?

Focus groups are group discussions organized to explore a specific set of issues. The group is *focused* in the sense that it involves some kind of collective activity — such as viewing a film, examining a single health education message or simply debating a particular set of questions. Crucially, focus groups are distinguished from the broader category of group interviews by 'the explicit use of the group interaction' as research data. (See Merton, *et al.*, 1956; Morgan, 1988.).

There is nothing new about focus groups. They are first mentioned as a market research technique in the 1920s (Basch, 1987; Bogardus, 1926) and were used by Merton in the 1950s to examine people's reactions to wartime propaganda (Merton *et al.*, 1956). In fact it is this last author, Merton, who is often credited with developing the *focused interview* with groups. (Although he never actually used the term *focus group* and would beg to differ from some contemporary uses of the technique, see Merton, 1987.)

Group discussions in their widest sense have continued to be popular as a method of data collection throughout the 1980s and early 1990s within specific niches such as in *communication research* (Philo, 1990; Schlesinger *et al.*, 1992; Corner, Richardson and Fenton, 1990) and for very specific purposes such as pre-testing questionnaires (see Roche, 1991; Watts and Ebbutt, 1987). However, group work has not been systematically developed as a research technique within social science in general, and there has been a failure to develop and exploit the full potential of focus group methods in particular. This chapter attempts to redress the balance through a detailed examination of the way in which focus groups were used in the AIDS Media Research Project.

## The AIDS Media Research Project: how and why we used focus groups

The AIDS Media Research Project was a three-pronged study of the production, content and effect of media messages about AIDS (see Beharrell, 1993; Miller and Williams, 1993; Kitzinger, 1993). Focus groups were used in order to examine the 'effect' element in this equation: to explore how media messages are processed by audiences. We wanted to know how people's understandings of AIDS were constructed. We were interested not solely in what people thought but in how they thought and why they thought as they did. What are the different components which make up what people *know* about AIDS? What forms does this *knowledge* take? How do people use the information that they possess? How are opinions shaped and consensus reached? How are views changed or confirmed? On what basis do people accept or reject new ideas and what role is played both by the media and by social interaction in this process?

Focus groups are particularly well adapted to exploring such questions because they allow one to observe social processes in action. Group discussion is also invaluable for *grounded theory* development — focusing on the generation rather than the testing of theory and exploring the categories which people use to order their experience (Glazer and Strauss, 1967). Listening to discussions between research participants gives the group facilitator time to acclimatize to, for example, their preferred words for speaking about sex and prevents the researcher from prematurely closing off the generation of meaning in his or her own search for clarification. Group work ensures that priority is given to the respondents' hierarchy of importance, their language and concepts, their frameworks for understanding the world.

### The Selection of Research Participants

The specific design of the focus groups used on the AIDS project involved pre-existing groups: groups of people who already knew each other through living, working or socializing together. We conducted a total of fifty-two different discussions, each group consisting of, on average, six research participants. The groups were selected in order to explore diversity of opinion (rather than to establish any kind of 'representativeness' which might reflect the distribution of those different opinions across the population as a whole). The sample included so-called 'general population' groups, such as a group of women whose children attended the same playgroup and a team of civil engineers working on the same site. It also included some groups who might be expected to have particular perspectives on AIDS (because of some professional or personal involvement): people such as prisons officers, male prostitutes, drug injecting users, gay men and lesbians.

---

*People who, as a group, have no obvious special interest in the issue:*
Retired people; residents living on the same Glasgow estate; school students; women with children attending playgroup; civil engineers; members of the Roundtable; American students; British students; office janitors; office cleaners; market researchers.

*People with some professional role or personal involvement or perceived high-risk status:*
Doctors; nurses; health visitors; prison staff; prisoners; teachers; drug centre workers and clients; NACRO and SACRO* workers and clients; social workers; young people in intermediate treatments; police staff; journalists; community council workers; gay men; lesbians; male prostitutes; family of a gay man.

---

*NACRO and SACRO are acronyms for the National and Scottish Associations for the Care and Resettlement of Offenders.

*Figure 10.1:* *Types of groups involved in the study.*

### Running the Sessions

Each session lasted about two hours and was tape recorded. On arrival, participants were asked to fill in an initial questionnaire giving personal demographic details and documenting their patterns of media consumption. They were then asked to write their own news bulletin about AIDS using a set of pictures provided by us (for discussion of this technique see Kitzinger, 1993).

Each participant then completed a second questionnaire exploring their knowledge about AIDS and asking them to rate a series of statements about risk of HIV transmission. The *news bulletins* were then read out and discussed in the group; this was followed by free-flowing debate.

Towards the end of the session participants were presented with the *card game*: a set of cards repeating the statements about risk which had been presented to participants in their individual questionnaires, but which now had to be responded to as a group (see below). Where there was time, participants were also asked to comment in detail on one particular advertisement (see Kitzinger, in press). Finally participants were presented with a third questionnaire which asked about the impact of the group session upon their own attitudes and understandings and gave them the opportunity to write down any information or comments that they did not wish to reveal to the group as a whole.

This chapter demonstrates the value of focus groups by comparing the data generated by the group discussion and exercises with those obtained by the two more common data collection techniques of questionnaires and individual interviews. Responses and comments from the group discussion can be compared to individual questionnaire responses by referring to the quasi-experimental data where we asked people the same questions about risk both on an initial questionnaire and then in the group discussion using the card game. The focus group can be compared to interviews by concentrating on the one factor which invariably distinguishes the two techniques of data collection, namely the interaction that exists in focus groups between the research participants themselves.[2]

## Comparing Focus Groups and Questionnaires

*Comparing responses to the questionnaire and the card game: misinterpretations and misinformation*

On their second questionnaire, research participants were asked to respond to a question taken from the British Social Attitudes (BSA) Survey: 'Here is a list of different kinds of people in Britain. Please indicate how much at risk you think they are from AIDS.' Respondents were presented with examples such as:

People who have sex with many different partners of the opposite sex.

| Greatly at risk | Quite a lot at risk | Not very much at risk | Not at all at risk |
|---|---|---|---|

Doctors and nurses who treat people who have AIDS.

| Greatly at risk | Quite a lot at risk | Not very much at risk | Not at all at risk |
|---|---|---|---|

Male homosexuals — that is, gays

| Greatly at risk | Quite a lot at risk | Not very much at risk | Not at all at risk |
|---|---|---|---|

(Brook, 1988)

We decided to reproduce the BSA question for two reasons. First, the question is phrased primarily in terms of risk groups rather than risk practices. Regardless of the respondent's knowledge of transmission as a biological process the information provided is an inadequate basis on which to assess risk. We were interested in exploring what kind of assumptions might influence people's responses. Second, the BSA question was of interest to us because, within the constraints of the question design, it seemed to highlight some peculiar inconsistencies. For example, current medical knowledge suggests that very few women have become infected as a result of lesbian sex, however 60 per cent of respondents in the BSA survey indicated that lesbians were 'greatly' or 'quite a lot' at-risk (Brook, 1988: 75).

Because of our interest in disjuncture between medical knowledge and popular perceptions we added in one new item: 'people who donate blood at a blood donor centre'. This is similar to the phrasing used in other surveys, such as that conducted at the Research Unit for Health and Behavioural Change (RUHBC). In their telephone survey they asked the question: 'In your opinion can people become infected with the AIDS virus by giving blood, for example, at a blood donor centre?' About a third of their respondents replied 'yes' (RUHBC, data update March 1990).

As expected, the questionnaire results from our study reflected some of the same apparent misunderstandings as had been revealed by the BSA and the RUHBC survey data. For example, over a third of our (non-random) sample gave responses indicating that lesbians were 'greatly' or 'quite a lot' at-risk and 4 per cent seemed to think that there was some risk of HIV transmission to 'people who donate blood at a blood donor centre'. Although surveys can highlight such apparent mismatches between medical knowledge and lay understandings they cannot explain *why* they occur. This is where focus groups can be of particular benefit and a technique such as the card game can be especially useful.

The card game consisted of a pack of cards each bearing a description of the people introduced in the BSA questionnaire. The cards were distributed to group members who took it in turn to read out a description and then the group as a whole debated where to place the card in one of the four categories of risk. This exercise demonstrated that part of the explanation for the apparent disparity between medical and some lay understandings of risk was that people did not necessarily interpret the questions in the same way as that intended by the researchers. For example, some people interpreted the question about blood donors as a question about whether or not blood donation could be a *route* of transmission, risky to the person receiving the blood. This only became clear during the course of debate between some participants who argued that the item should be placed in the 'not very much at-risk' category on the grounds that 'they heat-treat the blood now' and others who believed that it should be placed in the 'greatly at-risk category' because 'look at all the haemophiliacs'.

We were also able to observe that people did not necessarily give the 'right' answer for the 'right' reason. For example, on her questionnaire, one woman rated 'doctors and nurses who treat people who have AIDS' as 'not very much at risk'. However, during discussion it emerged that she had done so in the belief that medical staff are given injections to make them immune. In several other groups research participants asserted that 'you cannot tell by looking who has HIV'. However, when challenged by other members of the group, several people justified this point of view by saying that it was simply impossible to distinguish between someone who is HIV-antibody positive and someone who looks ill for some other reason (such as having flu or 'ordinary' cancer).

While these are useful insights, focus groups can do more than highlight whether or not people understand a question or what 'facts' influence their responses. Focus groups also generate data that allow an analysis of more fundamental questions, exploring people's assumptions, their models of thinking and the moral values they bring to bear on such questions.

### *Comparing responses to the questionnaire and the card game: exploring assumptions*

In the course of group discussion and negotiation people reveal their assumptions and rationales. For example, as we observed people talking to one another we could see that many research participants unquestioningly accepted the notion of risk groups. They readily spoke in terms of such categories and automatically made assumptions about the actual behaviour of, for example, the gay men versus the heterosexuals described in the BSA questionnaire.

When different groups of research participants placed the cards in different risk categories, this did not necessarily mean that they had different knowledge about the transmission process; it simply meant that they were drawing upon different models of how 'people like that' behave. A group of nurses and health visitors, for example, commented that when gay men were mentioned they assumed that they were promiscuous, whereas when assessing the risks for a 'married couple who only have sex with each other' they assumed that both partners were virgins before marriage. By contrast, a group of gay men consciously opposed the whole notion of risk groups and they rated 'people who have sex with many different partners of the opposite sex' as at higher risk than 'homosexuals — that is, gay men'. They did so on the grounds that the gay men would probably practice safer sex whereas the straight people would not.

At the other end of the spectrum from the gay men some research participants (mainly in the general population groups) thought entirely in terms of risk groups and were very resistant to the possibility that *any* gay person might not be at-risk. Some of the young, overtly heterosexual men repeated 'jokes', such as 'What does GAY stand for? Got AIDS Yet?', and were reluctant to admit that there was any safe way for men to have sex with each other. During discussion with a group of ex-prisoners, for example, one man stated that you could *not* generalize about the risk status of homosexuals. The other members of his group, however, insisted that all homosexuals were at-risk, an insistence which culminated in the assertion that 'all faggots have AIDS'. This was in spite of the fact that these young men were all aware of the information that, for instance, condom-use could reduce the risk. This insistence that all gay men were at-risk from AIDS was inextricably tied in with expressions of hatred against 'poofters' and assertions of their own masculinity. In fact, it seemed to have more to do with these young men's belief that homosexuality was 'sick' and 'disgusting' than with their knowledge of how HIV was transmitted. Indeed, similar criteria were used to assert that lesbians were a 'high-risk group': 'They are fagottesses'; 'they are leading the same life as what two men are'; 'God made two kinds of sex, male and female. They go together. He didn't mean males to go with males and females to go with females. And that's how they got it [AIDS]' (SACRO clients).

People's assessments about who is at risk of HIV infection are bound up with their taken-for-granted assumptions about reality, their presumptions about how different people behave, their moral values and models of thinking. The gay men who rated male homosexuals as at lower risk than 'people who have many different partners of the opposite sex' were deconstructing the question, and fitting information into a different framework which challenged many of the mainstream groups' common sense assessment of risk. Their ability to do this is not an automatic consequence of having particular knowledge (such as knowledge about the widespread adoption of safer sex practices by gay men). Some of the general population groups and many of the professional groups shared this knowledge, but none of them suggested rating the 'promiscuous' heterosexuals as at higher risk than the gay men. For example, when a group of doctors sorted the cards in a way which rated gay men as at greater risk than 'promiscuous' heterosexuals I informed them of the reasoning behind the different decisions taken by the group of gay men. One of the doctors immediately declared that he was well aware of the changes in behaviour among the gay community and he expressed surprise that he had not brought his knowledge to bear on his assessment of risk.

Similarly, in discussing why they might have rated lesbians as a high-risk group, some participants realized that this did not accord with any 'facts' of which they were aware. On reflection they decided that lesbians were not at particular risk and they were disturbed by the extent to which their original opinion differed from their preferred thought-out position. A group of research participants suggested that, in spite of their better judgement, they had a residual sense that lesbians did not deserve to be safer than straight women. 'It's just, I suppose, the way you've been brought up — you think that a man and a woman is more normal than two women. I don't know whether, risk of infection-wise, whether that it's true or not, it's just the way that you were brought up.' (Market Researchers)

Focus groups give researchers the opportunity to examine apparently perverse results generated by questionnaires and to unpack people's underlying presumptions. Where a questionnaire generates explanation by correlation — correlating items already built into the questionnaire — group discussions generate hypotheses through exploration. Such discussions keep the cultural context of information to the fore and make it very clear that factual information is not the only kind of knowledge that counts. Patterns of thinking, the categories we use to organize our ideas, the images and connections through which we conceptualize an issue, may be more important than the different *facts* that we *know*. It is in illuminating these dimensions that focus groups are of particular value; this applies not only in relation to questionnaires, but also in relation to individual interviews. The second half of this chapter compares focus groups to the individual interview method of data collection.

### Comparing Focus Groups and Interviews

The fundamental difference between an interview and a group discussion is the number and patterns of interactions. Whereas an interview is a two-way interaction (with interviewer and respondent taking alternate speech turns), group discussions involve multiple interactions between research participants themselves. In focus groups the co-participants act as co-researchers taking the research into new and often unexpected directions and engaging with each other in ways which are both complementary (such as sharing common experiences) and argumentative (questioning, challenging, and disagreeing with each other.) The research participants provide a sounding-board for each others' opinions and debates between them highlight group norms. The following discussion examines the different types of interaction which occur within groups in order to highlight the sort of data that can be generated by such interchanges.

#### *Tapping into different levels of knowing: brainstorming, jokes and story-telling*

The fact that group participants provide an audience for each other encourages a greater variety of communication than is often evident within more traditional methods of data collection. During the course of the AIDS project, group participants argued, boasted, made faces at each other, told stories and, on one occasion, sang songs. Group work is characterized by teasing, joking and the kind of acting out that goes on among peers. For example, some participants acted out the 'look of an AIDS carrier' (contorting their faces, squinting and shaking) and others took evident delight in swapping information about the vast quantities of saliva one would need to drink before running any risk of infection. (You'd need to swallow 'six gallons', 'eight gallons', 'ten gallons', 'dive into a swimming pool of saliva' or 'bathe in it while covered in open sores'.) Brainstorming and loose word association was another frequent feature of the research sessions. In several groups any attempts to address the risks HIV poses to gay men were drowned out by a ritual period of outcry against homosexuality:

*ITM:*   Benders, poofs
*ITM:*   Bent bastards
*ITM:*   Bent shops
*ITM:*   they're poofs, I mean I don't know how a man could have sex with another man it's . . .
*ITM:*   Its disgusting [ . . . ]
*ITM:*   Ah, Yuk!
(Young people in intermediate treatment, male (ITM))

A certain amount of similar brain-storming accompanied discussion of the idea that 'AIDS comes from Africa':

*ITF:*   Look at all the famine over there, all the disease coming off the dead cows and all that, they die and all that
*ITM:*   Dirtiness
*ITM:*   Filthy
*ITF:*   Blackness [ . . . ]
*ITM:*   It's just disgusting.[3]
(Young people in intermediate treatment, female (ITF)/male (ITM)

These sorts of interactions can make groups seem unruly (both at the time and when attempting to analyse the data) but such undisciplined outbursts are not irrelevant or simply obstructive to the collection of data about what people 'know'. On the contrary, the ebullience with which some people acted out 'the look of an AIDS carrier' vividly demonstrates the voyeuristic fascination of 'the face of AIDS' and the way in which some media images are reproduced, reinforced and reiterated through social interaction. The relish with which people swapped information about the vast quantities of saliva needed to pose any risk of infection highlights the potency of the 'yuk' factor in helping them to recall certain 'facts' about AIDS. The outcry provoked by any mention of homosexuality and the loose word association about 'blackness' reveal an essential element in how some people think about AIDS among gay men or in Africa. They form part of why people may believe that gay men (and lesbians) are inherently vulnerable to HIV or why they so readily accept that Africa is a hotbed of HIV infection (Kitzinger and Miller, 1992). In this sense focus groups reach the parts that other methods cannot reach — revealing dimensions of understanding that often remain untapped by the more conventional one-to-one interview or questionnaire.

Through observing the exchange of such information, and anecdotes, one gains insight into the social currency of such 'knowledges' and one is able to observe how people juggle contradictions. Indeed, focus group work highlights how people often hold contradictory beliefs which are brought into operation in different situations. For example, one of the young men who declared that all lesbians had AIDS subsequently boasted to his friends that two attractive lesbians had been up at his flat the previous night, and they certainly did not have the virus. The young man was drawing on two logically but not *ideologically* incompatible images of lesbians, each of which served his purpose at different points in the conversation.

During the course of the group session, then, the researcher can clarify the meaning of a 'fact', idea or story by witnessing how it is mobilized in social interaction, what ideological work it is employed to achieve. For example, group members often enthusiastically shared tales about the 'vengeful AIDS carrier' who sleeps with an unwitting stranger and departs leaving the message: 'Welcome to the AIDS club'. A health educator commenting on this phenomena suggested that such tales could do more for the prevention of HIV transmission than all the health education campaigns put together (*Guardian*, 30 October 1991). If these revenge tales do serve such functions it is certainly not all they do: in our general population groups such stories were not often used to advise people to take precautions during sex with anyone; instead they were used to justify identifying and isolating 'AIDS carriers'.

*Group norms: conformity, consensus and censorship*

In addition to the advantages discussed above, focus groups facilitate the collection of data on group norms, priorities and shared experiences. Often a particular phrase will mobilize an assertion of group consensus. A group of mothers, for example, discussing whether they had the right to know if another child in the play group had the virus asserted, 'you think of your own first'. It was this phrase, and these sort of sentiments, which seemed to capture their consent and resulted in nods of agreement round the group and assertions that 'that's right' and 'of course'.

Indeed, it was often the strength of the collective reaction that highlighted the specific context within which the research participants experienced AIDS information. When I asked one group of young women whether they had ever come across the advice that they could 'try sex which avoids penetration' they responded with initial bemusement followed by spontaneous protest:

> 'If you really wanted to prevent it everyone would end up locked up in their house.'

'It's sort of saying don't bother having sex, don't bother even going out in the first place.'

'It's [saying that sex is] a lost cause!'

(School students)

This apparently unanimous agreement underlined the extent to which young heterosexual women may experience such safer sex recommendations in terms of prohibitions. Advice to avoid penetration is seen as yet more constraints on, and attempts to control their sexual expression. This is not to say that on an individual level these women might not find most pleasure in what they would call foreplay — a subjective experience that might be more easily tapped by interview. However, the very lack of public discourse about non-penetrative sex contributes to the difficulties women face when attempting to establish the validity of such experiences or to secure safer sexual practices with men.

It is very hard for a group facilitator to ignore the issues which are important to the group — if only because the researcher is outnumbered! Indeed, the group dynamic can force the researcher to confront the context within which the research participants consider the issue. In one of the AIDS research sessions the participants started discussing nuclear power, Chernobyl and salmonella rather than HIV. They did not see this as going off the point, they were simply demonstrating their perspective on government AIDS information: we can't trust the government to give us the facts about pollution or food poisoning, why should we trust what they tell us about AIDS? Similarly, another group of women (who all lived in the same area of Glasgow) barely co-operated with the researcher in addressing questions about safer sex but quickly became animated discussing the dangers of needles discarded in the street by drug-users. This was the issue of primary importance to them and they resented the lack of information about this in the national campaign from the Health Education Authority based in England.

Sometimes the group process itself generates ideas which the individuals alone might not have articulated. Group sessions may encourage certain kinds of talk, particularly talk which is considered hostile to the interviewer or deviant from the majority culture (or the assumed culture of the researcher). This may be especially important when working with those who are oppressed or marginalized such as, in our case, injecting drug users and sex workers. It also may be particularly effective when it draws together people who have previously been unable to share their experiences or who are physically isolated from one another, such as those caring for elderly relatives, young children or workers doing piece work from home. Being with others who share similar experiences may also encourage critical comments from groups, such as pregnant women, who tend to be grateful and complementary about the services on offer. Indeed, some researchers have noted that group discussions can quickly become a collective 'moan session' as 'conversation seemed to feed on the climate of depreciation created' (Watts and Ebbutt, 1987: 31). Geis and his colleagues, in their study of the lovers of people with AIDS, found that:

> The group meeting experience evoked more angry and emotional comments about the medical community than did the individual interviews . . . perhaps the synergism of the group 'kept the anger going' and allowed each participant to reinforce another's vented feelings of frustration and rage . . .
>
> (Geis, Fuller and Rush, 1986: 48)

The group consensus can thus not only highlight norms and priorities, it can generate, or permit the expression of, particular perspectives. At the same time observation of how group members interact can expose how certain points of view may be overruled or silenced. For example, our group sessions highlighted the potential stigma some groups attached to knowing too much about AIDS. In several groups if one person revealed detailed information about how HIV was transmitted he or she was met with suspicion and cries of 'How come you know so much about this?' As one group of women commented:

> It's not the sort of subject that basically anybody's going to go to the library and say, 'Right, I want a book about this.'
>
> They'd look at you as if you were a les-pot! [General nodding and laughter]
>
> (Women whose children attended the same Playgroup)

In this context, wilful ignorance can, it seems, earn more respect than interest or knowledge, a fact which is, in itself, important to confront.[4]

Instead of generalizing about the effect of groups we need to pay close attention to the composition of groups in the research design and be aware of how the characteristics of any particular collection of individuals may influence what is said. The censorship of some experiences or the inclusion of group-generated ideas, does not invalidate the data but allows the researchers to explore how a group consensus can be reached with the systematic exclusion of certain items of stigmatized personal information, how assertive opinion leaders may make other people change their minds or how previously unarticulated points of view may be created by the group process.

### Debates and Differences

The group process however, is not only about consensus and the articulation of group norms and shared experiences or the straightforward group censoring of isolated individual opinions. The multiple differences between individuals within the group are equally important and, in any case, rarely disappear from view. Regardless of how they are selected, the research participants in any one group are never entirely homogenous. Participants do not just agree with each other they also misunderstand one another, question one another, try to persuade each other of the justice of their own point of view and sometimes they vehemently disagree. Mutual ridicule and cries of 'shut your gob or I'll thump you' can be somewhat alarming for the researcher who has been taught that interviewees need a 'wall-paper' or 'nodding-dog' interrogator who does nothing but smile to encourage them to talk. However, such conflict can be turned to the researcher's advantage.

During the course of the group the facilitator can explore such differences of opinion and encourage the participants to speculate about why such diversity exists. In our pre-existing groups people were sometimes surprised to discover how differently they thought about some things, especially when the group otherwise appeared relatively homogeneous — by gender, race, and class. Such unexpected dissent led them to clarify *why* they thought as they did, often identifying aspects of their personal experience which had altered their opinions or specific occasions which had made them rethink their point of view. For example, in a group of residents from the same Glasgow estate, two of the participants emphasized the need to carry on normally interacting with people who were sero-positive, whereas the other two women were extremely fearful of casual transmission and extra-vigilant (to the extent that one of them will not touch the button on a pelican crossing with her bare finger for fear of infection). When they were encouraged to explore why such a difference should exist between four women with very similar backgrounds and knowledge it was found that the first two (who were not worried about casual transmission) knew themselves to be in regular contact with individuals from so-called high risk groups: one had a brother who was an IV drug user, the other had a gay relative. This would suggest that routine exposure to people known to be in high-risk groups may be far more important in decreasing people's fear of casual transmission than knowledge in and of itself.

People's different assumptions are thrown into relief by the way in which they challenge one another, the questions they ask, the sources they cite, and what explanations seem to sway the opinion of other members of the group. When analysing the transcript of a group discussion it is well worth having special coding categories for certain types of interaction between participants such as 'questions', 'cited sources', 'deferring to the opinion of others' and 'changes of mind'.

When one person tells an anecdote or relates the plot of a TV programme, what line of questioning do the other members of the group pursue in order to decide, for instance, whether a particular person described in a story really is an innocent victim of AIDS? When participants describe an occasion when they think they might have been at-risk what queries are raised by the co-participants; how do they seek to reassure their friend?

When an argument breaks out, what sort of evidence seems to work in influencing the opinion of others? Why is it that someone who has the correct information may fail to convince his or her peers, and what is going on when people *do* change their minds in response to information presented by other members of the group? For example, when one schoolboy tried to explain to his friends that having the AIDS virus was different from having AIDS the argument clearly foundered for lack of vocabulary. Without the term *HIV* he was unable to persuade them that *carrying* it was not the same as *having* it (see Kitzinger, 1994). In another group, however, one individual was able to sway the opinion of all her friends by telling a single anecdote. In this group there was a great deal of initial scepticism about the view that HIV was created in a laboratory, but a story told by one of the research participants shifted the consensus:

> PP: My-holier-than-thou mother-in-law to put it politely, keeps informing me that it was a man-made disease . . .
> PP: well, my brother works in a lab . . . in America and when that all came out that it was a man-made virus I wrote and asked him and his letter was censured, what he answered to me was all blanked out . . . That made me think, 'aye, it is a man-made thing, there's something in that. Why should they blank out his letter?'
> JK: What do the rest of you think of this story?
> PP: It makes it more probable.
> PP: It makes me think it could be the way it started.
> PP: There must be something.
> (Women whose children attended the same playgroup)

This interaction was typical of many of the turning points in the groups. People commonly appeared to change their minds in response to personal evidence based on anecdotes or the perceived behaviour of professionals rather than information from leaflets or advertisements. There was a clear 'hierarchy of credibility' in operation between different types of sources (mother-in-laws coming rather low down on the list in western culture!)

### Conclusions

The focus group method is ideal for exploring social and communication issues, and examining the cultural construction of experience. It taps into people's underlying assumptions and theoretical frameworks and draws out how and why they think as they do. The data generated by this method confront the researcher with the multi-levelled and dynamic nature of people's understandings, highlighting their fluidity, deviations and contradictions.

This chapter is not arguing that the group data is inherently either more or less authentic than data collected by interview or questionnaire, instead it is based on the premise that 'all talk through which people generate meaning is contextual, and that the contexts will inevitably somewhat colour the meaning'

(Dahlgren, 1988: 292). It is a predictable sign of the dominance of the interview paradigm that when researchers have found differences between data collected by interviews and group discussion they have sometimes blithely dismissed the latter as inaccurate (e.g. Hoijer, 1990: 34). But differences between interview and group data can not be classified in terms of validity versus invalidity or honesty versus dishonesty. Comparing the effects of different methodologies when talking to heterosexual men about sex, for example, some researchers have noted that these research participants are more likely to express macho attitudes (with a male researcher) or to sexually harass (a female researcher) in group settings than in individual interviews (Wight, in press; Green *et al.*, 1993). The group data documenting macho or sexual harassing behaviour is no more invalid than that showing the research participants' relatively acceptable behaviour in interview situations. Instead of disregarding data from group settings we need to acknowledge the different types of discourses that may be expressed in the private and public arena, or with peers versus with an interviewer. The fact that particular groups facilitate the articulation of particular kinds of perspectives can then be consciously addressed and the importance of that context can be considered.

We are none of us self-contained, isolated, static entities; we are part of complex and overlapping social, familial and collegiate networks. Personal beliefs are not cut off from public discourses and individual behaviour does not happen in a cultural vacuum whether this is negotiating safer sex, sharing needles, campaigning for improvements in health care or going 'queer bashing'. We learn about the meaning of AIDS, (or sex, or health or food or cigarettes) through talking with and observing other people, through conversations at home, at work; and we act (or fail to act) on that knowledge in a social context. When researchers want to document people's understandings, or to influence them, it makes sense to explore all the levels of knowing and to employ methods which permit the examination of these social processes in action. Focus groups should encourage us to reflect critically on the dominance of individual interview methods in qualitative research. Perhaps, in many cases, researchers should not be asking, 'Why have focus groups?' but 'Why do individual interviews instead?'

### Acknowledgements

I would like to thank my colleagues, Peter Beharrell, David Miller, Kevin Williams and the grant holders Mick Bloor, John Eldridge, Sally Macintyre and Greg Philo for their contributions to this paper. I would also like to acknowledge the support of the funding body — the Economic and Social Research Council, grant no. XA44250006 and to thank Kay Weaver for lively debate on this issue.

## Notes

1  Part of this chapter first appeared in Kitzinger, J. (1994) 'The methodology of focus groups: The importance of interaction between research participants', *Sociology of Health and Illness*, 16, 1.

2  This paper does not address the relative merits of focus groups as opposed to participant observation. Although I was informally involved with some of the groups prior to the start of sessions (e.g. joining them in preparing a meal or sitting through the end of their business meeting) I do not have any way of systematically comparing such methods from my study. Morgan suggests that focus groups are particularly suited to the study of attitudes and cognition, whereas participant observation may be more appropriate for studies of social roles and formal organizations (Morgan 1988: 17).

3  Group discussions introduce an extra ethical dilemma for researchers. Many interviewers face dilemmas when listening to and documenting offensive (e.g. racist) comments; these dilemmas may be particularly acute for the group facilitator if such comments are directed at other members of the group even if unintentionally (such as in a group discussion about child sexual abuse disparaging comments being made about women 'asking for it' or being severely damaged by abuse). Such problems can be addressed through (a) thinking about the composition of the groups prior to running any such session; (b) using dissent within the group to challenge such attitudes, (c) being available to individual members of the group after the session. If necessary it may also be appropriate to intervene in the group as facilitator.

4  Some people suggest that group work is inappropriate for sensitive topics but this should not be assumed. In fact, depending on their composition, groups can sometimes actively facilitate the discussion of otherwise taboo issues because the less inhibited members of the group break the ice for shyer participants or one person's revelation of discrediting information encourages others to disclose. (See Kitzinger, 1994) It is worth noting that focus groups have successfully been used to elicit data from people who are perceived by researchers as 'difficult subjects' e.g. 'difficult-to-reach, high-risk families' (Lengua, *et al.* 1992) and 'high apprehensives' who are anxious about communicating (Lederman, 1983).

## References

BASCH, C. (1987) 'Focus group interview: An underutilized research technique for improving theory and practice in health education', *Health Education Quarterly*, 14, 4, pp. 411-48.

BOGARDUS, E. (1926) 'The group interview', *Journal of Applied Sociology*, 10, pp. 372-82.

BEHARRELL, P. (1993) 'AIDS and the British press', in ELDRIDGE, J. (Ed.) (1993) *Getting the Message*, London: Routeldge, pp. 210-52.

BROOK, L. (1988) 'The public's response to AIDS', in Jowell, R., WITHERSPOON, S. and BROOK, L. (Eds) *British Social Attitudes, the 5th report*, Aldershot: Gower.

CORNER, J., RICHARDSON, K. and FENTON, N. (1990) *Nuclear reactions: Form and response in public issues in television, a media research monograph 4*, London: John Libby.

DAHLGREN, P. (1988) 'What's the meaning of this? Viewers' plural sense-making of TV news', in *Media, Culture and Society*, 10, pp. 285-301.

GEIS, S., FULLER, R. and RUSH, J. (1986) 'Lovers of AIDS victims: psychosocial stresses and counselling needs', in *Death Studies*, 10, 1, pp. 43-53.

GLAZER, B.G. and STRAUSS, A. (1967) *The Discovery of Grounded Theory*, Chicago, IL: Aldine.

GREEN, G., BERNARD, M., BARBOUR, R. and KITZINGER, J. (1993) 'Who wears the trousers? Sexual harrassment in research settings', *Women's Studies International Forum*, 16, 6, pp. 627–37.

GREENBAUM, T. (1987) *The Practical Handbook and Guide to Focus Group Research*, Lexington, MA: Lexington Books.

HOIJER, B. (1990) 'Studying viewers' reception of television programmes: Theoretical and methodological considerations', *European Journal of Communication*, 5, pp. 29–56.

KITZINGER, J. and MILLER, D. (1992) 'African AIDS: The media and audience beliefs', in AGGLETON, P., DAVIES, P. and HART, G. (Eds) *AIDS: Rights, Risk and Reason*, London: Falmer Press, pp. 28–52.

KITZINGER, J. (1993) 'Understanding AIDS: Researching audience perceptions of acquired immune deficiency syndrome', in ELDRIDGE, J. (Ed.) *Getting the Message*, London: Routledge, pp. 271–304.

KITZINGER, J. (1994) 'The methodology of focus groups: The importance of interaction between research participants', *Sociology of Health and Illness*, 16, 1, January, pp. 103–121.

KITZINGER, J. (in press) 'The face of Aids', in MARKOVA, I. and FARR, R. (1994) *Representations of Health, Illness and Handicap*, Chur, Switzerland: Harwood Academic.

MERTON, R., FISK, M. and KENDALL, P. (1956) 'The focused interview: A report of the bureau of applied social research', New York: Columbia University.

MERTON, R. (1987) 'The focused interview and focus group: Continuities and discontinuities', in *Public Opinion Quarterly*, 51, pp. 550–66.

MILLER, D. and WILLIAMS, K. (1993) 'Negotiating HIV/AIDS information: Agendas, media strategies and the news', in ELDRIDGE, J. (Ed.) (1993) *Getting the Message*, London: Routledge, pp. 126–44.

MORGAN, D. (1988) *Focus Groups as Qualitative Research*, London: Sage.

MORGAN, D. and KREUGER, R. (1993) *Successful Focus Groups: Advancing the State of the Art*, London: Sage.

PHILO, G. (1990) *Seeing and Believing*, London: Routledge.

RESEARCH UNIT FOR HEALTH AND BEHAVIOURAL CHANGE, (RUHBC) (1990) *Data Update*, Edinburgh: Edinburgh University.

ROCHE, A. (1991) 'Making better use of qualitative research: Illustrations from medical education research', *Health Education Journal*, 50, 3, pp. 131–6.

SCHLESINGER, P., DOBASH, R., DOBASH, R. and WEAVER, K. (1992) *Women Viewing Violence*, London: BFI.

WATTS, M. and EBBUTT, D. (1987) 'More than the sum of the parts: research methods in group interviewing', *British Educational Research Journal*, 13, 1, pp. 25–34.

WIGHT, D. (in press) 'Boys' thoughts and talk about sex in a working class locality of Glasgow', *Sociological Review*, forthcoming.

*Evaluating Health Education Interventions*

## Chapter 11

# Theory, Utility and Stakeholders: Methodological Issues in Evaluating a Community Project on HIV/AIDS

*Ian S. Peers and Margaret Johnston*

It has often been argued that evaluation is useless, and at times worse than useless. Evaluation criteria that seem relevant at the outset may well prove more hindrance than help to a project that is breaking new ground and exploring ways of communicating on sensitive matters. By working closely alongside the various activities of a community youth education project on HIV, we have been able to find ways of tailoring our approach to their circumstance and needs. At the same time, in the course of evaluating an innovative and developing project, we have been obliged to reassess evaluation approaches. In consequence, our experience has highlighted several dilemmas and contradictions, and moreover we think we have gone some way towards devising an approach that combines the demands of objectivity and accountability with the need for a sensitive and adaptable response. In this chapter, we describe the project and the evaluation approach we adopted, and the discoveries we made in the course of our attempts to apply the latter.

## The Project

In 1988, the Health Education Authority (HEA) received four independent applications for programme funding, all concerned with HIV/AIDS education of young people in community settings. One was from a District Health Authority wanting to train and employ a team of paid peer educators to talk to young people in informal settings. The second was a joint proposal from two District Health Authorities and an agency supplying social action material for a commercial radio station, to employ a worker who would produce materials with young people. The third was from a national voluntary agency, to form an AIDS information team consisting of a paid project worker, two full-time volunteers, and local young people. The fourth application came from a voluntary agency who wanted funding to employ a worker to provide HIV/AIDS education for youth workers throughout a large urban area.

All four applicants were invited to resubmit their proposals stressing the peer education element, which they did, and the four were brought together as the HEA's Community Youth Project HIV/AIDS, though they were spread across England with none of them less than a hundred miles from the next. The project was set up in an atmosphere of urgency. Prompt responses were felt to be necessary to the problems posed by HIV/AIDS, and although provision for evaluation was made from the start, this took second place to getting the projects operational as quickly as possible. Consequently, it was some months after the contracts had been agreed, project workers had been appointed and the projects had started work, that the evaluation team was commissioned.

After a few months, the fourth project dropped out. The other three developed in ways not altogether foreseen at the outset. The funding of all three was extended for a year beyond the two years originally proposed, and the evaluation contract extended accordingly.

### Approaches to Evaluation

The evaluation team set out to work in a way that was appropriate to the structure and purpose of the project, and that would be useful both to participants within its life-time and to those undertaking similar work after it was completed. This, however, was no easy undertaking. According to the Joint Council for Standards in Education Evaluation (JCSE) standard of propriety, educational evaluations should be objective, accountable and fair (JCSE, 1981). In practice it is hard to combine these virtues. Too often, the quest for objectivity has led to the application of criteria which are not perceived to be fair by those carrying out the activity, and the claim to accountability then becomes meaningless, since the account is not accepted by those most closely involved.

The perception of evaluation as unfair and irrelevant has had the consequence that evaluation has seldom been used to good effect in education of any type. Since the early 1970s, the literature has been replete with comment on how evaluations have failed to have effectiveness (Zusman and Bissionette, 1973; Alkin, Daillak and White, 1979; Patton, 1987). It has been suggested that 'Good program evaluation studies fail more often than they succeed in having any impact on subsequent programs' (Davidson, 1980: 392). There have been many critiques of evaluation practices and procedures, and educational evaluators have been in the forefront of the criticism industry (House, 1989). These criticisms charged that many evaluations of social and education programmes were inappropriate in design (Patton, 1978; Rossi and Freeman, 1989), unrealistic (Schwarz, 1980), irrelevant (Cochran, 1980; Parlett and Hamilton, 1976) unfair, unused and politically naive (Weiss, 1986a).

Furthermore, HIV/AIDS education tends to be seen as a highly specialized area, requiring special evaluation approaches and even a special kind of evaluator.

> external evaluators working in the area of AIDS education may need a sensitivity, a wholeheartedness and a broadmindedness that is not always encountered amongst their counterparts working in more mainstream health education . . . Efforts to counter racism, homophobia and heterosexism, for example . . . may arouse strong emotions.
>
> (Aggleton, 1989: 233)

We selected our evaluation approach, then, not only aware that external evaluation can be viewed as useless, irrelevant, insensitive, intrusive and generally unfit to survive, but also realizing that the evaluation of a project set up by five independent bodies — involving representatives of several professions — to undertake work in assorted community settings on widely separated sites was likely to prove difficult. We also knew that the particularly sensitive subject-matter of HIV infection laid any evaluation procedure open to the charge of inappropriateness. We rejected the image of evaluators descending from some bureaucratic mountaintop with ready-made and irrelevant criteria, and the suggestion that HIV/AIDS education is somehow beyond the scope of objective evaluation. We believed it was possible to find an approach that would meet high standards of objectivity, that would respect the right of funders and the general public to know what was undertaken on their behalf, and which would be seen by those directly involved as fair and as relevant to what they were doing. Such an approach would have to take account of the full complexity of both the project and its environment, of the diverse and not always fully articulated hopes and expectations in which it was set up, of the fact that it was a unique venture, without exact precedent and never to be repeated in quite that form, and of its changing nature, generating different needs at different stages.

These requirements led to the adoption of three principles: (i) the intrepretation of project *theory* must be an integral part of evaluation; (ii) considerations of *utility* must inform all evaluation initiatives; and (iii) implementation of these principles depends on the identification and involvement of *stakeholders*. None of these principles are new in themselves. However, the way we have combined them into a responsive and participatory evaluation approach throws interesting light on their strengths and weaknesses, and particularly on the extent to which they are compatible with each other.

### Theory of Action

Theory is traditionally placed outside the scope of evaluation. The view has been widely accepted that educational evaluation is a judgemental decision-oriented assessment of the merit or worth of a programme (Alkin *et al.*, 1979; JCSE, 1981;

Guba and Lincoln, 1981). However, the notion that theory can usefully inform evaluation research is not new (Chen and Rossi, 1981; Bickman, 1987; Wholey, 1987; Shadish, 1987). Whereas the focus of many evaluations is to 'look down' from programme statements of intent to outcomes, we concur with Heileman's (1989) view that theoretically informed concepts and propositions can favourably affect the conduct of evaluation. We propose that evaluators should 'look up' to consider the theoretical legitimacy underpinning programme activity. We believe that deliberate consideration should be given to the questions of what problem is to be addressed, and what theory of action underpins the project's intended interventions. The role of evaluators is to make explicit the beliefs of sponsors and project implementers. These activities are what we call 'front-end' analysis. Subsequent decisions can be judged against programmatic theory of action, and theory by the utility of project intervention. It is preferable that front-end analysis take place during early conceptualization of a project. However, we show here that retrospective scrutiny of a project's theoretical basis can also be valuable.

### Utility

As we have indicated, many evaluations have no discernible impact on either programme functioning or subequent policy decisions. The utilization-focused approach to evaluation (Alkin *et al.*, 1979; Patton, 1986) addresses this problem by making the issue of utility central to both the design and the conduct of the evaluation. This emphasis on utility requires that potential users should be identified and involved from the outset and at every stage; that the content of the evaluation be determined by negotiation between the interests of the various users (or stakeholders); that evaluators make the quality of user participation their goal, and see their role as training stakeholders in the use of evaluation; that consideration be given to all the possible forms of evaluation impact, and that the cost of user participation in money, time and other resources, be accepted (Patton, 1986: 333–6).

A small, retrospectively-appointed evaluation must be less ambitious. We adhered to the principle of utility to the extent that we kept utility in the forefront of our own minds, that we ensured that stakeholders were consulted as soon as possible and as often as possible about what evaluation data would be of use to them, and acted upon their suggestions whenever we could, and that findings were not hoarded for a final report, but made available as soon as possible, while they could influence the development of the project.

### The Stakeholder Principle

The stakeholder principle follows logically from the principle of utility. In contrast to other evaluation persuasions this approach is democratic and participatory. The stakeholder approach is described by Weiss (1986a: 150) as

> involvement of people holding different positions in the social structure
> of programs, attention to their interests and utilities, representation of
> their priorities, emphasis on feedback and dissemination.

For any complex project, there is likely to be a long list of those involved or affected as agents, beneficiaries or 'victims': those actively involved in setting up and implementing the project, those who benefit from it directly or indirectly, and those whose interests are in some way damaged or threatened. (Guba and Lincoln, 1989). Evaluators are among the stakeholders, since their interests are involved.

Our approach was informed throughout by our awareness that the project consisted of numerous groups and individuals, each with their own background, interests, assumptions, hopes, needs and skills, and our belief that every viewpoint was to be taken into account and none was definitive. From this arose our commitment to a participatory, democratic mode of working. Projects were asked to specify what information would be of use to them, and draft reports were circulated and amended until they were agreed by all involved.

## Applying the Principles

In the course of applying these principles to an HIV/AIDS education project, we have discovered that they do indeed work. On the other hand, we have found that the concept of stakeholder is more complex and problematic than is sometimes recognized and that some of the difficulties and limitations of a stakeholder-oriented approach need to be more clearly understood.

It is an inevitable consequence of a participatory, stakeholder-oriented approach that conflicting pre-suppositions, arising from different implicit theories held by different stakeholders, will come to light as a project develops and so be available for further elucidation. In this section we will confine ourselves to one case where the evaluation set out to elucidate theory, one where a conflict of theory came to light unexpectedly, and an example where different theories were found to be co-existing without giving rise to problems.

### Rationale of Peer Education

The project was intended to be a demonstration of peer education in the community. We identified three possible motives for preferring peer education to the conventional, professional-led type:

1   Efficacy: young people may be perceived as ready-made experts in
    communicating with other young people.

2     Cost-effectiveness: peer education may be seen as a means whereby the effectiveness of a single trained educator may be multiplied.

3     Empowerment: it may be seen as right that young people should themselves control the process of education.

Careful consideration of the literature suggested that peer education is unlikely to fulfil all the hopes that it tends to inspire. There is evidence of some success in school and similar settings (Gartner, Kohler and Riessman, 1971; Gerber and Kauffman, 1981). In particular, peer-led education has been an element in many, but not all, successful school-based substance abuse prevention programmes (Flay, 1985).

However, the literature also indicates that benefits cannot be expected automatically. Research on school-based peer tutoring schemes strongly suggests that, provided schemes are properly thought out and administered, they are very good — for the peer tutors. Benefits to their tutees are more problematic. (Strodtbeck, Ronchi and Hansell, 1976; Gerber and Kauffman, 1981). Peer education in community work is a new phenomenon, and documentation tends to be informal. Despite voices claiming that it does work, published evaluations are apt to turn out to be evaluations of the training of peer educators, typically followed by a note to the effect that some peer-led education has taken place and it is hoped that more will follow (see Redman, 1987).

There are also consistent complaints that, far from being enabling, peer education delivers a dull, mechanical, top-down style of teaching (Gartner, Kohler and Riessman, 1971; Allen, 1976; Gerber and Kauffman, 1981). Peer educators have often been valued for their docility in adopting their trainer's methods exactly (Klepp, Halper and Perry, 1986). Moreover, it seems to be a mistake to look for savings. Proper training and organization are as costly as direct teaching. Levin, Glass and Meister (1987) found that peer tutoring was the most cost-effective of several interventions designed to improve performance in schools, but also one of the most expensive.

Thus it appears that evidence of success in schools is being used to promote the impression that this is a proven methodology, despite the lack of support for the assumption that it can be transplanted to the very different conditions of community settings. Moreover, evidence of benefits to peer educators has been accepted as evidence that the method works, even in contexts where any hope of an acceptable return on expenditure depends on benefits extending to the end-users, the pupils of the peer educators.

Ideally, all this wisdom should have been available at the planning stage. In practice, it was communicated to the projects about a year after they were set up. By this time, one project had dropped out, and the other three were all finding their briefs difficult to implement. One, alarmed at the prospect of employing young people to work unsupervised on the streets, had diverted its resources into a college setting, another was bogged down in disputes over what the worker was expected to do, and the third was almost at a standstill through recruitment problems. This confirmed the conclusion that could be drawn from the literature review: that peer education was much more difficult to practise successfully than was generally admitted.

The First Interim Report to the HEA argued that by deviating from their briefs and experimenting with different ways of involving young people in HIV/AIDS education of their peers, the projects were responding to their situation in the most constructive way possible. They should be encouraged to continue, and not expected to stick rigidly to unrealistic specifications. That conclusion was very useful to the sponsors, the HEA and the project teams. Morale within the projects and communications between them and the HEA improved in consequence of more realistic expectations.

### Attitudes to Training Peer Educators

One project came to an agreement whereby two part-time youth workers managed a team of peer educators, while overall responsibility remained with the Health Authority. Problems arose. Lines of communication were long and difficult, and the health promotion officer responsible for managing the project complained that it was hard to know what, if anything, was being achieved. The evaluation team responded to this situation by carrying out individual interviews with the two youth workers and as many of the peer educators as were available. A factual report was prepared, and submitted to the youth workers and peer educators for their comments. Then a 'discussion and recommendations' section was added, and the report sent to youth workers, peer educators, management both for the Health Authority and the Youth Service and the funders.

This concluding section noted the general high level of enthusiasm and commitment and the general agreement that after initial difficulties the team was now functioning well. However, it also pointed out that the young people seemed more aware than the youth workers of outstanding problems, particularly that the training seemed haphazard and disorganized, and highlighted two areas where there seemed to be a conflict between the youthwork tradition and the expectations of the Health Authority management.

One of these was the attitude to written records. The two youth workers appeared to have no concept of how frustrating the non-appearance of these was to their management. The other, more interesting problem concerned continuity and attitudes to young people. The report observes:

> The Youth Service tradition appears to rely heavily on aiming to provide a valuable experience for whoever happens to be present on a particular occasion. This is an appropriate goal in settings where people are attending voluntarily in their leisure time. However, the Information Workers are employees; they have been promised training and then

work, of an important nature; they are entitled to expect a structured, purposeful experience.[1]

The report goes on to note that the problem of reconciling empowerment with legitimate demands that peer educators should deliver acceptable education at reasonable expense has generally been evaded in the literature, but in this case:

> the task of defining objectives and planning the project seems to have been avoided by expecting the young people to take on more decision-making and planning than they could reasonably be expected to cope with, with disheartening results for the young people.

Thus the problem was traced to conflicting professional traditions, compounded by the unrealistic and incompatible expectations that flourish in the area of peer education and had already been elucidated by the evaluation.

### Theories of Networking

In the later stages of the evaluation, the evaluation team were engaged in drawing together various forms of information on networking. It occurred to them that the term was used with great confidence and enthusiasm, but without definition and possibly not always in the same sense. A letter was sent to six people, one manager and one worker on each project, asking how they would define the term *networking* and how it had contributed to their project. The replies were prompt, and in most cases quite lengthy, suggesting that this was a topic of considerable interest. There was agreement that networking involves making contacts between individuals and organizations with common goals, to share information and other goods for mutual advantage. However, the report also noted:

> there are two ways of understanding networking as an ideologically motivated activity; it can be seen as egalitarian and community-based as opposed to the authoritarian and hierarchical; it can also be understood as a means of effecting a shift in level of functioning from individual fragmented organisations to the super-organisation created by the network. This last approach assumes that objectives are shared, and that increased efficiency will be to the benefit of all.

> It seems likely that some people who are enthusiastic about self-publicity, or the more non-committal forms of co-operation, might have reservations about one or both of the last two objectives.

It must be admitted that so far we have no evidence that the discovery of divergent concepts of networking is of interest to anyone except ourselves.

Thus it appears that elucidation of theory, as one might expect, is of immediate utility only when differences or inadequacies of theory are giving rise to identifiable problems. Moreover, the problems must arise in such a way that theoretical elucidation can help towards a solution. In the case of networking, everyone was satisfied with their own practice and not concerned to interfere with anyone else's, so the discovery that some of them were working on different theories was of academic interest only. In the case of attitudes to training peer educators, the manager was in a position to respond to the evidence that the youth workers were functioning inadequately by appointing a person who seemed to him more likely to be effective; theories about why the youth workers were failing were therefore redundant. However, our work on theories of peer education was offered in a situation of complex but fairly evenly balanced tension between the HEA and some managers, who expected to see briefs carried out to specification, and project workers who felt that what they were doing was right and sensible (though in one case it was a manager who was in conflict with the HEA). The evaluation's analysis of the dilemma was sufficient to tip the balance and convince the HEA that it was better to let the workers follow their own intuitions.

### Findings that can be Utilized

By working closely with projects, and concentrating on small-scale evaluation initiatives closely linked to project activities, the evaluation team were able to produce findings that were of use in the life of the projects. This utility was chiefly in three areas, morale, organization and publicity.

### Morale

At an early stage in its development, one project appeared to be making no progress at all. Its attempts to recruit peer educators had met with little success, and such support as was forthcoming had rapidly fallen away. Since a solid team of peer educators was a prerequisite for all the other plans, this was very frustrating and discouraging.

At the suggestion of one of the evaluation team, this project started keeping *visual network charts* of all contacts made. This revealed a total of 296 contacts, in categories ranging from 'professional health groups' to 'personal friends'. This activity helped to change the perception of the worker and two full-time volunteers of their project as having had no success at all, and so may have been a factor in the successful recruitment that occurred soon after. It may be added that the new perception was not erroneous; once the project started to function successfully, the wide network of contacts already established proved useful in a number of ways, from facilitating access to hard-to-reach groups to offering opportunities for joint initiatives.

### Organization

One of the reports described above was written at the request of the Health Authority official responsible for managing the local project's funding. It recommended that the youth workers should receive additional support in the areas where they seemed most to need it: the keeping of adequate records and the provision of an organized and purposeful experience for the young people. This report, in conjunction with other events occurring around the same time, was partly responsible for a reorganization in which the agreement between the Health Authority and the Education Authority was terminated, the two youth workers were redeployed elsewhere, and the team of peer educators was reconstituted under the management of one of their own number, who was directly responsible to the Health Authority.

This episode shows that stakeholders, or at least some stakeholders, can identify information that would be of use to them, but it also illustrates the limitations of the stakeholder approach. The evaluators could be democratic in their choice of interviewees and in their insistence on checking that these were satisfied they were not being misreported. However, their findings were used within a power structure in which decisions are the prerogative of management.

### Publicity

One of the projects produced a magazine, *Sex: The Ins and Outs*, which was deliberately light-hearted and non-moralistic in approach, while providing sound information on such matters as safer sex and the availability of HIV testing facilities. Each copy contained a free condom. The object was to distribute this magazine free to as many as possible of the target age group in the area. The publication gave rise to a good deal of publicity, not all of it favourable. In particular, a newspaper headline, 'Condoms for Kids: 10,000 free with school sex mag', gave the impression that the magazine and its contents were being distributed to schoolchildren generally, not just to the over-sixteens. The evaluation team assessed the impact of the magazine on the target age group by carrying out focus group interviews in the area. The report on the responses, which were strongly favourable to the magazine and its approach, was used by the HIV Prevention Co-ordinator who had organized the production, to publicize the magazine and rebut the criticisms that had been made.

The peer education project, being multi-site, inchoate and characterized by emergent activities, was of the kind that Weiss (1986a: 155) suggests should be more amenable to the stakeholder approach than to conventional evaluation. Our stakeholder approach was not as formal as some authorities recommend. Guba and Lincoln (1989: 50), for instance, suggest written agreements with identified stakeholders. The circumstances under which we started work made a more tentative approach seem appropriate. However, we did make known from the start our hope that the evaluation initiatives could be co-operatively planned, that projects would suggest what information would be of use to them and that our commitment to the principle that findings were to be shared and revisions of drafts negotiated and agreed.

Our experience confirms our belief that we were right to adopt this approach. As the preceding sections make clear, we were able to produce findings, including theoretical findings, that were of real utility to other stakeholders. However, implementation was not straightforward and not totally successful. Not all of our findings were seen as what was needed at the time. We find ourselves with four questions that require careful consideration by anyone proposing to adopt a stakeholder approach.

*Is it possible to treat stakeholders democratically?*
It is implicit in the stakeholder approach that stakeholders can be identified, and when identified can each be given an equal voice, or at least a voice proportional to the size of their stake, in decisions about the conduct of the evaluation. In practice, we did not succeed in doing this, and would question whether it can be done.

The HEA, as funding body, was obviously a stakeholder, but in some respects it seemed to be several stakeholders. Three departments were involved in the management of the project and the evaluation. These groups were effectively outside the scope of the evaluation. They were stakeholders, but they were not part of the evaluation. Moreover, evaluation findings were used in the negotiations within the HEA that led to the extension of the Project, and this involved groups of which the evaluators had no knowledge. Thus there may be a class of stakeholder, in this and other evaluations, that is not accessible to the evaluation, yet has access to confidential findings and is able to use them in ways that seriously affect the interests of other stakeholders.

At the other end of the continuum, the public, the largest and arguably the most important stakeholder group, is too amorphous an entity to be consulted. This problem will arise with the evaluation of any project funded with public money for the benefit of the public. It is possible to list the public, or a section of the public, as a stakeholder; in practice it is not possible to give the public a voice in the sense that an individual or a small group can be given a voice. It is, of course, possible to sample those members of the public most affected, but even this presents difficulties, both practical and theoretical. Random sampling may miss the impact of a small project altogether; this was one reason why the idea of a formal, quantitative evaluation was abandoned at the outset. The alternative is to track down end-users who are known to have been in contact with the project, but this does not mean they are given a voice in the same sense as project workers, managers are given a voice for two reasons: there are powerful forces working towards systematic bias in the sample, and there are limitations on their ability to exercise their rights.

Marginalized groups by definition include the drifting and the inarticulate. The more marginalized a group is, the more dependent a researcher is on gatekeepers. In this Project, we were also dependent on project workers to put us in touch with suitable gatekeepers. In this situation, and working at a distance, it is not easy without hindsight to distinguish between a genuinely cooperative person who is scrupulously observing the rights of, for instance, children in care and someone who is skilled at sounding courteous and helpful without actually intending to do anything. Both entail numerous phone calls and long delays; you can only tell the difference when you eventually make an appointment or despair of making one.

The problem of inarticulate and uncooperative subjects is even harder to solve. We chose techniques — repertory grids and informal interview — that seemed least threatening and most likely to minimize differences in intelligence and verbal competence between subjects. Yet some of the interviewees found a request to make the comparisons which the grid method requires 'like school' and withdrew cooperation. So our findings are inevitably biased towards the more articulate and cooperative, because in the last resort it is impossible to give due weight to a point of view that is not expressed.

We also had to accept that participation is work, and work that cannot be expected of all stakeholders. Our stakeholders ranged from executives, who regarded reading, studying and commenting on reports as a normal part of a day's work, to illiterate and barely-literate young people to whom such an exercise would be unfamiliar and intimidating. In practice, we tailored our demands for participation to what seemed reasonable. We assumed that workers and managers could read reports and pestered them mercilessly for responses. When we interviewed peer educators, we sent drafts of our reports to gatekeepers, asked them to ensure that the young people saw them, and enquired later whether there were comments or corrections. When we tracked down end-users, we made sure that our report was seen by the gatekeepers, with a request to make it available to the young people, but we did not solicit comments. In fact, version A, the repertory grid we used, while it has built-in controls to ensure that the opinions recorded are those of the subject not the interviewer, does not readily allow checking by individual subjects once the results have been processed.

A further problem was that our stakeholders were not a closed group that could be listed once and for all at the outset. The community approach involves continual networking, so that new stakeholders were always appearing, as gatekeepers of young people's organizations, as volunteers, as collaborators, as co-funders, and in many other roles. No theoretically adequate way of dealing with this situation was found. In the last resort, it can only be said that the evaluators collaborated with as many stakeholders as they were able to identity and include.

Perhaps the most serious problem is that we were attempting to be democratic in an undemocratic setting. The example is discussed above (see *Findings that can be Utilized and Organization*) where youth workers were not providing adequate support and direction for a team of peer educators. Our report recommended that the youth workers should be given extra help and support, but instead they were taken off the project. The evaluation could attempt to be democratic, but they had no control over how their findings were used; this was determined by the existing power structure.

*Can evaluators and other stakeholders work cooperatively together?*
It was the declared and genuine intention of the evaluation to be responsive to the needs and wishes of the projects, but such an intention is not easily communicated in circumstances approximating an arranged marriage. Project teams and evaluators were obliged by the terms of their contracts to interact with each other, and the projects knew it was the function of the evaluation to report on them. At the beginning, our declared openness to suggestions was interpreted as reluctance to come clean about what we were really up to, and suggestions about what might be useful were interpreted as commands.

The process of establishing and developing good working relations continued throughout the lifetime of the project. After several months, we were sufficiently trusted for our requests for suggestions to be taken seriously, but then we discovered that stakeholders differed enormously in their ability to specify what would be useful information. One had a particularly positive view of the role of evaluation and took up the offer with enthusiasm. Most of the others, while being friendly to us, still seemed to take the understandable view that the less they saw of evaluators the better.

Even when projects were able to specify information, it was not always within the power of the evaluators to provide it when it was wanted. Moreover, the value to the projects was often more in the exercise of collecting the information than in anything the evaluation could provide by way of processed feedback. This was particularly true of evaluation suggestions that projects should trace networks of contacts and log telephone calls. The evaluators naively assumed that, since informal recording of networks had been found useful, more systematic recording and analysis of the same information would be even more welcome. The project workers found the exercises tedious and rightly complained that the evaluation reports of them were out of date and told them nothing that they did not know already.

When stakeholders know what question they want asked, they tend also to know what answer they want given. They are likely to be seeking confirmation of an optimistic hunch rather than objective information on a specific point. A happy example of this, concerning the report on the magazine readership, has already been given. Another case was less satisfactory.

The manager of one of the projects suggested that the project worker had influenced the intersectoral policy adopted for the area, particularly through a presentation he had given at one of a series of workshops, which were organized by the Health Promotion Unit with the expressed aim of establishing a community-wide HIV prevention strategy for the district. The evaluators duly identified those who had been at the presentation and asked for their recollections and reactions. The results of this exercise were highly favourable to the worker, who appeared to have given a star performance. This was not only remembered months afterwards but had influenced the day-to-day practice of several people. However, the report pointed out that through no fault of his own he could not be said to have influenced intersectoral policy, because the workshops did not attract the response that had been hoped for and no recognizable policy or strategy had emerged.

This led to a complaint that in addition to evaluating the impact of the worker we had evaluated the take-up of the workshops and done so unfairly; in reply we stressed we were not evaluating the Health Promotion Unit, but were obliged to explain why the worker had not fulfilled the claim made on his behalf. The issue was not satisfactorily resolved.

Another problem is how far the evaluation agenda can and should be shaped by the relative responsiveness of stakeholders to requests for suggestions. Evaluators have an obligation to attempt an overall assessment of the evaluant; where this cannot be exhaustive, it should as far as possible be balanced and representative of all relevant aspects. This can be difficult to reconcile with responsiveness.

One aspect of this problem emerged when the draft of the second interim report was compiled. In consequence of the different responses to the suggestion that projects should specify what information would be useful, the evaluators had distributed their time very unevenly; this was apparent in the unequal space devoted to reporting the different projects. This appears to be due to differences in individuals' perceptions of evaluation and in their confidence in their ability to formulate appropriate questions. Thus it seems that paradoxically the stakeholder approach may work against its own prime objective of empowering all stakeholders equally; in practice it may favour the confident and articulate, who already feel empowered.

Another aspect arose over timing. As has been explained, at first our efforts to be responsive met with little success. As time went by, more suggestions were forthcoming, but by now the evaluation was moving into its final, summative phase and had to consider what parts of its task were in danger of being neglected. Thus we moved from asking in vain for suggestions to finding ourselves unable to follow up all that were made.

The form taken by the problem of timing in the later stages arose partly from the nature of the project, with its bias towards community settings and disadvantaged or marginalized communities, and its emphasis on peer education. We found we had allowed these to cause an imbalance in our coverage of the project. Project workers necessarily keep in close touch with peer educators, training them and helping them to manage their work. The recipients of peer educators are relatively peripheral, sometimes meeting the educators for one or at most two workshops, sometimes contacted only through products such as magazines and videos. Thus it came about that, partly in consequence of our policy of working closely with projects, we found ourselves open to the criticism we had made of other evaluations: we were evaluating the process, the training and management of peer educators, while the outcome, the impact on end users, for the most part eluded us. This bias had to be corrected in the last stages of the evaluation by a strenuous and expensive attempt to track down and interview young people who had been exposed to project workshops.

We selected the repertory grid, supplemented by informal interviews, as the most appropriate tool for this purpose, and the difficulty of tracking down end-users was consequently increased by the need to do considerable work researching and piloting this method to adapt it to the particular needs of this project. This naturally exacerbated our problems of timing, so that at times it seemed as if our subjects would be lost beyond recall before we managed to interview them.

We found that consultation and co-operation with the projects was of real value, both in building good relations and in eliciting suggestions that we would not have thought of ourselves. On the other hand, a responsive evaluation requires continual planning, monitoring and replanning if it is to perform its task adequately, and this planning is obviously the proper job of the evaluation, not the other stakeholders. It follows that the obligation to produce a comprehensive, balanced evaluation, if accepted, must be seen as a constraint upon responsiveness.

*Does this approach result in findings that are owned by the stakeholders and derive credibility from the participatory process?*
Evaluators set out to be objective. This is not likely to be entirely compatible with giving people what they want. It is normal to want good reports about oneself and objective information about other people. On the whole, our reports seemed to be valued, not for the interactive labour that had been put into them, but insofar as they said what the recipients wanted to hear. Where there had been more than usual feed-back it was usually, as in the example above on intersectoral policy, because there was dissatisfaction.

Furthermore, it is not reasonable to assume that all stakeholders want evaluation findings equally. Weiss (1986b) points out that decision-makers, from the nature of their work, have uses for evaluation findings; other groups may be more concerned to check that they are not being misrepresented than to make any positive use of findings. It is no coincidence that the project that was most responsive to our utility-focused approach was the one where the key person was a manager, not a project worker.

The question of credibility is complex. It is a matter of debate what are the proper criteria for testing the findings of a stake-holder oriented evaluation. Guba and Lincoln argue that positivist criteria should be abandoned entirely, in favour of those arising out of the interactive process. 'It is the immediate and continuing interplay of information that militates against the possibility of non-credible outcomes' (Guba and Lincoln, 1989: 244). We have not gone so far, partly because we have not experienced the fierce interplay of competing interest that is implied here, but also because we believe that though absolute truth may be unattainable, the concept of objectivity still has meaning, and our findings can be measured against standards of wider and more enduring application than the consensus of those immediately involved.

Thus we would not concede that the credibility of our findings depends on the interactive process, but we would say that it is enhanced by it. At a detailed level, submitting reports to those described in them is the simplest and most reliable way of eliminating trivial inaccuracies. At a more important level, although we have not been able to adhere entirely to the principles of responsiveness and utility, we are confident we have kept in touch with what the projects are about. We know we have not been taking a tapemeasure to measure boiling point. The process of consultation has ensured that, though we have often had to take decisions that in theory should have been negotiated, those decisions have been informed by an understanding of what is relevant to the current activities of the projects.

*Is it possible for one team of evaluators to be as responsive as the stakeholder principle implies?*
It is normal practice for funders to select a team of evaluators whose skills seem appropriate to the evaluant. If a team offers a responsive, stakeholder-oriented approach, this is effectively an offer to place any reputable research technique at the disposal of the stakeholders. This is a bold undertaking both for the team and for the whole evaluation.

In the course of this evaluation we used quantitative and open-ended surveys, individual, focus-group and telephone interviews, participatory observation and repertory grids, as well as such activities as literature reviews, attending meetings and keeping site contact sheets. These occasions also had to be used as opprtunities for less structured observation and inquiry into the changing circumstances and activities of the projects.

Many of these skills and techniques had to be mastered before they were deployed. So much variety not only made the researcher feel that as soon as she was nearing competence in one activity she was reduced to a novice at another, but it exacerbated the problem of time-lag, as when the interviewing of end-users had to be delayed until preliminary work on the grid method was complete.

Moreover, the negotiation of a stakeholder-oriented evaluation is a skill in its own right, a skill more akin to facilitation than to research as conventionally understood, and this too had to be developed in the course of the project.

An alternative arrangement might be for responsive evaluators to confine themselves to a coordinating role, identifying evaluation needs and the skills appropriate to meet them, and delegating the actual performance to specialists in the particular skill required. There are two objections to such a solution. First, the recruitment and commissioning of an evaluation team is generally a lengthy business. Unless the relevant institutions changed a lot, recruiting experts might well entail more time-lag than the self-retraining we have undertaken. Second, such specialists would start without background knowledge of the project and take what they acquired away with them, so that, though there might be some gain in professionalism, it would be at the expense of the rich process of mutual education that has made this evaluation not only a satisfying experience to the participants but, we hope, a source of valuable insights to others.

## Conclusions

We feel we have justified our claim that this approach was appropriate to this project. Our decision to include theory within our brief was particularly valuable because of the circumstances under which the project was set up. Individual stakeholders varied enormously in their commitment to and understanding of peer education. It is no criticism of them to say that, seeing an urgent need for HIV/AIDS education, they consented to be huddled under a flag of convenience that promised speedy funding, but it is not surprising that many of them subsequently found themselves under pressure to do things they could not do or did not think it right to do. With hindsight, it seems possible that even more evaluation time might profitably have been spent elucidating the conflicting and often unreasonable expectations associated with peer education. Our utility-focused, interactive approach also fit in well with a project that was engaged in making a whole out of scattered and very diverse parts; the evaluation both profited from and contributed to this process.

Another strength of our approach was that it enabled us to track a moving target and tailor our activities to the projects as they developed, not as they were intended to develop. It would obviously not have been possible to plan to interview readers before the decision to produce a magazine had been taken or design the follow-up to a presentation when the event for which the presentation was prepared had not been considered. The fact that we were a small team undertaking many roles and many methodologies was a strength here, since it enabled us to gain intimate informal knowledge of the projects' circumstances and style of working. This was particularly valuable in view of the problems that have been associated with the external evaluation of HIV/AIDS education; trust could be built up over a long period and through many types of contact.

However, it will be clear that our approach is no ready-made solution. The requirement to be responsive is very demanding, for both stakeholders and evaluators. It has to be accepted that only an ideal stakeholder can specify information needs that translate into practicable evaluation procedures, and only an ideal evaluator could respond appropriately to every reasonable request.

Many of our dilemmas over utility and stakeholders arose from our attempt to combine approaches that appeared compatible or even inclusive of each other, but are based on opposing ideological assumptions. Though a utility-focused approach involves stakeholders and a stakeholder-oriented approach presupposes an emphasis on utility, the two differ profoundly in the attitude they take to power and hierarchical organization. If your priority is utility, you will look for 'quality participation' (Patton, 1986: 334). This implies that you will concentrate on securing the cooperation of the stakeholders most likely to supply it. If, on the other hand, our main concern is that all the interests that are affected should be justly represented regardless of relative power, then you will take positive steps to ensure that factors like lack of communication skills or lack of organization do not prevent individuals or groups from having an equal voice (Guba and Lincoln: 203). It will be clear that our practice was a pragmatic compromise between the two. We made all the effort we could to ensure that the inarticulate and inaccessible were heard. On the other hand, we accepted that not all stakeholders are equally able or willing to participate in evaluation, and our responsiveness necessarily depended on the extent to which the offer to be responsive was taken up.

Also, it must be sadly admitted that there is a certain unreality about attempting to be democratic in a hierarchical context. We are indebted to our funders, the HEA, for trusting us and allowing us to work in our own way, but we were working within a situation of centralized power, in which the projects were obliged to cooperate with us as a condition of their on funding. On the two occasions we know of when our findings were used by the HEA within the life of the project, the decision to terminate one contract and the decision to extend the other three conuacts, we were happy about the use to which our work was put, but nonetheless in both cases we were contributing to an exercise of power, not a democratic decision. The same applied within the projects, as in the case described above, when we recommended that workers should be given extra support, but instead they were taken off the project.

Nevertheless, there are two things to be said in favour of our method. First, it was feasible. The project had been turned down by more conventional evaluators as too small, too scattered and too diverse to be amenable to evaluation The fact that we were able to evaluate it at all says much for our approach. Second, to a remarkable degree, it worked, in the sense that it enabled us to deliver as much useful information as could reasonably be hoped for. Good relations were established with the projects, to the extent that they and the evaluation have been able to work collaboratively on a publication. Findings have been of real use within the life of the project. Last, the participatory method has ensured that our findings are relevant to what the projects have actually been doing. Their work has been so exploratory and innovative that any attempt to apply criteria that had been laid down at the outset would have been meaningless. Our way of working has obliged us to keep in close touch with the changing experience and development of the projects, and in consequence we are in a position to report on the strengths and weaknesses of what actually happened, unhampered by preoccupation with what was expected to happen three or more years earlier.

## Acknowledgements

The Community Youth Project HIV/AIDS and the evaluation, including the preparation of this chapter, has been funded by the Health Education Authority, London.

## Note

1  Quotations, unless otherwise attributed, are from the evaluators' final report to the Health Education Authority, by Ian S. Peers, Frank Ledwith and Margaret Johnston.

## References

AGGLETON, P. (1989) 'Evaluating health education about AIDS', in AGGLETON, P., HART, G. and DAVIES, P., *AIDS: Social Representations, Social Practices*, London: The Falmer Press.

ALKIN, M.C., DAILLAK, R. and WHITE, P. (1979) *Using Evaluations: Does Evaluation Make a Difference?*, London: Sage.

ALLEN, VERNON L. (ed.) (1976) *Children as Teachers: Theory and Research on Tutoring*, New York: Academic Press.

BICKMAN, L. (1987) 'The functions of program theory', in BICKMAN, L. (Ed.) *Using Program Theory in Evaluation: New Directions for Program Evaluation*, San Francisco, CA: Jossey-Bass.

CHEN, H.T. and ROSSI, P.H. (1981) 'The multi-goal, theory-driven approach to evaluation: A model linking basic applied social science', in FREEMAN, H.E. and SOLAMON, M.A. (Eds) *Evaluation Studies Review Annual Vol.6*, Beverley Hills, CA: Sage.

COCHRAN, N. (1980) 'Society as emergent and more than rational: an essay on the inappropriateness of program evaluation', *Policy Sciences*, 12, 2, pp. 113-29.

DAVIDSON, P. (1980) 'Evaluating lifestyle changes programs', in DAVIDSON, P.O. and DAVIDSON, S.M. (Eds) *Behavioural Medicine: Changing Health Lifestyles*, New York: Bruner/Mazel.

FLAY, B.R. (1985) 'Psychosocial approaches to smoking prevention: A review of findings', *Health Psychology*, 4, 3, pp. 449-88.

GARTNER, A., KOHLER, M.C. and RIESSMAN, F. (1971) *Children Teach Children: Learning by Teaching*, New York: Harper & Row.

GERBER, M. and KAUFFMAN, J.M. (1981) 'Peer tutoring in academic settings', in STRAIN, P.S. (Ed.) *The Utilization of Classroom Peers as Behaviour Change Agents*, New York: Plenum Press.

GUBA, E.G. and LINCOLN, Y.S. (1981) *Effective Evaluation*, San Francisco, CA: Jossey-Bass.

GUBA, E.G. and LINCOLN, Y.S. (1989) *Fourth Generation Evaluation*, London: Sage.

HEILEMAN, J.G. (1989) 'Theory driven evaluation: How conceptions of personal choice and organisational process can inform studies of everyday conversation', *Evaluation and Program Planning*, 12, pp. 113-20.

HOUSE, E.R. (Ed.) (1989) *New Directions in Educational Evaluation*, London: The Falmer Press.

JOINT COMMITTEE ON STANDARDS FOR EDUCATIONAL EVALUATION, (JCSE) (1981) *The Standards for Evaluation of Educational Programs, Projects and Materials*, New York: McGraw-Hill.

KLEPP, K-I., HALPER, A. and PERRY, C.L. (1986) 'The efficacy of peer leaders in drug abuse prevention', *Journal of School Health*, 56, 9, pp. 407-11.

LEVIN, H.M., GLASS, G.V. and MEISTER, G.R. (1987) 'Cost-effectiveness of computer-assisted instruction', *Evaluation Review*, 11, 1, pp. 50-72.

PARLETT, M. and HAMILTON, D. (1976) 'Evaluation as illumination: A new approach to the study of innovatory programs', in GLASS, G.V. (Ed.) *Evaluation Studies Review Annual 1979*, Beverley Hills, CA: Sage.

PATTON, M.Q. (1978, second edn. 1986) *Utilization-focused Evaluation*, Beverley Hills, CA: Sage.

PATTON, M.Q. (1987) *Creative Evaluation*, (second edition), London: Sage.

REDMAN, J. (1987) 'AIDS and peer teaching', *Health Education Journal*, 46, 4, pp. 150-1.

ROSSI, P.H. and LYALL, K. (1976) *Reforming Public Welfare*, New York: Russel Sage.

ROSSI, P.H. and FREEMAN, H.E. (1989) *Evaluation: A Systematic Approach*, (fourth edition), Beverley Hills, CA: Sage.

SCHWARTZ, P.A. (1980) 'Program devaluation: Can the experienced reform?' in LOVELAND, E. (Ed.) *Measuring the Hard-to-Measure, New Directions for Program Evaluation, Vol 6*, San Francisco, CA: Jossey-Bass.

SHADISH, W.R. (1987) 'Program micro- and macrotheories: A guide for social change', in BICKMAN, L. (Ed.) *Using Theory in Evaluation: New Directions for Program Evaluation*, San Francisco, CA: Jossey-Bass.

STRODTBECK, F.L., RONCHI, D. and HANSELL, S. (1976) 'Tutoring and Psychological Growth', in Allen (Ed.) (1976).

WEISS, C.H. (1972) 'Utilization and evelution: Toward comparative study', in WEISS, C.H. (Ed.) *Evaluating Action Programs: Readings in Social Action and Education*, Boston, MA: Allyn and Bacon.

WEISS, C.H. (1986a) 'The stakeholder approach to evaluation: Origins and promise', in HOUSE, E.R. (Ed.) *New Directions in Educational Evaluation*, London: The Falmer Press.

WEISS, C.H. (1986b) 'Towards the future of stakeholder approaches in evaluation', in HOUSE, E.R. (Ed.) *New Directions in Educational Evaluation*, London: The Falmer Press.

WHOLEY, J.J. (1987) 'Evaluation assessment: Developing program theory', in BICKMAN, L. (Ed.) *Using Program Theory in Evaluation: New Directions for Program Evaluation*, San Francisco, CA: Jossey-Bass.

ZUSMAN, J. and BISSIONETTE, R. (1973) 'The case against evaluation', *International Journal of Mental Health*, 2, pp. 111-25.

Chapter 12

# Assessing AIDS Preventive Strategies in Europe: Lessons for Evaluative Research

*Kaye Wellings*

Initial attempts at AIDS public education aimed at preventing further spread of HIV amongst the general population were energetic, extensive and often expensive. Because of the precipitate nature of the epidemic and the shortage of time in which to develop and evaluate campaigns, however, such campaigns were often steered more by art than science, and their success determined more by luck than judgement. The sudden onset of this new public health problem made it difficult to set in place the necessary evaluative procedures and often resulted in hasty preparation of evaluation work in most countries.

All too often, survey work in this area has been haphazard, *ad hoc* and piecemeal; necessary preliminary research has been neglected or omitted and piloting inadequate. The stages of evaluation often classified as *formative* (prior research designed to help the design of the most effective campaign) and *process* evaluation (research designed to measure aspects of dissemination) suffered most in this respect, being strikingly deficient in the evaluation attempts of many countries. The cautionary note of Fishbein and Middlestadt that 'the AIDS epidemic is much too serious to allow interventions to be based on some communicator's untested and all too often incorrect intuitions about the factors that will influence the performance or non-performance in a given population' went largely unheeded at the start of the epidemic.

These, and other difficulties, are amply illustrated in the context of the assessment of HIV/AIDS preventive strategies in Europe. More positively, a review of evaluative techniques in different European countries serves to point up possibilities for overcoming difficulties and generates new ideas for evaluative research. AIDS is now rightly seen as a chronic public health problem rather than an acute national crisis, and as such is in need of sustained prevention efforts. Future public education programmes may lack the urgency and the creative energy of early efforts, but they will hopefully benefit from adjustments made possible by a critical review of past initiatives, so that evaluation will be increasingly important. Assessment of the efficacy of ongoing activities is essential if possibilities are to be created for improvements in the future. The task facing us now is to develop innovative techniques which will redress past problems and to help to establish a climate of open exchange between policymakers and researchers.

The term *general population* is used here in the sense of a heterogeneous mass, undifferentiated in terms of groups or behaviours, so the focus is chiefly on broad spectrum approaches to public education (the main emphasis being on interventions through the mass media). Illustrations are drawn from the EC Concerted Action *Assessing AIDS Preventive Strategies* set up to compare and contrast HIV/AIDS public education approaches, and the methods used to assess them, in order to arrive at a better understanding of how public education in this area might optimally be effected and evaluated. To this end, data have been collected on interventions and their evaluation for selected European countries. The cross national comparison holds valuable lessons for both campaigns and their evaluation, but the concern here is with the latter.

This chapter explores some salient issues in outcome evaluation research, including the methods used and agencies involved and the possibilities for advancing this area of research.

## Outcome Evaluation: Effects, Effectiveness and Efficacy

Examples of some of the shortcomings of evaluative research in the area of AIDS public education are not hard to find. Often, what has passed as outcome evaluation is more properly described as monitoring the *effects* of campaigns, rather than measuring their *effectiveness* or *efficacy*. Inadequately formulated campaign objectives and targets, and a disregard for possible unintended consequences of interventions, have made it difficult for researchers to select valid indicators of effectiveness. A major problem in relation to assessing efficacy has been the perennial one of attributing outcome to intervention, exacerbated in the case of AIDS by the problem of 'background noise' and the impossibility of setting up quasi-experimental 'dose-controlled' methods of evaluation in the context of a serious epidemic. In addition, an over-reliance on studies of knowledge, attitudes and beliefs (KAB) focuses too narrowly on the individual and neglects to assess changes wrought in the social context.

What has passed as outcome evaluation to date in the context of AIDS is probably more properly described as monitoring. In many cases what have been measured have been the *effects* of campaigns (whether they achieved any results at all) rather than their *effectiveness* (whether an intervention achieved its objectives) or *efficacy* (whether it achieved its objectives more effectively than an alternative course of action, or none at all) — this last seen by many as being at the heart of the evaluative process.

*Effectiveness — goal-directed evaluation*

In terms of assessing effectiveness, the formulation of campaign objectives is of utmost importance because they determine not only the campaign components, but also the performance indicators and outcome variables. Evaluation of the effectiveness and efficacy of campaigns requires the use of variables or indicators which provide measures by which the outcomes of interventions and programmes can be assessed, the selection of which is fundamentally dependent on the objectives of a campaign (Heymann and Biritwum, 1990). The primary outcome variable — incidence of HIV infection — is not as yet considered a sensitive indicator for the general population, partly because of the nature of the virus and its long incubation period and partly because of the vagaries of the collecting process, though the time may rapidly be approaching when such a view may need to be revised. In many instances, therefore, intermediate goals of national programmes have constituted the indicators themselves, an increase in condom use, for example, lessening of discrimination against people with HIV. In the case of AIDS and HIV, the proximate outcome variable most relevant to reducing HIV transmission in most situations will be the adoption and maintenance of behaviours that protect uninfected individuals from contracting HIV and prevent infected individuals from transmitting it. Some of the difficulties inherent in this process are listed below:

*Objectives may not be specific and no targets may be set*
Lack of clarity over the scope of the objectives has led to confusion over the measurement procedures in some instances. Alternately, or additionally, haste and a feeling of working in the dark has in some cases prevented the formulation of specific objectives. Effectiveness evaluation requires that targets are set so that success in achieving them can be systematically measured (Valdiserri, 1989). Yet the absence of baseline data from which to measure change has made it difficult to envisage what might be appropriate and relevant targets, for example, 'By the end of the current campaign, to reduce by 25 per cent from base line, the proportion believing that receiving blood transfusions puts one at risk of HIV infection' or 'to reduce to fewer than 10 per cent the number of people who are unaware of the protective effects of condom use'.

Ideally, it would have been beneficial to have been able to draw on an existing stock of knowledge about the sexual behaviour of the general population, yet there was a dearth of relevant surveys to use for this purpose. In the future, projects such as the EC Concerted Actions on Sexual Behaviour and the Risks of HIV Infection and on Assessing AIDS Preventive Strategies should be remedial in this respect.

*The objectives may not be shared by all responsible for the intervention*
With regard to objectives, a consensus has not always existed amongst those involved in interventions. In some countries — in the UK, for example, and in Sweden — AIDS was initially treated as a national emergency. This had

important implications for the manner in which the campaigns were conducted. In such countries, the government retained far more direct control over the interventions, at least initially. Because of a lack of direct practical expertise in the area, civil servants were more likely to defer to the ideals, principles and strategies of the (generally commercial) agencies chosen to execute the campaigns.

As a result, a different set of criteria were applied in judging the success or failure of the campaigns. Generally speaking, commercial agencies earn their accolades as a result of producing advertisements which achieve high levels of impact, awareness and recall, and may have less regard for securing longer term objectives of motivating action and changing attitudes. Such campaigns present difficulties in terms of follow-up and sustainability. Because the primary objective was initial impact rather than sustainability, research instruments used for evaluation failed to measure the campaign's potential for encouraging long term changes in attitudes and behaviour.

*The intervention may result in consequences which are unintended as well as intended*
Surveys using indicators based on official objectives will answer the question 'Did the interventions achieve the intended effects?' but not the question 'Did they achieve other effects?' Common to the aims and objectives of public education in all countries has been the *primary* prevention of HIV — the provision of information on ways in which HIV is and is not transmitted, and on the means by which one can protect oneself. There has been more variation in the emphasis placed on *secondary* and *tertiary* prevention — the removal of unfounded fears and anxieties which would lead to social disruption and the elimination of negative attitudes towards those already affected which could create an unfavourable climate in which prevention and care are effected.

In many countries, change in the social environment to facilitate the prevention and treatment of HIV and AIDS was an explicit aim of the campaigns. In such countries, for example, Germany, Norway, Switzerland, Sweden, France and the Netherlands, solidarity campaigns have been set up to achieve such ends. Even countries in which the emphasis is on primary prevention depend on changes in the social climate in relation to TV advertising, condom availability, etc., for their success. This needs to be taken account of in the evaluation process. The absence of explicit measures of change in the social context has resulted in unforeseen and unintended outcomes (whether favourable or unfavourable), going unrecognized and unrecorded. Evaluative efforts need also to pick up these more felicitous unintended consequences.

The aim of raising awareness and creating an impact have sometimes been at odds with that of creating a facilitative climate in which AIDS prevention and the care and treatment of those with HIV and related illness could be provided. The first British campaign achieved unprecedented success in raising public awareness. This was shown in the survey work following the campaign in which more than 90 per cent of the British public recalled the campaign components.

This survey, however, was not designed to investigate the side effects of this level of concern which were largely unanticipated. In the month following the campaign, attendance for HIV testing at clinics and surgeries increased to unmanageable levels, as letters to the medical journals were to testify. Facilities for neither pre- nor post-test counselling were in place to cope with the deluge which ensued.

Survey methods are not best suited to the task of measuring such an outcome, and efforts must be made to imaginatively exploit other sources. HIV testing data have been used to measure response to public education (Beck *et al.*, 1990) but they also offer a useful proxy measure of such unintended outcomes of campaign initiatives as levels of anxiety. The potential use of routine data to pick up this sort of effect is illustrated in Figure 12.1, and shows the value of broad based surveillance of outcome measures.

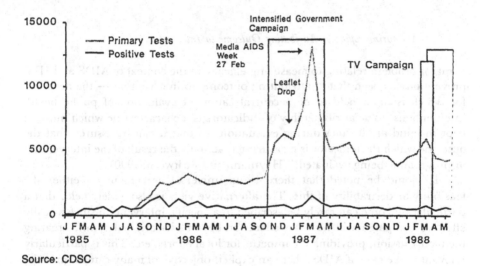

Source: CDSC

*Figure 12.2: HIV antibody tests in England and Wales, January 1985–June 1988*

Not all unintended consequences of interventions are undesirable. The social context in which AIDS public education has been carried out has placed restrictions on what can and cannot be done, but it has, in turn, been influenced by the AIDS epidemic. In particular, AIDS has had implications for health education and sex education in general. For example, as a result of AIDS publicity, the ruling on television advertising of condoms was changed in several countries, including France, the UK and Ireland. In Belgium, in the Netherlands and in the UK, AIDS has had an enabling effect on the provision of sex education.

Where the programme objective of changing the social environment was explicit, evaluation efforts were more likely to take the effect on social context into account. The Swiss, for example, acknowledged the importance of the 'multiplier effect' — the political function of the campaign to persuade teachers, parents, opinion leaders, etc. to play their part in raising awareness, and so have attempted to evaluate this by measuring how many actions have resulted from each campaign. In general, however, this has been a neglected area of evaluation.

Research designed to evaluate campaigns must evaluate the campaign objectives themselves, in addition to whether or not they were successfully achieved. In the past the neglect of this area of research has perhaps been understandable, given that those responsible for the interventions are often also responsible for commissioning the research. If the results of intervention studies are to be used to guide future interventions, attention must be paid to this task in the future.

### Measuring Efficacy: Attributing Outcome to Intervention

A major problem relating to measuring efficacy in the context of AIDS and HIV prevention has been that of attributing outcome to intervention — the necessity for which is often held to be a central canon of evaluation of public health interventions. 'The attributability of indicators is a characteristic which must be kept in mind at all times during evaluation, so that it can be assured that the outcome which the indicator is measuring is actually the result of the intervention or programme being evaluated.' (Heymann and Biritwum, 1990)

It should be noted that there is no universal agreement on either the feasibility or desirability of this. The alternative view is also widely held, that a particular outcome can rarely be ascribed to a specific intervention since a really effective campaign will have an effect far beyond its original remit, creating media discussion, providing the impetus for local efforts, etc. This is particularly relevant in the case of AIDS where an explicit objective of many campaigns was, as stated above, to create a favourable climate in which interventions could be received. The objective of changing the social environment made it especially difficult to disentangle the effects of specific interventions designed to improve knowledge and change attitudes and behaviour in individuals from those aimed more broadly at facilitating a favourable climate in which AIDS public education could take place.

Nevertheless, the policymaker, charged with the task of cost-effective utilization of public resources, understandably wants to know which of the interventions have greatest impact and effectiveness. The researcher's role must be to devise methods of achieving this objective. Methods relying on respondents' retrospective reports of gains in knowledge, changes in attitudes or modifications of behaviour as a result of the campaign in question have often been the only available ones, because of the absence of base line data, yet suffer seriously from the biases introduced by the desirability response, by recall difficulties, and a lack of specificity in terms of meaning. Pre- and post-test surveys and tracking surveys (involving repeating the same set of questions at intervals of similarly selected samples) offers some improvement but provides no assurance that what is being measured is the effect of a particular intervention and not a generalized response to the AIDS epidemic.

The more rigorous quasi-experimental methods, using phased implementation, randomized field experiments, the application of media weight bias, or simple random assignment of individuals to one group or another (by which one group exposed to the intervention is compared with a control group with no such exposure) have, to date, been contra-indicated in the case of AIDS-preventive strategies. Initially, there were definite practical, political, ethical and, in some cases, economic obstacles to the implementation of these strategies. The 'dose-controlled approach' requires time to implement and so was contra-indicated by the precipitate nature of the epidemic and the urgency and haste with which response needed to be made. In addition, the urgent need for the data made it morally indefensible to deny people interventions in the interests of scientific accuracy. Further, quasi-experimental designs are difficult to apply to mass media campaigns because ideally, and by definition, virtually everyone is exposed to them. Most important, the success of the experimental approach depends on being able to ensure that observed differences in outcomes between treatment and control group do not arise from any other factors than the intervention under investigation.

In the case of the AIDS epidemic, the usual problem of interference was heightened. Public knowledge was accumulating, through media coverage, commercial advertising, etc., at such a pace that even a short time lag could result in a change in measures with or without intervention. Not only has it been difficult to separate out the effects of national campaigns from the effects of national news coverage, but overspill between countries has made it difficult to separate out the effects of one national campaign from another. In Ireland, for example, 75 per cent of households receive British TV and so the Irish public had been heavily exposed to British campaigns before the start of their own in 1987 (Harkin and Hurley, 1988). Similarly, in the Dutch campaign, the impetus for a general campaign came in part from the public who had seen the British campaigns on their TV screens, and, questioning the absence of such a campaign in the Netherlands, put pressure on the authorities for a similar intervention in their country.

Clearly there have been very real difficulties in prospectively controlling for intervening variables in the evaluation of AIDS-preventive activities. Nevertheless, although experimental design was not feasible, imaginative analysis and interpretation of results has compensated in some cases. Attempts have been made in several countries to attribute outcome to intervention retrospectively. One method of effecting this has been to partially disaggregate the data at the analysis stage using outcome variables to discriminate between those exposed to campaigns and those not. The evaluation of the Dutch 'excuses' campaign designed to encourage condom use, for example, (de Vries *et al.*, 1989), compared responses of those who claimed to have recalled the campaign with those of others who did not. A statistically significant higher level of endorsement of the messages of the campaign, amongst respondents who claimed to have seen the campaign, provides some support for attributing the effects to the campaign. Similar techniques have been used in evaluation of the French campaign to investigate the effect of education on discriminatory attitudes (Moatti *et al.*, 1988). Alternatively, it has been possible to select and measure retention of items of information attributable only to the campaign, for example, in the UK campaigns (Wellings and Orton, 1988).

An essential caveat here is the lack of certainty that some other explanatory variable, such as perception of personal risk, may not be responsible for both sensitizing people to the public education materials, thereby facilitating recall and absorption, at the same time as predisposing them to a change in behaviour. Determinants of variations in exposure, therefore, need to be introduced as explicitly as possible into the analysis and interpretation of results to eliminate the possibility of spurious associations.

Now that the pace of events allows a more considered approach, we are likely to see greater and more widespread application of quasi-experimental approaches to evaluation. These are most likely to take the form of small scale studies isolating one variable, the message of the campaign — for example, the agency selected or the approach adopted. An example is to be found in the work of Canadian researchers in this area who have tested response and reaction to condom leaflets using fear, or humour or a neutral approach (Dube *et al.*, 1993).

### Choice of Research Methods

The methods used to date in the evaluation of AIDS public education campaigns, for the time and urgency reasons already mentioned, have tended to be the old stalwarts. The stock-in-trade of evaluation of public education in relation to the general population, particularly interventions deploying the mass media, has been the knowledge, attitude and behaviour (KAB) survey. Typically, the KAB survey investigates exposure to, recall and comprehension of campaign messages and self reported behaviour change. The methods used, however, have not been wholly appropriate or adequate to the task of measuring these objectives.

KAB surveys have drawbacks in terms of both their theoretical foundations and inherent problems of validity and reliability. In terms of explanatory models for determinants of behaviour, the dominant framework of the KAB survey remains the Health Belief Model, with its attendant drawbacks in terms of neglect of the social context in which health-related behaviour occurs (Fishbein and Middlestadt, 1989). A major disadvantage, as already mentioned, is that since the investigative unit is the individual, such surveys fail to monitor changes wrought in the social environment. In particular they neglect to explore the influence of social, political and ideological factors which may either impede or expedite AIDS public education. Used alone, KAB surveys are not appropriate instruments for the evaluation of changes in the social context, and ideally their findings should be synthesized with those from studies using other approaches, such as work exposing barriers to preventive action.

The main methodological problem of KAB surveys are those of validity and reliability. Most surveys use quota samples which, like all surveys using this selection method, present problems of reliability, since those most likely to be willing to disclose details of their personal opinions and behaviour cannot be taken to be representative of the population as a whole. Nor can they be relied upon to produce responses which always correspond totally with the objective reality of their actions. Surveys of this kind are useful for assessing the impact of campaigns and the knowledge gleaned from them, but they are less reliable in the case of assessing attitudes and behaviour changes, being particularly susceptible to the influence of the social desirability response.

These difficulties were exacerbated in relation to the assessment of HIV/AIDS preventive strategies. One consequence of the sudden onset of the AIDS epidemic was that many evaluations had to be prepared simultaneously with the interventions, leaving little time to develop and pilot research projects. In the panic of the moment, research seemed to abandon established empirical rules and failed to draw on the body of knowledge previously accumulated. Simple methodological principles, those relating to order-effect in question formulation, for example, seemed to be overlooked. Part of a Norwegian survey had to be repeated because of failure to take account of the biasing effect of question order (Kraft and Rise, 1988) and in Sweden inadequate piloting failed to reveal difficulties of understanding certain questions (Brorsson, 1989).

One solution to the problem of bias in the collecting process has been to attempt to triangulate results, to check against other data sources which might provide more objective measures of behavioural change. In this respect, a number of sources have proved useful, condom sales figures have provided a rough and ready guide to trends in condom use, and have been profitably used in France, Switzerland, the UK, Netherlands and the GDR (Figures 12.2–5). Although it cannot be assumed that condom sales figures are necessarily a more reliable source of data, they at least provide a check on self-reported data.

The changing volume of calls to AIDS Helplines has also provided a rough and ready indicator of the level of public interest and involvement in the AIDS issue (Wellings and Orton, 1988). Routinely collected data on the nature of calls to AIDS Helplines has provided information on the target groups reached by the intervention, the need for information and the messages received, the source of information on AIDS and HIV (Danish Health Board, 1988). The use of STD surveillance as surrogate measures of sexual behaviour and in validating self-reports of sexual behaviour also warrants further exploration and exploitation (Renton, 1991).

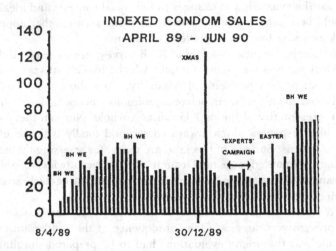

INDEXED CONDOM SALES
APRIL 89 - JUN 90

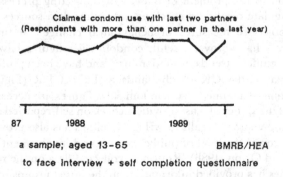

Claimed condom use with last two partners
(Respondents with more than one partner in the last year)

a sample; aged 13–65          BMRB/HEA

to face interview + self completion questionnaire

Figure 12.2:   *Practice of condom use in the UK*

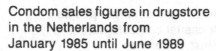

Condom sales figures in drugstore
in the Netherlands from
January 1985 until June 1989

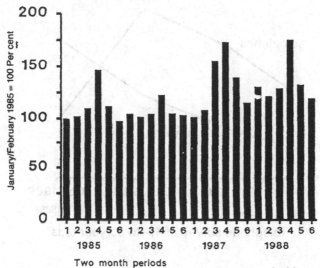

de Vroome *et al.*, 1990

Percentage of respondents who
claim to have used a condom
in the previous six months

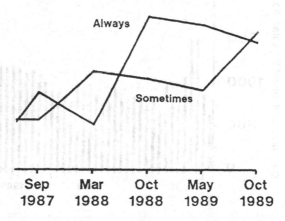

random sample; men and women aged 15–45 years
telephone interviews
de Vroome *et al.*, 1990

*Figure 12.3:  Condom usage in Netherlands*

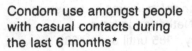

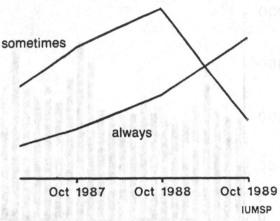

Condom use amongst people
with casual contacts during
the last 6 months*

sometimes

always

Oct 1987     Oct 1988     Oct 1989

IUMSP

Telephone survey of 17- to 30-year-olds

Condom sales in Switzerland
since 1986

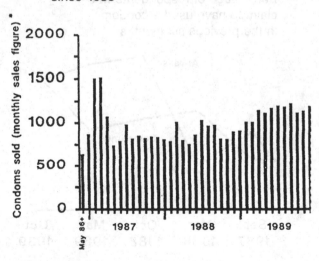

*6 manufacturers representing more than 80 per cent
of the market

+ 1986 figure is a yearly average: IUMSP/GES 199

*Figure 12.4: Knowledge and practice of condom use amongst Swiss youth*

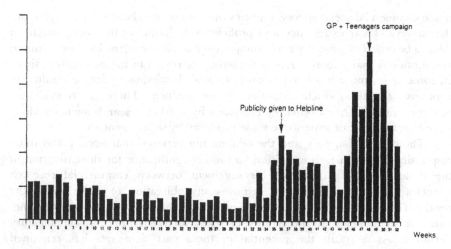

*Figure 12.5:   Call taken per week by Belgian AIDS Helpline, 1989*

Media analysis has also provided a valuable indicator of changes in the social context and interesting projects have been carried out in this area (Paluosa, 1987; Birchmeier and Richard, 1988) though inadequate communication has sometimes prevented the results from being of as much practical use as they might have been.

## Selection of Agency

The choice of agency to carry out the evaluations has proved pivotal in determining the quality of the data produced, the manner in which it was used and its impact on future campaigns. Several models emerge from a survey of different European countries. In the first, those responsible for the campaigns, generally Governmental agencies, have directly commissioned survey work of commercial social research agencies who are required to report directly back to them. This pattern is to be found in the UK, Spain, Denmark and Germany.

A second pattern to emerge is one in which relevant research has been carried out generally by an academic agency, independently of campaign originators and resources, which has formed the basis of evaluation, such as in Sweden (Brorsson, 1989) and in Flemish speaking Belgium (van Hove *et al.*, 1989). A third pattern combines elements of both of these. Those responsible for funding campaigns and programmes also fund an independent evaluation survey; data is collected by a commercial company but the survey is designed and the data analysed and interpreted by academic teams of behavioural scientists as in France, Norway, the Netherlands and Ireland (Moatti *et al.*, 1988; Kraft and Rise, 1988a, 1988b, 1988c; de Vroome *et al.*, 1990, Harkin and Hurley, 1988).

The urgency with which data was needed in the context of HIV prevention made commercial social survey agencies the obvious candidates for carrying out the surveys. Their experience and proficiency in handling the sheer weight of data to be collected gave them advantages over academic agencies. The common assumption is that scientific rigour is thereby sacrificed to the demands of time. In some cases, more haste did mean less speed. Inadequate piloting resulted in expensive mistakes which took time to be rectified. There is no evidence, however, that the questionnaires produced by market research agencies alone were either inferior or superior to those produced by other agencies.

The choice of agency and the relationship between that agency and those responsible for campaign execution had more significance for dissemination of the data. A direct contractual arrangement between commercial research agencies and campaign funders removes any obligation to make public the results. Generally, social research companies are required to produce 'top line' data, or frequencies at the aggregate level, analysed only by classificatory variables. As a result the potential of these vast data sets has remained unexploited in many cases, (as in the case of the UK British Market Research Bureau (BMRB) data, and that produced by Intomart in the Netherlands) and they have either failed to enter the public domain or taken an inordinately long period of time in which to do so. The involvement of academic research teams in data processing, as in France and the Netherlands (the University of Utrecht for the Safer Sex Foundation) has generally resulted in more sophisticated analysis and more useful explanatory insights. In addition, the usual channels of dissemination, through publication in journals or presentation at conferences, ensured that findings have emerged with greater certainty and speed.

There is clearly a political dimension of evaluation since the results may show projects as not as effective as the originators believed they would be. Inevitably, where those commissioning the evaluation and controlling the dissemination have also been responsible for the campaigns, it has been difficult to ensure impartiality.

### Comparability Across Countries

In the context of the measurement of efficacy, the European context might seem to present a kind of laboratory in which evaluation can take place. Cross national comparisons, at first sight, present tempting opportunities for the assessment of different intervention strategies. Yet the constraints of time and budget have prevented the kind of controlled implementation and evaluation which would permit a thorough comparison of the relative effectiveness of different interventions within countries. The multiplicity of different social, cultural, political and health factors operating in the different countries has limited controlled analysis. The practical frustrations of dealing with secondary data quickly become apparent in the context of European comparisons. Direct comparisons are difficult, not only because of different fieldwork dates, but also because of methodological differences between surveys and measurement effects within each. Just as the interventions used in different countries are context specific, so too are the methods used to appraise them. Social and cultural factors play a major part in the selection of methods. Postal surveys amongst the more socially obedient Swedes and Norwegians, for example, dependably produce response rates of 60 per cent or more, while in Britain and Germany response rates of 30 per cent are nearer the norm. Similarly, telephone surveys can be conducted in Switzerland and France safe in the knowledge that more than 95 per cent of the population have a telephone, but the same assumption cannot be made for many other European countries. Differences in wording of questions are substantial and are not simply eliminated by translation. Some of these difficulties are illustrated by looking at the extent of measurement bias in findings from surveys conducted by three different agencies at roughly the same time within the UK.

*Table 12.1: Knowledge of ways in which HIV is transmitted: UK, January 1987.*

|  | MORI<br>Fieldwork:<br>4 Jan 1987<br>*n* = 1004 | GALLUP<br>Fieldwork:<br>24 Jan–3 Feb 1987<br>*n* = 1115 | BMRB<br>Fieldwork:<br>26 Jan–7 Feb 1981<br>*n* = 708 |
|---|---|---|---|
| Coughs and sneezes | 5 per cent | 12 per cent | 3 per cent |
| Insect bites | 40 per cent | 24 per cent | 30 per cent |
| Kissing | 40 per cent | 19 per cent | 10 per cent |
| Sexual intercourse | 94 per cent | 99 per cent | 86 per cent |
| Sharing needles | 98 per cent | 98 per cent | 75 per cent |

MORI: Quota sample; aged 16–54; face-to-face interview in home.
GALLUP: Quota sample; aged 16+ ; face-to-face interview in home.
BMRB: Quota sample; aged 13–59; face-to-face interview in home.

Difficulties of eliminating bias in the research instrument are magnified when comparison is extended to different countries, and make it difficult to make valid comparisons. A further difficulty lies in the fact that there has been no standardization of wording in the KAB surveys conducted in the context of HIV/AIDS prevention in the European countries. There is no guarantee that differences between countries shown in Table 12.2 are real and not an artefact of the methodology.

The ideal solution might seem to be to implement a standard universal cross-national protocol for use in every country, so that methodological differences can be controlled and measurement effect minimized. There are, however, major difficulties involved in developing a common research methodology, some of which are illustrated by efforts in 1987 by Gallup International to achieve this (Gallup, 1988). Despite the best efforts by the parent

Table 12.2: Knowledge of transmission routes in selected European countries.

| | FRA Jun 1987 per cent | GER Feb 1987 per cent | IRE Feb 1987 per cent | NOR Jan 1986 per cent | SPA Jul–Sep 1987 per cent | SWE Mar–Apr 1986 per cent | SWI Apr–May 1986 per cent | UK Feb 1986 per cent |
|---|---|---|---|---|---|---|---|---|
| Sexual intercourse: man and woman | 93.5 | 96.0[1] | 97.0 | 85.0 | 78.0 | — | 88.0 | 62.0 |
| Sexual intercourse: two men | } | } | } | 95.0 | 90.0 | — | } | 95.0 |
| Sharing needles for drug use | 75.4 | 83.0 | 96.0 | 93.0 | 90.0 | — | — | 63.0 |
| Kissing | 10.5 | 41.0 | — | 33.0 | 46.0 | 30.0 | 26.0 | 21.0 |
| Being bitten | 10.0 | 21.0 | — | 21.0 | — | 29.0 | — | 33.0 |
| Shaking hands | 0.5 | 1.0[1] | — | 3.0 | 6.0 | — | 32.0 | 2.0 |
| Sharing drinking and eating utensils | 9.0 | 15.0 | 15.0 | 13.0 | 25.0 | — | } | 11.0 |
| Public toilets | 9.5 | 19.0 | 26.0 | — | 27.0 | 30.0 | 21.0 + + | 7.0 |
| Giving blood | 37.3 | — | 73.0 | 32.0 | — | — | — | 44.0* |
| Receiving blood | — | 87.0 | 91.0 | 95.0 | 89.0 | — | 54.0 | 92.0 |

} Question mentioned only sexual intercourse and did not make distinction between sex with a man and sex between two men.
* Question first asked in November 1986.
- Spontaneous mention.
+ + Question included mention of saunas and swimming pools.

FRA = France: AGORAMETRIE Research Institute (Moatti et al. 1988).
GER = Germany: IfD commissioned by Zeitschrift 'Ja',[1] FORSA 1988, commissioned by Central Office of Health Education.
IRE = Ireland: Irish Marketing Surveys for Health Education Bureau.
NOR = Norway: Markedsog Mediainsitutet for Health Directorate, (Kraft and Rise, 1988b).
SPA = Spain: Centro de Investigaciones Sociologicas (CIS).
SWE = Sweden: Institute for Social Medicine, Uppsala University, (Brorsson, 1989).
SWI = Switzerland: IPSOS
UK = United Kingdom: British Market Research Bureau for Central Office of Information, (DHSS and Welsh Office, 1987).

company to gather standardized data for each country, local survey agencies were ultimately responsible for carrying out the surveys for Gallup, and there were limits to the extent of control which Gallup could exercise in the field. As we have seen, there can be substantial differences attributable to the variation in research agency in any one country and these differences are further exaggerated between countries.

Even when a standard protocol is applied, there is no certainty that its translation will be precise enough to ensure that measurement effects resulting from differences in the attribution of meaning have been controlled. Differences in wording of questions are not simply eliminated by translation. It may be possible to use sexual vernacular in the Netherlands or Denmark, where sexual terms do not double as terms of abuse, but the same words may offend in other countries and could risk reducing the response rate. The difficulties of ensuring standardization and replicability, eliminating bias in the research instrument and in ensuring that populations share a common meaning in order to obtain valid or comparable results in one country are magnified when comparison is extended to different countries.

### Conclusions

What seems clear is that the challenge of evaluation is likely to be best met by collaborative efforts and diverse approaches. It should be the sole responsibility of neither those responsible for implementing preventive interventions nor researchers skilled in evaluating them. Researchers involved in the evaluation of an intervention should be involved from the earliest inception of the campaign intervention, should be informed of its objectives and should carefully devise ways of measuring progress made towards them. Additionally though, they must devise methods to evaluate the objectives themselves, if evaluation is to inform and improve future efforts. They must also look beyond short term goals to the potential for sustained adoption of risk reduction measures in the population.

Although the primary objective of preventive interventions is to achieve a reduction in the number of new HIV infections, and ultimately cases of AIDS, neither of these two goals can as yet be used to develop direct indicators of effectiveness or efficacy. Interim measures — changes in level of knowledge, attitudes and lifestyle — must therefore suffice as proxies. Whatever their defects, surveys are the primary method of evaluating such changes and, if conducted carefully, permit the determination of fundamental trends. Indirect data can be useful in augmenting and validating data from these sources. Among these data are condom sales, helpline data, STD prevalence data and data on HIV testing. By piecing together these data on a national and international comparative basis, evaluative research can make a contribution to the selection, design and execution of appropriate preventive strategies in the general population.

## References

BECK, E.J., DONEGAN, C., KENNY, C. *et al*, (1990) 'An update on HIV-testing of a London sexually transmitted diseases clinic: Long-term impact of the AIDS media campaigns', *Genitourin Med*, 66, pp. 142–7.

BIRCHMEIER, B. and RICHARD, J.E. (1988) SIDA — MEDIA, Rapport Final 1988, Cah Rech Doc IUMSP.

BRORSSON, B. (1989) *Allmanheten och HIV/AIDS; Kunskaper, attityder och beteende 1986–1989*, Rapport Nr 9, Uppsala University.

DANISH HEALTH BOARD, September 1989; Unpublished research report.

DUBE, L., READI, G.B. and DESCOMBES, C. (1993) 'A field study on community efficiency in promoting condom use for AIDS prevention, Poster presentation (POC 22) at the IXth International Conference on AIDS, Berlin.

FISHBEIN, M. and MIDDLESTADT, S.E. (1989) 'Using the theory of reasoned action as a framework for understanding and changing AIDS-related behaviours', in MAYS, V.M., ALBEE, G.W. and SCHNEIDER, S.F. (Eds) *Primary Prevention of AIDS*, Beverley Hills, CA: Sage.

GALLUP REPORT No. 273, (1988) *AIDS*, June.

HARKIN, A.M. and HURLEY, M. (1988) 'National survey on public knowledge of AIDS in Ireland', *Health Education Research*, 3, 1, pp. 25–9.

HEYMANN, D.L. and BIRITWUM, R. (1990) *Evaluation of the Effectiveness of National AIDS Programmes*, GPA, WHO Geneva, 15.01.90.

VAN HOVE, E., KNOPS, N., NEUWINCKEL, S. and POPPE, E. (1989) *Jongeren en AIDS*, Antwerp: Universitaire Instelling Antwerpen.

KRAFT, P. and RISE, J. (1988a) 'AIDS public knowledge in Norway 1986', *NIPH Annals*, 11, 1, June, pp. 19–28.

KRAFT, P. and RISE, J. (1988b), 'AIDS-sources of information and public opinion in Norway 1986', *NIPH Annals*, 11, 1, June, pp. 9–17.

KRAFT, P. and RISE, J. (1988c) 'Public awareness and acceptance of an HIV/AIDS information campaign in Norway', *Health Education Research*, 3, 1, pp. 31–9.

MOATTI, J.P., MANESSE, L., LE GALLES, C., PAGES, J.P. and FAGNANI, F. (1988) 'Social perceptions of AIDS in the general public; a French study', *Health Policy*, 9, pp. 1–8.

PALUOSA, H. (1987) 'AIDS and the media in Finland', paper presented to the 10th International Conference on Social Science and Medicine, Leuwenhorst, The Netherlands.

VALDISERRI, R.O. (1989) *Preventing AIDS: The Design of Effectiveness Programmes*, New Brunswick, Rutgers University Press, p. 250.

DE VROOME, E.M.M., PAALMAN, M.E.M., SANDFORT, Th.G.M. *et al*. (1990) 'AIDS in The Netherlands: The effects of several years of campaigning', *International Journal of STD and AIDS*, 1, pp. 268–75.

WELLINGS, K. and ORTON, S. (1988) 'Evaluation of the HEA public education campaign', Feb–Jun, London, Health Education Authority, *HEA AIDS Programme Information Pack*.

WELLINGS, K., WADSWORTH, J., JOHNSON, A.M., FIELD, J. and BRADSHAW, S. (1990) 'Safer sex practice in a general population sample', Paper presented at International Conference, 'Assessing AIDS-Preventive Strategies', Montreux.

*A Feminist Approach to Social Research on HIV/AIDS*

Chapter 13

# Methodological Issues in Researching Young Women's Sexuality

*Janet Holland, Caroline Ramazanoglu, Sue Scott, Sue Sharpe and Rachel Thomson*

The Women, Risk and AIDS, Project[1] was conceived in the late 1980s when fear of AIDS in the UK was escalating. Public concern focused on contamination by members of high-risk groups — homosexual (and bisexual) men, injecting drug users, sex workers, and those who had been treated with blood containing HIV in the early stages of the epidemic. The key policy issue was that of containing the *risky* few, in order to protect the *innocent* public. Most women were considered to be innocent of AIDS and to have a low risk of infection. Reports from parts of Africa, the USA and elsewhere, however, made it clear that HIV was spreading through *normal* heterosexual sexual practices (Gross, 1988; Heyward and Curran, 1988, *AIDS Newsletter*, 1990b: 5).

Although numbers were small, there was evidence of a steady growth in heterosexual transmission of HIV in the UK (Department of Health Quarterly Statistics; Johnson, 1988; The Collaborative Study Group, 1989; Donoghue, Stimson and Dolan, 1989; *AIDS Newsletter*, 1990a: 2). The notion of high-risk groups produced during the moral panic of the 1980s was not useful for explaining how HIV/AIDS was spreading, how women might be affected, and how the epidemic might be limited. The first investigations of the social aspects of AIDS began to suggest that heterosexuality was inadequately understood. It was clear that research was needed to explore sexual practices and relationships rather than sexual identities. Watney (1987) marked a shift in thinking when he argued that anyone embarking on a sexual career now stood in a different relation to risk than was previously the case.

Government health education campaigns in the UK at the time, targeted high-risk groups and concentrated on promoting condom use as protection against sexually transmitted infection. Women whose behaviour was taken as risky were sex workers, the 'promiscuous' and injecting drug users. These were taken to be deviant and overtly sexual women. The majority of women were defined in terms of their relationships either to men or to children, and not in terms of their sexual desires or needs. There was no sense, in the fears of AIDS expressed in the mass media, that 'decent, normal women' constituted a sexual risk, nor that such women were at risk from 'decent, normal men' (except for the partners of seropositive men given contaminated blood products). A focus on male heterosexual behaviour and male dominance of heterosexual relations was lacking in understandings of risk-taking (Wilton and Aggleton, 1991).

The advances in contraceptive methods in this century have served to put the onus of responsibility more firmly on women; many men (and women) had grown up assuming that these female methods (diaphragm, cap, IUD, the pill) were the most appropriate (Pollock, 1985). In promoting men's condom use as a safeguard against the spread of AIDS through heterosexual intercourse, the government campaigns assumed that sexual encounters between women and men could be negotiated as matters of rational choice. If women routinely asked men to use condoms, then couples could choose safer sex.

Public and official responses to the AIDS epidemic drew attention to a lack of knowledge about sexual practices in western cultures and to ignorance of the ways heterosexual sexual practices are negotiated. Connections between sociological understandings of sexual behaviour and policies for promoting safer sex were not well established and were particularly lacking in the case of young women.

It was unlikely that there would be a widespread heterosexual epidemic immediately in the UK, but very little was known of the sexual practices of young women, the ways they become sexually active, how they negotiate their sexual encounters, what risks they are aware of and what risks they take. We wanted to extend the challenge to the concept of *risk groups* by arguing that young women's sexuality should be understood through analysis of their sexual practices rather than the type or number of partners (Holland, Ramazanoglu and Scott, 1990). While private sexual practices could not be accessed directly, it was possible to ask young women to talk about their sexuality.

By sexuality we understand not only sexual practices, but also what people know and believe about sex, particularly what they think is natural, proper and desirable. Sexuality includes people's sexual identities in all their cultural and historical variety. While sexual intercourse is a meeting of bodies, these bodily practices are given meaning by ideas and values, and situated in social relationships.

As feminist sociologists, we shared the assumption that an imbalance in the relative power of men and women generally in British society has been well established, and so an imbalance was to be expected in sexual relationships and the negotiation of sexual practices (Sharpe, 1976). Men's ideas about women, women's ideas about men, and their expectations of each other, could then be a critical factor affecting the negotiation of safer sex. The well documented extent of sexual violence, and unwanted pregnancies experienced by women, suggest that young women cannot simply choose effective control over safer heterosexual sex (Kelly, 1988; Stanko, 1985). The prevalent definition of *proper sex* as the act of vaginal penetration and male orgasm, relegates much safe-sex to the category of foreplay. A study of young women's sexuality seemed a valuable contribution to knowledge about how safer sexual practices might most effectively be promoted.

### The Women, Risk and AIDS Project: a Feminist Study

The Women, Risk and AIDS Project was planned as an investigation of the role of young women in influencing the spread or containment of AIDS in Britain, focusing on their sexual behaviour, their knowledge and understanding of the disease and their interpretations of risk and safety. We considered that without knowledge of young women's understanding of pleasure and danger in sexual activity, and their ability to communicate effectively their ideas on safety within relationships, any attempt to educate young people on the nature of AIDS and its control was likely to be ineffective and irrelevant to their practice.

A study of young women's sexuality need not necessarily be a feminist project. Our project was feminist in the sense that we sought to investigate gendered power relations as a structural feature of young women's sexual relations, and justified this perspective from numerous existing feminist studies of social relationships.[2] We assumed, as Joan Acker (1989: 238) has put it, that 'gender is implicated in the fundamental constitution of social life'.

We expected both to add to knowledge on sexual risk-taking, and safer sex, and also to establish the value of taking gender to be central to any understanding of heterosexuality. Our framework of feminist theory was complemented by reflection on appropriate methods for accessing sexuality and concern for the ethics of our research practice. In this chapter we attempt to explain the links between studying young women's sexuality within a framework of feminist assumptions and methods, and the conclusions we have drawn from the data. Young women's accounts of their sexuality gave us a particularly rich source of data, but also a number of problems about how to interpret interview accounts. We state briefly the aims of the project before setting these problems in the context of feminist method.

### The Aims of the Project

The project was planned as a systematic investigation of the sexual practices, beliefs and understanding of young women in two large cities. Specifically, the aims were:

1 to interview young women in London and Manchester in order to document and interpret their understanding of HIV and sexually-transmitted diseases; their conceptions of risk and danger in sexual

activity; their approaches to relationships and responsibility; their ability to communicate effectively their ideas on safety within sexual relationships and marriage. The interviews were to enable us to build up detailed accounts of the sexual practices, beliefs and expectations of the young women in the samples;

2    to provide policy-oriented information to contribute to the education of young people on sexual risk and safety; to consider the extent to which health education programmes have influenced behaviour, and what factors are likely to constrain or to encourage change towards safer sexual practices. It was our intention to consider the relevance of existing AIDS education programmes to the lives of the young women in our sample, to identify the factors which are likely to constrain or encourage the use of safer sexual practices and to feed these findings back into future education initiatives.

3    to develop a theory of the social construction of sexuality, identifying the processes and mechanisms through which young women construct, experience and define their sexuality and sexual practices; to examine the relationship between these processes and broader gendered power relations.

## Feminist Method and Young Women's Experience

In approaching this project as feminist sociologists we did not always agree on all aspects of feminist methodology. Feminists have characterized the dominant methodologies of twentieth century social science research as sexist and as unable to grasp the ways in which women's experiences of life differ from those of men. This critique of male-centred knowledge has pushed feminists into new ways of thinking about how we know what we know, about the relations between subjectivity and objectivity, empiricism and realism, modern and postmodern theory, and so about how knowledge can be validated. The problems of how to take account of gender relations when women and men are socially divided by class, racism and ethnicity and other divisions have been critical.

These developments have produced a flood of feminist empirical research and a series of debates on methodology and epistemology (Kelly, 1978; Mies, 1983; Clegg, 1985; Harding, 1987; Collins, 1990; Stanley and Wise, 1993). We do not have space to review the diversity of these developments and their implications here, but have focused on the ways in which a feminist perspective shaped our study and influenced our conclusions.

The adoption of feminist methodology implied a commitment to the grounding of our study in women's experiences of sexuality. This valuing of subjective experience is probably the most contentious feature of feminist research, and has been much debated within feminism (Stanley and Wise, 1990, Harding, 1991). Feminists have questioned whether our gendered social positions (our everyday social positions and experiences as women or men) make a difference to what we can see, or what we want to see as sociologists. We claim that taking people's everyday experience of sexuality seriously is particularly productive in enabling researchers to grasp both the complexity of the connections between individuals and the structures and ideas that constitute forms of male dominance and substantially shape heterosexual relationships.

Young women's subjective accounts of their experience as they understood it would not, however, provide us with factual reports of sexual activity or direct access to actual safe and unsafe practices. Our research could not be a description of a sample of sexual behaviour from which we could simply generalize, since interview transcripts do not simply speak for themselves. Interviews are social interactions to which researchers bring themselves and their ideas, and when we interpret interviews we bring ideas to the interpretation (Holland and Ramazanoglu, 1994). As feminist researchers we conceptualized the interview accounts as situated within a framework of ideas and structures of which the young women themselves may or may not have been aware (we return to this point below).

Throughout the project, we had to make sense of how young women talked about their experience in the light of feminist conceptions of gendered power relations. This meant taking systematic note of our own process of theorizing in order to show how we moved between questionnaire responses or interview transcripts and our general conclusions on factors which promote or inhibit safer sexual practices. Our research could only be as good as the questions we asked and the assumptions we made.

By drawing on feminist theory in framing our questions, we identified key assumptions in dominant beliefs about sexuality and took a stand against them. The patriarchal paradigm within which theories of young women's sexuality were framed is so powerful that our approach had to take it into account and disrupt it in order to make it visible. The key assumptions that we considered had been produced within a patriarchal framework of thought and should be challenged were: the focus on individual behaviour; the 'rational-choice' model of health promotion; the idea that men and women are equal partners in negotiating sexual practices.

The official conceptions of sexuality and models of behaviour that informed public health education in the 1980s were largely based on a view of behaviour as a matter of choice by free individuals. Individuals could make rational choices (for example, to protect their own health) or could fail to make such choices. In understanding rates of unintended pregnancy among young women, the patriarchal focus was on the behaviour of the individual and her failure to make a responsible choice.

By emphasizing inequalities of gender and the extent of men's dominance in heterosexual relations, we challenged the rational-choice concept of safer sex. Women's ability to choose safer sexual practices, or to refuse unsafe (or any other) sexual activity, was not a question of free choice between equals, but one of negotiation within structurally unequal social relationships.

A feminist view would see young women who are exposed to the risks of pregnancy, HIV or sexually-transmitted disease, as situated in social relationships (Sharpe, 1987; Lees, 1993). Young women do not have unprotected sexual intercourse alone, and they have to communicate their needs and desires within social structures that systematically privilege the male over the female (Fine, 1988; Lesko, 1988). Our focus on young women's expressions of their experience, rather than on the facts of their behaviour, gave us qualitatively and politically different access to how and why young women take sexual risks, and accept risky practices.

This difference in approach was based on the claim, first, that sexuality is socially constructed, and second, that this process of social construction has defined heterosexuality in terms of male sexual practice and male sexual needs. It is support for these claims that disrupts the patriarchal conception of heterosexual relations. We were able to draw on feminist research on female sexuality and women's bodies which had been developing since the 1960s (see Jackson, 1978, 1982; Coveney *et al.*, 1984; Vance, 1984; Fine, 1988; Lesko, 1988; Martin, 1989; Thompson, 1990; Jacobus *et al.*, 1990). Social theories outside feminism have taken little account of this feminist work on the gender relations within which heterosexual relations are embedded. Feminist knowledge of women's sexuality has had a limited effect on the medical establishment or on health education policy. As a result, social factors affecting the connections between heterosexual beliefs and practices, the production of sexual identities and safe or unsafe sexual practices were largely unexplored.

We were concerned that women were being positioned within AIDS discourses in ways that legitimated and reinforced male sexual dominance. Attributing sexual risk to group membership, rather than to actual sexual practices, ignored the fact that men and women could gain different reputations from the same sexual behaviour. What gained a man status as a 'bit of a lad', condemned a young woman as a 'slag'. Defining so-called promiscuous women as a high-risk group reinforced existing gender stereotypes, leaving the 'double standard' of male and female sexual conduct unchallenged. In spite of its tragic consequences, the AIDS epidemic has provided an opportunity for opening up discussions of sexuality and examining these gendered differences.

Once we started to analyse young women's accounts of their sexuality, it became clear that they had absorbed conceptions of heterosexuality in which men and women have different value, and play very different roles. Men are taken to have an active, driving sexuality that needs physical satisfaction. Women in this construction are the passive objects of men's desires, whose satisfaction lies mainly in satisfying a male partner. Female sexual identities are defined through this passive role primarily in terms of women's social relationships to men. An empowered, independent woman with her own active sexual desires, who seeks sexual pleasure on her own terms, is not a 'normal', feminine woman, but a sexual deviant and a social danger.

The example of producing a condom in a sexual encounter and asking a partner to use it illustrates this point. The rational-choice model of individual behaviour does not grasp the social meanings of condom use that young people have to manage. The message expressed by a man producing a condom is potentially that of a caring and responsible partner who offers protection. A man who is embarrassed, can then be understood as sexually inexperienced or incompetent, or as one who is taking the woman to be untrustworthy, a source of infection. If it is the woman who produces the condom, then the message is that she is a sexually knowing and experienced woman who takes risks and so does not trust the man she is with. Her condom challenges his masculinity and her subordination to him. Her embarrassment would be a properly feminine response to her unfeminine behaviour (Holland *et al.*, 1991).

The meanings of asking a man to use a condom can be seen as reinforcing a particular aspect of heterosexual practice and reifying its importance. Condoms offer the least disruptive solution to HIV transmission in accordance with definitions of heterosexuality that privilege male experience. AIDS, it has been argued, offers opportunities for new definitions and understandings of sexual practice (Coward, 1987; Scott, 1987; Segal, 1987) but there has been little evidence of such changes in heterosexual practices.

In planning the study, the complexities of managing sexual behaviour seemed more accessible through young women's accounts of their sexual experiences, than through an examination of the successes and failures of risk-taking individuals. We started from an assumption of gendered inequality in sexual relationships, and this assumption was amply supported in the data. Since we assumed inequality, we had an initial focus on power.

Far from men and women being equal sexual partners who could choose to control risks, we took sexual relations to be social sites in which men routinely have power over women, whether or not they know this, or want, or intend to exercise such power.[3] Women can and do resist male power, but it is hard for them to identify it, or to see how their own feminine beliefs and practices often constitute a form of collusion with male dominance. Conventional femininity constructs women as subordinate to men. In order to show this, it was central to our method that we should account for what Foucault (1991: 28) has called 'the micro-physics of power' in young women's sexual relationships.

Foucault did not conceive gender as a source of power, nor see men as possessing power. He saw a 'network of power relations' as 'forming a dense web that passes through apparatuses and institutions, without being exactly localized in them' (Foucault, 1984: 96). Although Foucault largely ignored gendered power relations, Jana Sawicki (1991: 24) comments that, 'by utilising this ascending analysis, Foucault shows how mechanisms of power at the microlevel of society have become part of dominant networks of power relations.' Our problem was to identify what mechanisms drew both men and women into such a strongly entrenched system of male dominance of heterosexuality, and, if safer sex is to be promoted, how this dominance can be resisted (Ramazanoglu and Holland, 1993).

Feminists have claimed that there is something distinctive in feminist research even though feminists use techniques used by others. The distinctiveness of feminist approaches lies not in the details of technique, but in how the research process is understood, and in the conclusions drawn from the research. Feminist knowledge differs from knowledge produced by other methodologies.

In the rest of this chapter we discuss three problem areas in trying to grasp the different ways in which young women's sexual encounters are negotiated. First, feminists have to select research techniques and identify appropriate data; second, they have to consider the ethics of interviewing on sensitive topics; third, having produced the data, they have to decide how to draw conclusions from them.

## Research Techniques and Sample Selection

There has been much discussion in recent years about the most appropriate techniques and tools for feminist research. In the 1970s and 1980s, feminist method came to be associated with the use of qualitative methods and informal interviews as a means of accessing experience, but not without critical reflection on these methods (Roberts, 1981; Bowles and Duelli Klein, 1983). We would argue, however, that the distinctive character of feminist research lies in asking questions that render the 'everyday world' problematic (Smith, 1988). For example, asking how the context and process of heterosexual interaction restricts the negotiation of safer sex practices allows for the problematization of the institution of heterosexuality.

When we began to design this project there was a dearth of information available about the sexual behaviour of young people; this meant that we had no adequate, up to date, baseline from which to work. In order to understand the social construction of sexuality and how safer sexual practices might be promoted, we needed a methodology and research instruments to enable us to explore, with the respondents, the meanings which attach to their behaviour.

In pursuit of our aims, we had to find young women willing to talk at some length about their sexuality. This gave us three immediate problems. First, it restricted the size of the sample since this is a labour-intensive method of producing data; second, we had no sampling frame of young women willing to talk; third, we wanted a sample that could be representative of young women more generally.

Our first decision was to target young women in central areas of London and Manchester. It was not possible in a small study to cover the whole of the UK, so we picked two urban areas where the heterosexual spread of HIV might reasonably be expected.

The lack of a sampling frame meant that simple random samples were not possible, and the sensitivity of this topic meant that respondents would of necessity be volunteers. In order to ensure that the young women were representative of the main social divisions within the UK, we constructed two purposive samples (one for London and one for Manchester). This enabled us to select young women on the basis of criteria that we considered to be of direct relevance to the investigation. The samples were stratified by: age, into three age groups (16–17, 18–19, 20–21); social class (based on parents' or guardians' occupation); power (based on educational and/or labour market attainment or aspirations); ethnic origin; and degree of sexual experience. The study was carried out between 1988 and 1990. Eighty-two per cent of the young women interviewed had had some sexual experience, and 98 per cent of the 20–21 year-olds were sexually active. Eighty-two per cent of the sample were classified as English, Scottish or Welsh, and 18 per cent as Asian, Afro-Caribbean or other.

The characteristics of the sample generated in this way were compared with the characteristics of comparable studies (see Bowie and Ford, 1989; Ford and Morgan, 1989; Johnson *et al.*, 1989; Kent *et al.*, 1990; Ingham *et al.*, 1991; Woodcock, Stenner and Ingham, 1992). Our results were similar in terms of sexual experience and age of first sex to random samples of young people gathered by Ford and Morgan, and Bowie and Ford (Holland, 1992).

To facilitate the construction of the sample we decided on a two-stage strategy which enabled both the team and the young women to select for the informal interviews. We used an initial questionnaire, covering a range of demographic variables, and basic information on sexual knowledge, sex education, contraception and numbers and types of sexual relationships. These questionnaires could be completed anonymously or the young woman could provide a contact address, if she was willing to be interviewed. We agree with many of the criticisms of the survey method, such as Graham, 1983, but felt that quantitative methods can render useful information within a framework of feminist theory, and that it is possible to ask young people detailed and sensitive questions about sex using a questionnaire format (Abrams *et al.*, 1990; Roberts, 1990; Kelly, Regan and Burton, 1991). We received completed questionnaires from 500 young women (including those who were later interviewed in depth).

We gained access to these young women in a wide range of settings: schools, colleges, youth clubs, young mothers' groups, a range of workplaces and through magazines aimed at the relevant age group. We had difficulties of access largely at the level of the organization. Gatekeepers wanted to protect their young women from our intrusion into their private activities. Sex was often considered too sensitive a topic for us to take into the organization. If we were able to come face-to-face with the young women, tell them what we wanted and administer the questionnaire ourselves, we had a better response.

From the questionnaires, the team was able to select 150 young women who were both willing to be interviewed and who fitted the categories of the purposive sample design. These were interviewed in depth. The interviews were tape recorded, transcribed, and then analysed with the aid of The Ethnograph package for qualitative data analysis.[4]

A 20 per cent sub-sample was drawn from the original sample and followed up with a second interview approximately one year later. These second interviews introduced a longitudinal element into the design to enable us to explore any changes in the respondents' lives, particularly with regard to their sexual practice in the year following the first interview. Second interviews were carried out with sexually active young women who had either expressed a wish in the first interview to change their behaviour, whose sexual practices meant that they might be at-risk in relation to HIV, or who had some particular experience which meant that they were going through a period of transition in relation to sexuality. We wanted data that illustrated the ways in which young women *talk* about their sexuality and sexual practice, including the ways in which they express and understand contradictions, as well as a survey of their reported behaviour. For this reason we decided that in-depth interviews would be the central method of data collection.

The interviews were informal and intensive, covering sensitive areas and exploring what the young women knew about sexuality, contraception and safer sex, STDs and HIV/AIDS; how and what they learned about sex and sexuality; their ideas about risk, danger and control in sexual encounters; their conceptions of trust and of a double standard; their ideas of sexual pleasure, and the ways in which they negotiated their social and sexual relationships. General topics were included, such as their household situation, relationships, friendships, lifestyle, education, employment, religion, their image of themselves and their hopes and plans for the future. The format of the informal interview allowed young women to use their own definitions of sex and of risk and pleasure. We did not set out to define sexual activity as heterosexual vaginal intercourse, nor to specify safer sexual practices, but to accept and explore each young woman's own definition of what it meant to be sexually active.

## The Ethics of Interviewing on Sexuality

Feminists have paid considerable attention to the issue of the rights of the researched, and appropriate relationships between researcher and researched (Cook and Fonow, 1986; Eichler, 1988; Harding, 1987) and have identified some of the problems of exploitation of women as subjects of research, particularly those in studies of women by women. Women who are exploited themselves in the research process might exploit the women they research. A young woman research assistant, without power in the research context may be sent out to interview women, and then find the data she collects removed entirely from her control by whoever it is who runs the research project of which it is a part (Kay, 1990). Even an aware feminist researcher potentially has power in the research context — power to define the situation. She may be older, more educated, from a different social class than the woman she interviews, who may in turn defer to her, or feel relatively powerless on one or other of those grounds.

We were fully aware of the complexity and sensitivity of the subject of the research and of the imbalance of power between ourselves and the young women we interviewed. There was potential for the exploitation and objectification of respondents inherent in the research process (Ramazanoglu, 1989). We discussed the means of minimizing the likelihood of this occurring and were agreed that the young women should understand that they were being taken seriously and that the information which they gave could be useful in developing better education for young people in the future. To this end we produced leaflets about the project which indicated to the young women how they could be part of the research.

Issues of anonymity and confidentiality are particularly important when dealing with sensitive topics and we made every effort to assure our respondents that their identity would be protected. Researchers can never be entirely confident that they are proceeding on the basis of informed consent, especially when their respondents have little or no knowledge of the business of research. While most of the respondents seemed grateful for the assurance, we did have some surprising reactions. Far from wishing us to protect their privacy some young women were of the opinion that if we were writing a book about them then they should be named in it. We have, however, chosen to protect their anonymity.

Some feminist researchers have argued for the empowerment of women through the research process suggesting that findings should be fed back to, and negotiated with co-researchers (Acker *et al.*, 1983; Mies, 1983). They seek reciprocity in the research relationship through sensitivity to the researcher's intrusion into women's lives. They want to realize the meanings, the lifeworld of the women they research, in ways that make sense for the women themselves. Some have attempted to involve the researched in the entire research process, from setting the agenda for research, undertaking it in a reciprocal relation, to interpreting and writing up (or producing some statement) of the results (Graham, 1984). Here the attempt is to *empower* the women who are the object of research.

This approach is not without its problems and may result in a bland consensus, lacking in sociological insight (Poland, 1985). In particular it can suggest that it is the role of the researcher to act as a channel for the experiences of others. We return to this point in the next section. While we felt a responsibility not to exploit or objectify our respondents, we could see no realistic way of empowering the young women directly through the research process when our contact was, in most cases, a single interview. It was our intention that any benefits from the research should be fed back to young women via the provision of policy-oriented information contributing to the development of more appropriate information and education for young people in relation to HIV/AIDS and sexuality in general. This is the policy we have followed through presentations, publications and contacts with practitioners, feeding our data into training for practitioners and educational materials for young people.

We were aware that many of our respondents would have little experience of talking about sex, particularly with strangers. We hoped that the fact that the interviewers were women, and we were unlikely to meet again outside the interview, would facilitate rather than inhibit disclosure. The *naturalistic* interview, conducted with empathy by a woman, can lead women into considerable revelation. This has ethical and political implications relating to the exploitation of women's vulnerabilities for the sake of career advancement (Finch, 1984: 80). A number of the young women did say that they had never spoken of certain things before, but most seemed to find this useful rather than threatening. Some appeared to use the interview as a means of reflecting on their sexual behaviour and relationships. For example, one young women, who reported engaging in potentially risky sex with a number of partners, told us in the second interview that the first interview had helped her change her understanding of her experience.

We were asked by one HIV/AIDS worker whether we had undertaken counselling training in order to carry out the research (cf Kelly *et al.*, 1991; Bergen, 1993). She clearly felt that this was not only appropriate but necessary. It was our view, however, that while there may be elements of the therapeutic encounter in an in-depth interview, and while sociological research may be an extension of the panoptic gaze (Foucault, 1991), and to have inherited some aspects of the confessional, a sociological interview is not a counselling situation. We felt strongly that it would be irresponsible and unethical to enter into a counselling discourse as we were not trained or resourced as counsellors.

We were prepared, though, for our respondents to ask questions back (Oakley, 1981), and did our best to respond to such questions at the end of the interview. Being asked such questions as 'Is oral sex dangerous?' raised a number of issues both about the nature of research and about the nature of knowledge. We did not feel it proper to take on the role of sex educators or experts on HIV and AIDS, but we did feel that our respondents had the right to the same information as we had ourselves. We dealt with this by directing young women to the best available sources of information and/or advice, rather than advising them ourselves. There were however, occasions when we were unwittingly doing sex education simply by asking questions. In some interviews it became obvious that just hearing that oral sex or masturbation were possibilities for women was a revelation to the respondents.

This decision was not in itself a protection from the effects of listening to our respondents speak about difficult experiences and we had to develop strategies both to support them, and to sustain ourselves on occasions when interviews were particularly disquieting or emotionally charged. What the respondents said, or might have said if they could have talked about it, could be psychologically, emotionally, personally or socially problematic for them. In a number of the interviews, accounts of sexual intercourse in response to pressure from men, sexual violence, rape or child sexual abuse emerged (Holland *et al.* 1992b). Our agreed strategy was to allow the respondent to define the situation and how far these experiences should be talked about, but to suggest sources of information and support if this seemed appropriate.

Each of us had experiences of distressing interviews but the support of the rest of the team and a shared understanding of the tensions and difficulties in many women's lives made it easier to see such experiences as part of the research process. We were concerned about the potential for voyeurism in producing explicitly sexual data. Talking about sex is part of the realm of the sexual, and we felt that for this reason we should not push our respondents to express themselves explicitly unless they were obviously comfortable doing so. The implications of reflexivity in the relationship between researchers, respondents, research topic and the process of data production should, we feel, be made explicit in all good sociological research, but has been a particular concern of feminist research in recent years (Williams, 1993).

## Interpreting Interviews — Making Sense of Experience

Our interview transcripts together with the interviewers' field notes on their observations and interpretations of each encounter gave us our raw data. With these data, and our framework of theory, we set out to draw conclusions. The first stage of analysis was that of familiarizing ourselves with the content of the interviews. Four out of the five of us had conducted interviews, and we all read our own and others' transcripts and discussed our responses to them with the rest of the team (that is, within a general framework of feminist assumptions). We interrogated the data for support (or the lack of it) for our initial concepts, and for those generated in this process. This means that the absence of data could itself be data. As there is no shared language of sex that gives positive expression to women's embodied experience (Holland *et al.*, 1994a) the lack of explicit terminology in much of our data leads to gaps and silences that are themselves a topic for analysis.

Our starting assumptions that sexual relationships were both unequal and gendered were substantially supported by the data, but it was our attempts to account for the unexpected and for absences and silences that led us to our main conclusions. We were confronted with material that could not simply be 'read' either from the data or from our starting assumptions. This raised specific problems about what we were doing when we interpreted interview transcripts. Specifically, we had to draw conclusions from interview talk in which the respondents give varying meanings to their experiences, and offer understandings in different terms from those of the research team. This could put us in the position of deciding whose interpretation was the correct one. However sensitive feminists are to the relations between the researcher and the researched, ultimately the researcher runs off with the data and makes her own interpretation of it. Dorothy Smith comments:

> For while we have developed methods of working with women that are
> fully consultative and open, a moment comes after talk has been

inscribed as texts and become data when it must be worked up as
sociology. (Smith, 1989: 35)

In making feminist sociology out of talk, we explicitly rejected the idea that the
researcher's interpretation is 'truer' than that of the respondent. But, because we
started from feminist assumptions about the existence of gendered inequalities,
we rejected a relativist position that would make any interpretation 'true' in its
own terms. We had a number of instances that illustrate this problem. For
example:

1   A young woman claimed that she was having 'good sex', but as the
    interview proceeded it became clear that sex was now 'good' because it
    did not hurt any more. Her view of 'good sex' differed both from that of
    the research team, and from that of many other young women.
2   A number of young women gave accounts of sexual intercourse under
    pressure from men that the research team understood as rape. Some
    young women did identify their experience as that of rape, but some of
    these reported that this was in retrospect, or after counselling. Others
    specified that the experience was not rape, because they felt that they
    could have stopped it, or should not have let it start, or should not have
    been drunk, or were in some other way responsible.

Within this process of interpretation, we located ourselves as fallible, subjective
people. We could not then simply decide whether or not sexual experiences were
'really' good, or 'really' rape. But as feminists, we thought that how sex and rape
are defined is politically important, and not simply relative. We had then to make
explicit what the young people who agreed to be interviewed contributed to the
research in their own understandings, and what we have made of these
contributions. Their interpretations and our interpretations, and the reasons for
differences between them, belong in the research.

We approached this problem by making explicit that in coding and
analysing the transcripts we were drawing on three levels of meaning:

1   the language and meanings used by the young women and explicit in
    the interview transcripts;
2   interviewers' fieldnotes, which entailed some preliminary interpretation
    of meanings in the interview;
3   team discussion, interpretation and coding of the data, in the light of
    feminist and sociological theories.

Researchers who analysed these transcripts without sharing our assumptions on
theory and methodology would not come to the same conclusions. Teamwork
helped to make our process of interpretation explicit, in that individual readings
of the data had to be explained and justified to colleagues, and made us

constantly attentive to questions of validity. We have endeavoured to utilize differences in the interpretation of data as a strength.

While most young women predictably reported difficulties in asking sexual partners to use condoms, some did not (Holland *et al.*, 1991). In interpreting the complexities of women's successes and failures in introducing condoms into sexual encounters we felt it necessary to extend the analysis beyond the level of reported condom use (Thomson and Scott, 1990). In exploring the minority of cases where condom use did not appear as a problem, we were led to compare the kinds of relationships in which young women felt able to communicate their desire for safer sex, with those in which they did not. This led us to the conclusion that there were contradictory pressures on young women both to take responsibility for their own safety, but also to take feminine roles in responding to men's desires. Where men defined condoms as incompatible with male sexual needs ('like washing your feet with your socks on'), young women had to accept unprotected sex, or had to be assertive (and so unfeminine) or be prepared to abandon the relationship. The 'rational' discourse of safer sex, promoted as official information, was antithetical to the ideology of femininity that constructs sex as the relinquishment of control in the face of love. Young women must constantly work through these contradictions in sexual encounters.

In order to reach this conclusion, we had to unravel the variability in women's accounts of using and not using condoms. We positioned their accounts within a framework of gendered power relations that silences female desire and needs. If young women do not derive much pleasure from penetrative sex then condoms may make little difference to their own enjoyment of sex, but this may not be a point they see as relevant to negotiation about condom use. The differences in expressions of their experience, and between their understandings and feminist concepts, illustrate the lack of a discourse of pleasure for women within which young women can both develop and locate their own sexuality. The conflicting social pressures that constitute the social context of sexual risk and safety explain the differences between the research team's theoretical framework and young women's varying expressions of their experience.

These examples indicate a general problem for social researchers of how to take account of respondents' experiences and subjectivity while still claiming some general validity for their conclusions. This has been both a particularly open problem in feminist research (Harding, 1987) and a focus of criticism (Hammersley, 1992; Williams, 1993). We intended to make explicit the problems of both grasping women's experience, and also transcending it in order to reach general conclusions.

If respondents have no sense of the centrality of gendered power relations in the shaping of their sexual relationships, they do not experience 'gender'. Our problem was how to balance our interpretation of young women's sexual relationships and practices as male-dominated, against their own varied understandings and meanings. We would agree with Dorothy Smith (1986:6) that women's own experiences are not a sufficient means to explain social practices and processes and that there is a complex process of negotiation between data and analysis. Personal experience can be valid as a source of knowledge, but circumscribed by the limits of personal ideas and practices. We were able to show, by analysing their own accounts of sexuality, how young women might be aware that their romantic hopes had not been fulfilled as they expected ('all lads are bastards') but yet have no critical consciousness of the structural inequality of their sexual relations. But we have taken experience seriously because it does constitute a starting point which is otherwise missing from the production of sociological knowledge (Cain, 1986; Stanley and Wise, 1993). Analysis was also affected by the fact that some young women were influenced by feminism and had reflected critically on their experience.

Our method committed us to a complex process of moving between data, theory and our own, differing and changing, understandings of sexuality which are both part of the data and part of the theory. It was necessary to interpret contradiction and diversity in the young women's accounts, rather than acting as a conduit through which they simply speak for themselves, but we have tried to make this process of interpretation explicit.

Some of the differences between women's accounts and our interpretations are illustrated through our conception of empowerment (Holland *et al.*, 1992a). We developed a concept of intellectual empowerment to explain the way in which some of the young women made sense of the situations in which they found themselves. A minority of young women had a critical consciousness of male dominance of sexuality and wanted to take more control, but were not able to act consistently on their knowledge. In a few cases, young women did seem able to recognize male dominance and to empower themselves in their own sexual relationships. We used the concept of experiential empowerment to explain this successful negotiation. Sometimes, however, empowerment was confined to specific situations, for example, a respondent might have a relatively equal and openly negotiated sexual relationship with one partner but find that in her next relationship she was unable to insist on safer sex.

We were concerned that no matter how much knowledge and intent young women might have, the most significant factor seemed to be the position taken by male parters. We found only a very small group of young women who appeared to have a strong sense of autonomy and to be relatively empowered on both an experiential and an intellectual level. These young women did give accounts of transferable skills in sexual negotiations. By looking at the detail of young women's experience with the insights of existing feminist theory, we were able to identify both general, structural aspects of gender relations and the variable meanings, agency and practices in young women's accounts.

One young women, who was strikingly different from most others, had a highly developed sense of her own sexual self. She was willing to end relationships that she felt were not what she wanted, and did not feel that it was up to her to satisfy a man physically on his terms. But she had developed good communication skills, and expected to have to educate men in how to enjoy a safe sexual relationship. This level of critical consciousness could not be achieved through adopting a respectable feminine sexual reputation, nor in a conventional feminine role. Her case showed how necessary it is to educate not only young women about their own safety, but also to target men. Making men aware of their social power, and the dangers to both men and women of its exercise, would constitute a breakthrough in public health promotion and provide the groundwork for greatly improved communication and shared understanding in sexual relations.

We reached our conclusions through grasping women's experience as they expressed it, interpreting their experience in the light of feminist conceptions of gendered relationships, and explaining the differences. This required a critical understanding of the research process, and of our own place within it.

## Conclusions

Most of the sexually active young women reported at least some unsafe sexual practices. Our main conclusion was that the pursuit of conventional femininity is an unsafe sexual strategy for young women. For sex to be safer they need to be empowered to express their own sexual desires, manage risks and to be able to insist on their own safety. This is unfeminine behaviour and challenging to conventional masculinity. Change will be less a matter of disseminating knowledge than of transforming social and sexual relationships. Sexual practices cannot be altered simply through education about sexual risks. Young women need positive messages about their sexuality with which they can identify; a positive conception of the possibilities of sex as both enjoyable and safe, so that they can have the confidence to resist sex on other terms. Emphasis is needed, not only on how relationships are negotiated, but also on problematizing men's power and women's submission. Insistence on informed consent to sexual activity confronts men's sexual beliefs and expectations. There is an urgent need to challenge young men to think about how men's behaviour and expectations of women might be changed.

It is perhaps one of the contradictions of the late twentieth century that it has taken the perception of AIDS as a social crisis for issues of power in heterosexual sexual relations to be taken seriously by policy makers. Existing feminist work, and our own experience, suggest that women are not simply passive victims of male power. They are, to differing extents, aware of complexities and contradictions within their situation and adopt strategies to manage these. Research which does not take questions of gender and the importance of women's lived experience into account can tell us little about these strategies, or about factors that might shape safer sexual practices. Grasping young women's contradictory understandings of their own experience, in the context of the gendered nature of heterosexual practice, is more useful as a basis for developing policy to promote safer sex, than data collected and presented according to more traditional methodological rules, that see subjectivity as a problem to be controlled.

## Notes

1 The Women, Risk and AIDS Project is staffed by the authors working collectively, and has been financed by a two-year grant from the ESRC. It has also received grants from Goldsmiths' College Research Fund and the Department of Health. The Leverhulme Trust gave a further one-year grant for a comparable study of young men (1991-2) and for comparison of the two studies. Tim Rhodes was a team member on this project.

2 The feminist literature establishing the central place of gender in social life is too great to review adequately here. In this chapter we deal with the consequences of adopting this assumption.

3 From our later study of young men (the Men, Risk and AIDS Project) it is clear that many young men are not fully aware of male power and do not wish to exercise power over women, but as they struggle to attain masculinity, and defend themselves against emotional pain or sexual failure, they are drawn into the reproduction and reinforcement of their power over women (Holland *et al.*, 1994b).

4 We used The Ethnograph to construct systemic networks as a way of organizing our concepts, coding and data. A systemic network is an analytic device developed in the field of linguistics that is particularly suitable for the organization of qualitative data, since it preserves and represents some of the original essence of these data (in this case, the understandings of the young women that were expressed in the interview transcripts). A network is an instrument for enabling theory to be tested, translating the language of the interview transcript into the language of the theory. This helps both with the interpretation of patterns and meanings in the data (see Bliss *et al.*, 1983); and also with tracing the process of theory construction, from the expressions used in the interviews to the researchers' conclusions.

## References

ABRAMS, D., ABRAHAM, C., SPEARS, R. and MARKS, D. (1990) 'AIDS invulnerability; relationships, sexual behaviour and attitudes among 16-19 year-olds, in AGGLETON, P., DAVIES, P. and HART, G. (Eds) *AIDS: Individual, Cultural and Policy Dimensions*, London: The Falmer Press.

ACKER, J. (1989) 'The problem with patriarchy', *Sociology*, 23, 2, pp. 235-40.

ACKER, J., BARRY, K. and ESSEVOLD, J. (1983) 'Objectivity and truth: Problems in doing feminist research', *Women's Studies International Forum*, 6, pp. 423-35.

*AIDS Newsletter* (1990a) 'HIV and AIDS in Scotland', 5, 5, p. 2.

*AIDS Newsletter* (1990b) 'European statistics', 5, 5, p. 5.

BERGEN, R.K. (1993) 'Interviewing survivors of marital rape', in RENZETTI, C.M. and LEE, R.M. (Eds) *Researching Sensitive Topics*, London: Sage.

BLISS, J., MONK, M. and OGBORN, J. (1983) *Qualitative Data Analysis for Educational Research*, London: Croom Helm.

BOWIE, C. and FORD, N. (1989) 'Sexual behaviour of young people and the risk of HIV infection', *Journal of Epidemiology and Community Health*, 43, 1, pp. 61-5.

BOWLES, G. and DUELLI KLEIN, R. (Eds) (1983) *Theories of Women's Studies*, London: Routledge and Kegan Paul.

CAIN, M. (1986) 'Realism, feminism, methodology and law', *International Journal of the Sociology of Law*, 14, pp. 255–67.

CLEGG, S. (1985) 'Feminist methodology: fact or fiction', in *Quality and Quantity*, 19, pp. 83–97.

COLLABORATIVE STUDY GROUP (1989) 'HIV infection in patients attending clinics for sexually transmitted diseases in England and Wales', *British Medical Journal*, 298, pp. 415–8.

COLLINS, P.H. (1990) *Black Feminist Thought: Knowledge, Consciousness and the Politics of Empowerment*, London: Harper Collins Academic.

COOK, J. and FONOW, M. (1986) 'Knowledge and women's interests: issues of epistemology and methodology in feminist social research', *Sociological Inquiry*, 56, pp. 2–29.

COVENEY, L., JACKSON, M., JEFFREYS, S., KAYE, L. and MAHONEY, P. (1984) *The Sexuality Papers: Male Sexuality and the Social Control of Women*, London: Hutchinson.

COWARD, R. (1987) 'Sex after AIDS', *The New Internationalist*, March 1987.

DONOGHOE, M., STIMSON, G. and DOLAN, K. (1989) 'Sexual behaviour of injecting drug users and associated risks of HIV infection for non-injecting sexual partners', *AIDS Care*, 1, 1, pp. 51–8.

EICHLER, M. (1988) *Nonsexist Research Methods: A Practical Guide*, London: Allen and Unwin.

FINCH, J. (1984) 'It's great to have someone to talk to: The ethics and politics of interviewing women', in BELL, C. and ROBERTS, H. *Social Researching: Politics, Problems, Practice*, London: Routledge and Kegan Paul.

FINE, M. (1988) 'Sexuality, schooling, and adolescent females: the missing discourse of desire', *Harvard Educational Review*, 58, 1, pp. 29–53.

FOUCAULT, M. (1984) *The History of Sexuality: An Introduction*, (translated by HURLEY, R.) Harmondsworth: Penguin.

FOUCAULT, M. (1991) *Discipline and Punish: the Birth of the Prison*, (translated by SHERIDAN, A.) Harmondsworth: Penguin.

FORD, N. and MORGAN, K. (1989) 'Heterosexual lifestyles of young people in an English city', *Journal of Population and Social Studies*, 1, 2, pp. 167–85.

GRAHAM, H. (1983) 'Do her answers fit his questions? Women and the survey method', in GAMARNIKOW, E., MORGAN, D., PURVIS, J. and TAYLORSON, D. *The Public and the Private*, London: Heinemann.

GRAHAM, H. (1984) 'Surveying through stories', in BELL, C. and ROBERTS, H., *Social Researching: Politics, Problems, Practice*, London: Routledge and Kegan Paul.

GROSS, J. (1988) 'Bleak lives: women carrying AIDS', *New York Times*, Aug 17.

HAMMERSLEY, M. (1992) 'On feminist methodology' (and replies by RAMAZANOGLU, C. and GELSTHORPE, L.), *Sociology*, 26, 2, pp. 187–218.

HARDING, S. (Ed.) (1987) *Feminism and Methodology*, Bloomington, IN: Indiana University Press.

HARDING, S. (1991) *Whose Science? Whose Knowledge: Thinking from Women's Lives*, Milton Keynes: Open University Press.

HEYWARD, W.L. and CURRAN, J.W. (1988) 'The epidemiology of AIDS in the US', *Scientific American*, 259, 4, pp. 52–9.

HOLLAND, J. (1992) *Sexuality and Ethnicity: Variations in Young Women's Sexual Knowledge and Practice*, London: Tufnell Press.

HOLLAND, J. and RAMAZANOGLU, C. (1994) 'Coming to conclusions: Power and interpretation in researching young women's sexuality', in PURVIS, J. and MAYNARD, M. (Eds) *Researching Women's Lives from a Feminist Perspective*, London: Taylor & Francis Ltd.

HOLLAND, J., RAMAZANOGLU, C. and SCOTT, S. (1990) 'AIDS: from panic stations to power relations: sociological perspectives and problems', *Sociology*, 24, 3, pp. 499–518.

HOLLAND, J., RAMAZANOGLU, C., SCOTT, S., SHARPE, S. and THOMSON, R. (1991) 'Between embarrassment and trust: young women and the diversity of condom use', in AGGLETON, P., HART, G. and DAVIES, P. (Eds) *AIDS: Responses, Interventions and Care*, London: The Falmer Press.

HOLLAND, J., RAMAZANOGLU, C., SCOTT, S., SHARPE, S. and THOMSON, R. (1992a) 'Pressure, resistance empowerment: Young women and the negotiation of safer sex', in AGGLETON, P., DAVIES, P. and HART, G. (Eds) *AIDS: Rights, Risk and Reason*, London: The Falmer Press.

HOLLAND, J., RAMAZANOGLU, C., SHARPE, S. and THOMSON, R. (1992b) 'Pleasure, pressure and power: Some contradictions of gendered sexuality', *Sociological Review*, 40, 4, pp. 645–74.

HOLLAND, J., RAMAZANOGLU, C. SHARPE, S. and THOMSON, R. (1994a) 'Power and desire: The embodiment of female sexuality', *Feminist Review*, 46.

HOLLAND, J., RAMAZANOGLU, C., SHARPE, S. and THOMSON, R. (1994b) 'Achieving masculine sexuality: Young men's strategies for managing vulnerability', in DOYAL, L., NAIDOO, J. and WILTON, T. (Eds) *AIDS: Setting a Feminist Agenda*, London: Taylor & Francis Ltd.

INGHAM, R. WOODCOCK, A. and STENNER, K. (1991) 'Getting to know you . . . young people's knowledge of their partners at first intercourse', *Journal of Community and Applied Social Psychology*, 1, pp. 117–32.

JACKSON, S. (1978) *The Social Construction of Female Sexuality*, London: Women's Research and Resources Centre.

JACKSON, S. (1982) *Childhood and Sexuality*, Oxford: Blackwell.

JACOBUS, M., FOX KELLER, E. and SHUTTLEWORTH, S. (Eds) (1990) *Body/Politics: Women and the Discourses of Science*, London: Routledge.

JOHNSON, A. (1988) 'Heterosexual transmission of human immuno-deficiency virus', *British Medical Journal*, 296, pp. 1017–20.

JOHNSON, A., WADSWORTH, J., ELLIOTT, P. *et al.* (1989) 'A pilot study of sexual lifestyle in a random sample of the population of Great Britain', *AIDS*, 3, 3, pp. 135–41.

KAY, H. (1990) 'Research note: Constructing the epistemological gap: gender divisions in sociological research', *Sociological Review*, 38, 2, pp. 344–51.

KELLY, A. (1978) 'Feminism and research', *Women's Studies International Quarterly*, 1, pp. 225–32.

KELLY, L. (1988) *Surviving Sexual Violence*, Cambridge: Polity Press.

KELLY, L. REGAN, L. and BURTON, S. (1991) *An Exploratory Study of the Prevalence of Sexual Abuse in a Sample of 16–21 year-olds*, London: Polytechnic of North London.

KENT, V., DAVIS, M., DEVERELL, K. and GOTTESMAN, S. (1990) 'Social interaction routines involved in heterosexual encounters: Prelude to first intercourse', Paper presented at the 'Fourth Conference on the Social Aspects of AIDS', April, London, Southbank Polytechnic.

LEES, S. (1993) *Sugar and Spice: Sexuality and Adolescent Girls*, London: Penguin.

LESKO, N. (1988) 'The curriculum of the body: lessons from a Catholic high school', in ROMAN, L.G. and CHRISTIAN-SMITH, L.K. with ELLSWORTH, E. *Becoming Feminine*, London: The Falmer Press.

MARTIN, E. (1989) *The Woman in the Body*, Milton Keynes: Open University Press.

MIES, M. (1983) 'Towards a methodology of feminist research', BOWLES, G. and DUELLI KLEIN, R. (Eds) *Theories of Women's Studies*, London: Routledge and Kegan Paul.

OAKLEY, A. (1981) 'Interviewing women: A contradiction in terms', in ROBERTS, H. (Ed.).

POLAND, F. (1985) 'Breaking the rules: Assessing the assessment of a girls' project', in *Studies in Sexual Politics*, 4, University of Manchester, Department of Sociology.

POLLOCK, S. (1985) 'Sex and the contraceptive act', In HOMANS, H. (Ed.) *The Sexual Politics of Reproduction*, Aldershot: Gower.

RAMAZANOGLU, C. (1989) 'Improving on sociology: Problems in taking a feminist standpoint', *Sociology*, 23, 3, pp. 427–42.

RAMAZANOGLU, C. and HOLLAND, J. (1993) 'Women's sexuality and men's appropriation of desire', in RAMAZANOGLU, C. (Ed.) *Up Against Foucault: Explorations of Some Tensions Between Foucault and Feminism*, London: Routledge.

ROBERTS, H. (Ed.) (1981) *Doing Feminist Research*, London: Routledge and Kegan Paul.

ROBERTS, H. (1990) *Health Counts*, London: Routledge.

SAWICKI, J. (1991) *Disciplining Foucault: Feminism, Power and the Body*, London: Routledge.

SCOTT, SARA (1987) 'Sex and danger: feminism and AIDS', *Trouble and Strife*, 11, pp. 13–17.

SEGAL, L. (1987) 'AIDS is a feminist issue', *New Socialist*, April.

SHARPE, S. (1976) *Just Like a Girl: How Girls Learn to be Women'*, Harmondsworth: Penguin.

SHARPE, S. (1987) *Falling for Love: Teenage Mothers Talk*, London: Virago.

SMITH, D. (1986) 'Institutional ethnography: a feminist method', *Resources for Feminist Research*, 15, pp. 6–13.

SMITH, D. (1988) *The Everyday World as Problematic*, Milton Keynes: Open University Press.

SMITH, D. (1989) 'Sociological theory: methods of writing patriarchy', in WALLACE, E. (Ed.) *Feminism and Sociological Theory*, London: Sage.

STANKO, E.A. (1985) *Intimate Intrusions: Women's Experience of Male Violence*, London: Routledge and Kegan Paul.

STANLEY, L. and WISE, S. (1990) 'Method, methodology and epistemology in feminist research processes', in STANLEY, L. (Ed.) *Feminist Praxis: Research, Theory and Epistemology in Feminist Sociology*, London: Routledge.

STANLEY, L. and WISE, S. (1993) *Breaking Out Again: Feminist Ontology and Epistemology*, London: Routledge.

THOMSON, R. and SCOTT, S. (1990) *Researching Sexuality in the Light of AIDS: Historical and Methodological Issues*, London: Tufnell Press.

THOMPSON, S. (1990) 'Putting a big thing into a little hole: teenage girls' accounts of sexual initiation', *The Journal of Sex Research*, 27, 3, pp. 341–61.

VANCE, C. (Ed.) (1984) *Pleasure and Danger: Exploring Female Sexuality*, London: Routledge and Kegan Paul.

WATNEY, S. (1987) *Policing Desire: Politics, Pornography and AIDS*, London: Methuen.

WILLIAMS, A. (1993) 'Diversity and agreement in feminist ethnography', *Sociology*, 27, 4, pp. 575–90.

WILTON, T. and AGGLETON, P. (1991) 'Condoms, coercion and control: Heterosexuality and the limits of AIDS education', in AGGLETON, P., HART, G. and DAVIES, P. *AIDS: Responses, Interventions and Care*, London: The Falmer Press.

WOODCOCK, A., STENNER, K. and INGHAM, R. (1992) 'Young people talking about HIV and AIDS: Interpretations of personal risk of infection', *Health Education Research: Theory and Practice*.

*Looking Forward*

## Chapter 14

# Towards the Mainstreaming of HIV/AIDS Research

*Mildred Blaxter*

The body of research within the social sciences on HIV/AIDS of the past seven or eight years has in fact been an experiment in itself. If there is a concerted attack on a topic, made in an atmosphere of urgency, with the greatest possible openness to different disciplines and new approaches, and an unusual lifting of the dead hand of the conventional in academic research: what is the result? It might easily be no more than a mishmash, with pointless repetition and inexplicable contradiction. In fact, the result has been a remarkably coherent whole. The first lesson about social science research which can be learned is perhaps that this method — a purposive, largely problem-driven, sometimes acrimonious, but often energetically collaborative research attack — can achieve as much, and sometimes more, than the conventional measured advance of scientific knowledge.

It was the need for quick answers to policy-relevant questions which released funds and encouraged research into areas which had previously been seen as too difficult, or not proper for public funding, or unwarranted intrusion into people's lives. Methodologically, the perceived importance and urgency of the subject permitted a range of methods, which, whether because of their expense, their novelty, or their breaking of conventional rules, might otherwise have found difficulty in funding or legitimation. The innovations have not necessarily been to do with the topic, but with the opportunity that the topic raised. In particular, medical and epidemiological interests came to appreciate and collaborate with various methods of social science, including qualitative methods, as never before: in this respect a considerable revolution has taken place in less than a decade.

It is not, however, the purpose of this conclusion to summarize the special methodological contributions which HIV/AIDS research has made, much less to attempt to make a case for their successes. Rather, the purpose is to ask, in a very speculative manner, what lessons may be learnt for the sociology of health and illness generally. It could be argued that the first enthusiasm among research administrators and funders is — for whatever reasons — coming to an end: earmarked research money is not now so liberal, projects viewed as gambles are less likely to be accepted. Consolidation rather than experimentation is the theme. This is perhaps a good moment to ask about the integration of this research with other areas. One criticism sometimes levelled at the HIV/AIDS research community is that it has been inward-looking and disassociated from other fields of work in the relevant disciplines. Perhaps this has been inevitable: it should not, however, now continue. The trend towards mainstreaming of HIV/AIDS services is currently much discussed among planners and administrators — the disappearance of earmarked budgets, or the use of generic rather than specialized services. Research, too, will have to enter the mainstream.

## Models of Health Behaviour and Behavioural Change

There is no doubt that the major contribution which HIV/AIDS research has most obviously made is in the area of the theory of health behaviour and the practice of health promotion. Here, the research is of course part of a general and wider trend. In many areas, evidence has been accumulating that models such as the Health Belief Model, with their focus on intentions, beliefs, knowledge, and norms, and their assumption of individual rationality, are in fact poorly predictive of health-related behaviour (RUHBC, 1988). In the past, this type of model has underlain much of formal health education, including public campaigns and school-based education. The contribution of HIV/AIDS research — perhaps because much has been conducted outside conventional health education, perhaps because of the unusual coming together of different disciplines — has been to add considerable weight to attacks on an already shaky theoretical edifice.

It may be of interest to consider a few of the issues in the context of other sorts of behaviour. First, there is the question of health as a value and whether any particular behaviour is seen as essentially a health issue anyway. We do know that health is an important value, but others may be equally or more so. Coping as a mother may be more important to overburdened working-class women than any health risk attached to smoking; complying with a husband's tastes more important than the healthiness of diet; sexual reputation more important to young women than making sure they have condoms available. Moreover, the extent to which different publics agree about what *is* a health issue is variable. For those who take most exercise, for instance, predominantly young men, the motivations often have very little to do with health. Issues of body image are more important to young women than healthy diets. Choosing partners and safer sex are bound up, among young people, with couple formation, love, growing up: a rather remote health risk comes a long way down personal lists of priorities. Again, the nature of the behaviour has to be considered. Is it a single, purposive action and a positive message such as 'Have your child immunized' or 'Go for breast screening', or is it a behaviour difficult to alter either because of some addictive component or because it is embedded in social life? Can behaviour be changed by the will of the individual, or are there others involved?

There are some particular topics where HIV/AIDS research has made particular contributions, and where explicit comparisons with other health-related behaviours might be profitably researched. Consideration of the meaning of *rationality*, and study of perceptions of vulnerability and risk, have been particularly fruitful. The move beyond the individualistic approach, to a view of health-related behaviour as social action and as relationships, might well be more clearly made in other fields such as diet. The way in which behaviours which are disapproved of are pathologized — as evidenced by the vocabulary of *relapse*, or *recidivism* applied to safer sex habits (Weatherburn and Project SIGMA, 1992) — is another area where comparative work with other health-related behaviour would be useful. This type of vocabulary is derived from the area of addictions, where originally it was associated with the laudable intention of the medicalization, and hence de-moralization, of behaviours. It is now ironic that it is seen as an imposition of moral attitudes. There has long been work in the field of alcohol use which moves away from a disease model, or a 'loss of control over the body' model, towards a view of lifestyle habits as socially constructed and contextually embedded. There are other areas of health behaviour where these approaches would be useful.

### Theory and Method

Theory and method cannot really be separated, as several papers in this volume note. These new models of health behaviour require different methods of research, as Ingham, Woodcock and Stenner (1992: p. 171) have summarized elsewhere:

> . . . a shift away from an obsession with individual knowledge or attitude scores on questionnaires towards the elucidation of meanings, powers, liabilities and constraints, from simple concepts of illness avoidance towards an acknowledgement of the importance of social relations, and from crude frequencies towards the dynamic processes involved in creating and maintaining identities.

Similarly, as Kitzinger suggests in Chapter 10, the recognition that personal behaviour does not happen in a cultural vacuum invites some critical reflection on the dominance of individual interview methods, and encourages the use of other ways of examining attitudes or knowledge in a social context.

Larger-scale surveys will always be considered appropriate for the purposes of comparison and generalization, and the attempted quantification of behaviours of interest. These theoretical considerations profoundly affect both the way in which questions are framed, however, and the form which analysis takes.

To guide these questions and analysis and to offer explanation and understanding, other methods for 'the elucidation of meaning' are required. These have ranged from the use of personal biographies as case-studies to show how understandings are 'anchored' by individuals and tied to other aspects of their experience (Stephenson, Breakwell anf Fyfe-Schaw, 1993) to the use of focus groups to study how meanings are socially created and shared (Chapter 10). Holland *et al.* (Chapter 13) demonstrate particularly clearly how theory, data collection, and analysis all interact in this interpretive type of work, where the researchers' readings of the data have to be balanced against the understandings and meanings of the subjects:

> . . . a complex process of moving between data, theory, and our own, differing and changing, understandings of sexuality which are both part of the data and part of the theory.

These issues were brought to the fore because of the nature of the topic of HIV/AIDS and sexuality, highlighting the problem of the researchers' location of their interpretations within a feminist framework, when the young women who were their subjects might not have any 'critical consciousness of the structural inequality of their sexual relations' (ibid.). This careful analytic stance can provide wider lessons, however. It is less obvious, but probably equally true, that analysis of doctor-patient interaction can ignore the fact that for some of the subjects the concepts of imbalance of power, or conflicting models of disease, may be outside their 'critical consciousness'. There is evidence that the concept of 'inequality in health' is perceived differently by researchers and researched. These issues, grounded in theoretical approaches, have clear consequences for the forms of questions as well as the interpretation of their answers.

### Methods of Eliciting 'Behaviour'

At the most practical methodological level, there is no doubt that HIV/AIDS research has made a marked contribution to behavioural enquiry. It is perhaps a caricature to say that for other forms of health-related behaviour where information has necessarily to rely on self-reports, research has tended to adopt one of two equally crude and extreme positions. Either self-reports have been treated as if they were unquestioned hard data (consumption of chips has reduced by 9.6 per cent) or not taken seriously at all, since of course 'everyone will lie'. Because of the special scepticism which reports of sexual behaviour have attracted, it has been necessary for researchers to consider questions of reliability and validity of the data with extra care.

Details of the methods, often innovative and scrupulous, employed to assess the reliability and validity of self-reports have been discussed in Chapter 1 and will not be repeated. The use of diary methods, and an emphasis on the reliability of *coding*, are points which might be specially noted. An important general point made by Breakwell and Fife-Schaw (Chapter 2) is the demonstration that a critical mass of studies is required before concern about replicability and reliability can be laid to rest.

Cumulatively, this work has provided lessons for other areas of enquiry. Yes, it can be shown that for various reasons respondents will offer accounts of behaviour which are not necessarily true. But it is not assumed, in any case, that definitions of the behaviour in question are unproblematic, or that everyone will mean the same things by the terms used. Nor, although respondents will courteously make up answers in reply to interviewers' demands, can they really be expected to remember, quickly and accurately, for example, the number of lifetime sexual partners — any more than they could remember accurately the exact quantity of last week's alcohol consumption.

Many of these concerns for the accuracy of the data could well be applied to other areas of behavioural research, where methods and measures have become conventional through long use and are unexamined. In population samples, care for representativeness is often confined to a few mechanical considerations. As Breakwell and Fife-Schaw (Chapter 2) note, there has to be caution about automatic weighting procedures applied for non-response, if there is any doubt about the relationship of population characteristics to the phenomenon being examined. In the type of population survey conducted for health education purposes, how often is weighting automatically applied for non-response, or when samples are deliberately non-representative in quantitative terms, without consideration of whether those not included are likely to be — for instance — those who are in fact ill, or those who are most likely to smoke, or those whose diets are the poorest? How commonly are the lower bound incidence estimates used by Breakwell and her research team employed?

### Categories and Definitions

A central theme of this search for validity has been a major concern for the meaning of categories. This has, perhaps, been one of the major contributions of this research. A range of ideas came to the fore in this context, at first at least partly as methodological considerations, which have considerable potential for the rejuvenation of other topics in medical sociology.

As noted in Chapter 1, this research has had to take particular care with its definitions. What a *sexual partner* or a *sexual act* are, and what they are understood to be by respondents in research, have had to be specially considered. As described by Davies (Chapter 4), behavioural units of analysis have required particular attention. As Silverman notes in Chapter 5, serious questions must be asked about the operational definition of a concept like *safe sex*. The ambiguity of language, especially in this area of sexual behaviour, has been highlighted. This close examination of the meaning which an activity actually has, in everyday situations, might profitably be undertaken similarly in other areas of research: categories such as *consultation*, or *sickness absence*, or *prescription* can certainly be used unthinkingly in analysis, as if their exclusiveness and facticity were unproblematic.

In the same way, and perhaps even more importantly, a central message of AIDS research has been the rejection of unthinking categorization of people. The concept of *risk categories* — the suggestion that there are those who are at-risk simply because of who they are — has been firmly rejected, and a great deal of empirical evidence offered to demonstrate that the use of categories such as homosexual, bisexual, prostitute, is not useful. This has profound implications for methodology, first because of what it says about units of analysis, and second because it makes clear that assumptions must not be made about either/or identities. As Watney (1991) suggested: 'Academic methodology has been threatened by what we have learned: that sexual and drug-using behaviours are not immutably fixed and static, with clearly defined and identifiable social groups.' In other areas of research in health and illness where the stereotypes are not so stigmatizing, or where the conventional labels are legitimized by long clinical or administrative practice, the misleading nature of these labels may not be so obvious. Nevertheless, it is very possible that categories of research subjects, or analytic descriptions, such as *diabetic* or *single parent* would equally merit closer examination.

### Hard-to-Reach Groups: Research Ethics

Questions of sampling and the categorization of subjects raise the question of hard-to-reach groups. There has of course been, since the 1960s, one tradition in sociology which uses ethnographic techniques or participant observation to uncover very private groups or describe milieux not usually open, for example, Whyte, 1955. Of more recent years there have been few studies to match these classics: they have had problems finding funding, perhaps being seen as self-indulgent or voyeuristic, and slightly suspect.

There is no doubt that AIDS research has included a new flowering of this type of ethnographic work and has won for it a new acceptance. Medical interests, in particular, have acknowledged that it is essential to know about these populations who cannot easily be sampled. Many of the populations of interest, or behaviours which are particularly relevant, are very difficult to observe or elicit: as McKeganey, Barnard and Bloor (Chapter 7) note, '. . . in this area as in many others related to AIDS we are working at the very margins of what is possible'.

Thus, as described in Chapter 6 by Power, the use of insiders as key informants or researchers has become more acceptable. There has, in the past, been considerable resistance to this among funding bodies (despite the few classical examples), especially when the groups involved were stereotypically thought deviant, or less reliable or organized. The gradual acceptance of those with street credibility and personal knowledge as contacts and interviewers does not represent new methods, but it does involve a new legitimation. As part of that legitimation, methodological issues (as in the study described by Power) of reliability, validity and consistency, the control of interview procedures, and the use of triangulation of sources, have all received particular attention. Ethnographic methods such as those of McKeganey, Barnard and Bloor have not only emphasized 'entering the worlds of others', but have incorporated a concern, new in this context, for hard data also.

Research on hard-to-reach groups, the use of indigenous informants, and ethnographic methods generally, all raise important issues of research ethics. It is perhaps notable that McKeganey, Barnard and Bloor have been the only authors in this volume to consider this explicitly. There is no doubt, however, that the impetus given by AIDS to research into some of the most hidden aspects of people's lives ought to bring the ethics of these intrusions into debate.

In fact, such debates are common wherever AIDS researchers gather. It could be suggested that this is one area where AIDS research certainly can, and ought to, contribute to medical sociology more generally. Ethical questions have been raised here because of the emotive nature of the topics of sex, and death. Are those who are ill over-researched? What rights have insider groups and the subjects themselves to dictate what research shall be done and how? What obligation is there on anyone to allow researchers into intimate areas of their lives? How far do researchers want to give publicity to some attitudes which they may uncover, such as racist or homophobic beliefs? How far is it proper to retain an objective, non-interfering stance in tragic situations? To what extent is our research essentially exploitative? Such questions as these, brought into the open in AIDS research, are equally relevant to many other topics in health and illness.

There seems as yet to be little sign of spill-over into the wider arena. However, it can be argued that (despite some active consumer views in the fields, for instance, of disability and of maternity care) medical sociological research has commonly taken quite cavalier attitudes to the rights of subjects. Most researchers will share slightly guilty memories of the way in which a medical legitimation has fostered respondents' submissiveness to calls upon their time, energy and privacy, and of occasions when 'the advance of knowledge' or 'this may help other people' has not really seemed sufficient justification. If debate about the ethics of research can be extended from the topic of AIDS to other severely ill, seriously troubled and often powerless subjects, then a service will be done to the sub-discipline as a whole.

### Issues of the Sociology of Health, Medicine and Medical Practice

Finally, there is a set of issues which have come to the fore in the AIDS research of the 1990s, which potentially have much wider application. For the most part they have not as yet been taken into the mainstream. In some cases, there is parallel but different work which AIDS research has not sought to connect with. They can be no more than listed.

Medical self-management is one: not simply *illness behaviour*, or the way in which uninformed lay people define and react to their diagnoses or manage their day-to-day symptoms, but the informed, independent, dialogue of those who need medical treatment with their professional advisers. There has, of course, been some study of certain other groups of patients with chronic conditions, but for the most part issues of personal choices in treatment and the self-management of serious disease have been neglected. Responsibility for the health of others, not just self-responsibility, is another theme which has emerged: something which has been ignored elsewhere, even in the field of STDs. There are also other issues in the field of medical practice — notably those of confidentiality, and of the attitudes of professional staff to particular groups of patients — where questions have been raised which merit wider consideration.

Perhaps most importantly of all, AIDS research has raised questions of health as a societal value, and health and illness as metaphors by which anxieties about the place of the body in the social order have been expressed. Sontag (1983, 1988) has, of course, considered other diseases — cancer, TB — as metaphors, as well as AIDS, and the relationship between a society and its diseases has been well explored by Herzlich and Pierret (1984). There is, however, little else to match the very many sophisticated analyses that have been published on the meaning of AIDS in cultural and societal perspective. Are there not others which might be similarly revealing? What is the meaning, in Western society at the end of the twentieth century, of 'heart disease'? How is it that a disease such as lung cancer is becoming the new venereal disease — shameful, the victim's own fault, not to be publicly named, perhaps even to be treated reluctantly? What of the diseases seen as deriving from disequilibrium with a modern environment: allergies, asthma? Herzlich and Pierret have noted, in a French population, the clear sense which people have of illness as actively determined by the conditions of modern urban life.

In the area of health policy and health promotion, the ways in which the public's perceptions change, or could be changed, is another topic to which AIDS research can contribute to existing bodies of work. Beliefs among the target populations of the motivations of those promulgating a message are, of course, important. If all the experts are giving the same message, that breast milk is best for small babies, for instance, it may be perceived that paediatricians are on the whole knowledgeable and devoted to the wellbeing of babies, and to be believed. On the other hand, what are perceived as moral campaigns on health issues have been almost universally unsuccessful, especially if seen as part of the eternal battle of the older generation against the younger. And, of course, any disagreement among the experts is anti-education of a powerful kind. Processes of social diffusion have been shown to effect various changes in general health-related behaviour: how may these processes operate in the area of sexual behaviour? It can be noted that the climate of opinion has undoubtedly changed in some ways — in the acceptability of talking about condoms, for instance.

These are all topics, not methodologies. However, as noted earlier, theoretical approaches and methods cannot easily be separated, and as Silverman notes in Chapter 5, *analytic* issues are central. The nature of the issues has fostered appropriate methods — for instance, media and policy analysis, or the use of focus groups to understand the way in which public representations are formed — less used in other areas of medical sociology.

## Conclusion

Finally, it may perhaps be noted that one of the special characteristics of this field is that research practitioners have tended to engage in it with personal passion and conviction. Different disciplines and approaches, theoretical interests and action research, have all come together because of a real involvement. It is difficult to think of another field in which, in the past, this has been so marked. A simple lesson which may be learnt is the value of a coalition of concern.

## References

HERZLICH, C. and PIERRET, J. (1984) *Malades d'hier, malades d'aujourd'hui*, Paris: Payot.
INGHAM, R., WOODCOCK, A. and STENNER, K. (1992) 'The limitations of rational decision-making models as applied to young people's sexual behaviour', in AGGLETON, P., DAVIES, P. and HART, G. (Eds) *AIDS: Rights, Risk and Reason*, London: The Falmer Press.
RESEARCH UNIT IN HEALTH AND BEHAVIOURAL CHANGE (RUHBC) (1988) *Changing the Public Health*, London: Wiley.
SONTAG, S. (1983) *Illness as Metaphor*, Harmondsworth: Penguin.
SONTAG, S. (1988) *AIDS and its Metaphors*, Harmondsworth: Penguin.
STEPHENSON, N., BREAKWELL, G. and FYFE-SCHAW, C. (1993) 'Anchoring social representations of HIV protection: the significance of individual biographies', in AGGLETON, P. DAVIES, P. and HART, G. (Eds) *AIDS: Facing the Second Decade*, London: The Falmer Press.
WATNEY, S. (1991) 'AIDS: the second decade: "Risk", research and modernity', in AGGLETON, P., HART, G. and DAVIES, P. (Eds) *AIDS: Responses, Interventions and Care*, London: The Falmer Press.
WEATHERBURN, P. and Project SIGMA (1992) 'On relapse: recidivism or rational response?' in AGGLETON, P., DAVIES, P. and HART, G. (Eds) *AIDS: Rights, Risk and Reason*, London: The Falmer Press.
WHYTE, W. (1955) *Street Corner Society*, Chicago, IL: University of Chicago Press.

# Notes on Contributors

*Marina Barnard* is a Research Fellow at the Public Health Research Unit, University of Glasgow. Her interests lie somewhere between sociology and anthropology. For the past six years she has researched the links between injecting drug use, prostitution and HIV/AIDS. She is co-author with Neil McKeganey of *AIDS, Drugs and Sexual Risk: Lives in the Balance*, Open University Press, 1992. More recently she has begun to look at young people's experimentation with drugs and the various routes into drug use.

*Mildred Blaxter* is Honorary Professor of Medical Sociology in the School of Economic and Social Studies, University of East Anglia. She was Co-ordinator of the ESRC's Programme of Behavioural Studies in HIV/AIDS, and Convenor for the Department of Health of the Working Group on the Dissemination of Research on HIV/AIDS, and is a member of the MRC Committee for Epidemiological Studies on AIDS.

*Michael Bloor* is a Senior Lecturer in the School of Social and Administrative Studies and is Director of the Social Research Unit at the University of Wales, Cardiff. His current research interests embrace HIV, health services research, problem drinking and steroid use.

*Mary Boulton* is a Senior Lecturer in Sociology as Applied to Medicine at St Mary's Hospital Medical School, University of London. She was Honorary Secretary of the MRC AIDS Behavioural Research Forum and a member of the Steering Group of the ESRC's Programme of Behavioural Studies in HIV/AIDS. Her current research interests include the sexual behaviour of gay and bisexual men in relation to HIV/AIDS, the experience of families with an HIV-infected child, and social aspects of genetic screening.

*Glynis M. Breakwell* is Professor of Psychology and Head of Department of Psychology at the University of Surrey. Her research interests include identity dynamics and social representations; political and economic socialization; attitudes towards science and technology; sexual attitudes and activity in adolescence; environmental change; risk perception. Her recent books include *Coping with Threatened Identities*, Methuen, 1986; *Facing Physical Violence*, BPS/Routledge, 1989; *Social Psychology of Identity and the Self Concept*, Academic Press/Surrey University Press, 1992; and *Empirical Approaches to Social Representations*, Oxford University Press, 1993.

*Stefano Campostrini* is a Research Fellow and Lecturer at the Department of Statistical Science at Padua. He holds a doctorate in statistics from the University of Padua in Italy where his thesis was on measurement and analysis issues in continuous surveys. During 1990 and 1991 he was a research fellow at the University of Edinburgh where he worked exclusively on the analysis of the CATI-based lifestyle and health survey at RUHBC.

*Anthony P. M. Coxon* is a Research Professor in Sociology at Essex University and Emeritus Professor of Sociological Research Methods of the University of Wales. He is a Principal Investigator of Project SIGMA and has been involved in research on gay men and AIDS since 1982, including the co-ordination of the WHO seven-nation Homosexual Response Studies. Particular areas of current research include the validity and use of sexual diaries, belief systems about HIV and other STDs and the social context of gay men's virological status.

*Peter Davies* is Director of Research at the School of Health Studies, University of Portsmouth. His research interests include gay men, particularly in relation to HIV/AIDS and aspect of research methodology. He is a Principal Investigator of Project SIGMA and co-editor (with Peter Aggleton and Graham Hart) of *Aids: Social Representations, Social Practices*, Falmer, 1989; *AIDS: Individual, Cultural and Policy Dimensions*, Falmer, 1990; *AIDS: Responses, Interventions and Care*, Falmer, 1991; and *AIDS: Rights, Risk and Reason*, Falmer, 1992.

*Chris R. Fife-Schaw* is a Lecturer in Psychology at Surrey University. He was Senior Research Fellow on the Social and Behavioural Consequences of HIV/AIDS for 16–21 Year-Olds Project and has published research findings from this project in the *Archives of Sexual Behaviour, AIDS Care* and *The Journal of Community and Applied Social Psychology*. He has also published research on political attitudes and behaviour and on young people's responses to the new technologies.

*Janet Holland* is a Senior Research Officer in the Social Science Research Unit, Institute of Education, University of London, and Lecturer in Education at the Open University. She has general interests in the area of youth, gender and class and is currently researching family interactional practices. She is a member of the Women, Risk and AIDS Project team and a contributor to the Men, Risk and AIDS Project.

*Margaret Johnston* is currently based at the School of Education, University of Manchester. She has done research in child language, language in schizophrenia and methods in HIV/AIDS education, and has contributed to publications on peer education in HIV/AIDS, and on the influence of learning context on attainment. She is at present preparing distance-learning materials in research methodology.

*Jenny Kitzinger* is a Research Fellow at the Glasgow University Media Group. She is currently working on the media coverage of sexual violence against children. Her other research interests include the politics of sexuality and women's health.

*Neil McKeganey* is a Senior Research Fellow in medical sociology at the Public Health Research Unit, University of Glasgow. For the last six years he has carried out research into the social determinants of risk taking of drug injectors and female prostitutes. He is co-author with Marina Barnard of AIDS, Drugs and Sexual Risk: Lives in the Balance, Open University Press, 1992 and is currently writing a book on female prostitution and AIDS. In 1994 he will direct a programme of research on the various routes into, and out of, dependent drug use.

*David McQueen* is Chief of the Behavioural Surveillance Branch in the Centre for Chronic Disease Prevention and Health Promotion, Centers for Disease Control, Atlanta in the USA. He was founding Director in 1983 of the Research Unit in Health and Behavioral Change at the University of Edinburgh, Scotland. As a Professor at the University of Edinburgh he oversaw many health research projects but was principally involved with a CATI-based lifestyle and health survey.

*Ian S. Peers* is a Lecturer in Quantitative Research Methods in the School of Education, University of Manchester. He has directed research programmes in the areas of education and human service evaluation including the HEA-funded Peer Education Evaluation Project. His other major interests are in psychometrics, cognition and learning, and the teaching of statistical methodologies.

*Helen Pickering* is currently the Senior Social Scientist at the Medical Research Council/Overseas Development Administration project on HIV/AIDS in Uganda. Previously she worked on an AIDS project at the Medical Research Council in The Gambia.

*Robert Power* is a Senior Research Fellow at the Centre for Research on Drugs and Health Behaviour. His recent research has concerned the coping strategies of drug users not in contact with treatment services. His main interests lie in qualitative and action research and the advancement of peer education which utilizes idigenous fieldworkers. He has published widely in both the academic and popular press.

*Caroline Ramazanoglu* is a Senior Lecturer in Sociology at Goldsmiths' College, University of London. Her interests are in the area of gender, racism, power and methodology. She is a member of the Women Risk and AIDS Project team and a contributor to the Men, Risk and AIDS Project. Recent publications include *Feminism and the Contradiction of Oppression*, Routledge, 1989; and as editor, *Up Against Foucault: Explorations of Some Tensions between Foucault and Feminism*, Routledge, 1993.

*Sue Scott* is a Senior Lecturer in Sociology at the University of Stirling. She was previously lecturer in sociology at the University of Manchester and a member of the Women, Risk and AIDS Project team. Her interests are in the sociology of the body and sexualities, theorizing risk and feminist theory and methodology. She is currently developing a programme of research on Sex Education in Scotland.

*Sue Sharpe* is a freelance writer, researcher and consultant, whose main interests are the lives and experiences of young women, but include work on young men and heterosexuality. Her books include *Just Like a Girl*, Penguin, 1976 (second edition 1994); *Falling for Love*, Virago, 1987; *Voices from Home*, Virago, 1990; *Fathers and Daughters*, Routledge, 1993. She is currently working on a study of boys, and is a contributor to the Men, Risk and AIDS Project.

*David Silverman* is Professor of Sociology at Goldsmiths' College, University of London. His research interests are in qualitative methodology and the organization of professional-client encounters. He has researched outpatient interviews in paediatric cardiology, cleft-palate and diabetic settings and worked extensively on HIV counselling. His most recent books are *Communication and Medical Practice*, Sage, 1987; and *Interpreting Qualitative Data: Methods for Analysing Talk, Text and Interaction*, Sage, 1993.

*Rachel Thomson* is Senior Development Officer for the Sex Education Forum at the National Children's Bureau with general interests in sexuality, young people and policy. She is a member of Women, Risk and AIDS Project team and a contributor to the Men, Risk and AIDS Project.

*Kaye Wellings* is a Senior Research Fellow at the London School of Hygiene and Tropical Medicine. She has worked in the field of education and sexual health for fifteen years and has had extensive experience in evaluating public education on HIV/AIDS in the UK and Europe. She was part of the team which conducted the National Survey of Sexual Attitudes and Lifestyles, and is co-author, with Jane Wadsworth, Anne Johnson and Julia Field of *Sexual Behaviour in Britain*, Penguin, 1994; and *Sexual Attitudes and Lifestyles*, Blackwell, 1994.

# Index

Note: 'n.' after a page reference denotes the number of a note on that page.

accountability of evaluation 180
acquiescence 45–7
Advisory Council on the Misuse of Drugs (ACMD) 97
age
  behavioural changes 25–38
    longitudinal cohort-sequential studies 28–30
    cohorts 25–6
    effects 35–6
    and high-risk behaviour 142–4
agency-based studies 6–7
  naturally-occurring data 87–8
AIDS Media Research Project 160–2
anal intercourse 138–44
analysis of data 35–7
analytic induction 89
anthropological research 12, 149–50, 157
assertion of knowledge 80
asymmetry of sexual acts 63
awareness-raising campaigns 202–3

baseline surveys 42
behaviour
  health 244–5
  sexual
    analysis 57–68
    change 3–4, 8–9, 25–8, 39–55
    diaries of 125–48
    feminist perspective 223
    high-risk 6–7
behavioural risk factor surveillance system (BRFSS) 40

bias 34
  diaries 129, 136
  evaluating AIDS-preventive strategies 213, 215
  indigenous interviewers 102
  KABP surveys 207
  longitudinal cohort-sequential designs 33, 36
bisexual men 61
  see also gay men
blood donation and risk 163
brainstorming 167

capture/recapture studies 8, 112, 113–14, 121
case-study research 89
categories 247–8
censorship, focus groups 170
Christian spirituality 60
clients of prostitutes 154, 155–6
coding, sexual 132
cohort effects 36
cohort studies 3, 25–6
  longitudinal sequential designs 3, 25–38
collection of data 8–13
  continuous 39–55
  periodicity 29–31
  from prostitutes 120
combined research methods 12, 150, 152–4, 156–7, 194
commercial agencies, AIDS-preventive campaigns 202

communication during sexual interaction
60
*see also* negotiation of sexual practices
community guides 99–100
community health education project
179–98
comparative research 89
computer assisted telephone interviewing
(CATI) 39, 40, 41–2
condom use
advertisements 203, 206
anal intercourse 138–9, 141–2
acceptability of questions 31
changes 50–1
evaluating AIDS-preventive strategies
207, 208–10
feminist perspective 219–20, 224–5
prostitutes 151, 154
women's experience 233
confidentiality 103
conformity, focus groups 168–70
consensus, focus groups 168–70
consistency, data
continuous data collection 45
computer assisted telephone
interviewing (CATI) 41
drug users 101
longitudinal cohort-sequential
designs 32
constant conparative research 89
contact tracers 99
contactability of prostitutes 114–15,
116–17
content analysis 132
contextuality, sexual acts 62
continuous data collection 39–55
conversation analysis 72–82, 90
cooperation, stakeholders 190, 191–3
cost-benefit analysis, behavioural change
58–9
costs of research 105–6
counselling, HIV
analysis of naturally-occurring data
69–93
and sociological interviews 230
credibility of evaluation 193–4
cross-cultural variations, HIV counselling
71, 76–9
cross-sectional surveys 3, 25–7, 42
acquiescence 46
cultural aspects
focus groups 166, 169

HIV counselling 71, 76–9
sexual sessions 63–4, 66

debates, focus groups 170–2
debriefing, indigenous interviewers 103,
106
decision-making and rationality 60–1
definitions 247–8
delays in HIV counselling 72, 74, 75, 77
democratic evaluation 189–91, 196
design, research 3
continuous data collection 39–55
longitudinal cohort-sequential designs
25–38
deviant-case analysis 89
diaries, sexual 10–11
gay men 85–6, 125–48
prostitutes 150–1, 152, 153–6
differences, focus groups 170–2
discussion groups 106
*see also* focus groups
discussions about AIDS 45, 46
dispreferred answers 90n.1
divine orthodoxy 70
dominant sessions 139
drop-out rate 32–3, 36
drug users
data validity 9
hidden population estimation 8
indigenous interviewers 7, 97–109
prostitutes 112, 119

economic monitoring, prostitutes 154–5,
156–7
education *see* health education
interventions
effectiveness of campaigns, evaluation
200–4
effects of campaigns, evaluation 200
efficacy of campaigns, evaluation 200,
204–6
ejaculation, and risk 139–40
embarrassment, HIV counselling 71,
72–6
empowerment of women 234–5
through research 229
ethical issues
focus groups 174n.3
hard-to-reach groups 248–9
indigenous workers 100, 103–4
prostitutes 119–21, 154
sexual diaries 134, 145n.7

sexuality interviews 228–31
ethnography 249
indigenous interviewers 102, 103, 107
evaluation
    community education project 179–98
    European preventive strategies 199–216
explanatory orthodoxy 70

face-to-face interviews *see* interviews
fairness of evaluation 180, 181
false identifiers, prostitutes 116
feminist approach, social research 14–15,
    219–39
field research
    indigenous workers 7, 97–109, 249
        combined research methods 12
        data validity 10
    reliability of data 88–9
    social science study methods 150–7
focus groups 13, 159–75
    community education project 188
    indigenous interviewers 106
formative evaluation 199
front-end analysis 182

Gallup International 213–15
Gambia, The 149–58
gatekeepers 98, 190–1, 227
gay men
    analysing sexual behaviour 61–3
    focus groups 164–5
    response to HIV/AIDS 125–48
gendering of sexual acts 63, 65–6
general population surveys 5–6, 53, 200
    continuous data collection 40
    data validity 32
    response rates 33–4
generalizations 73
glosses 73, 74, 75, 77–8
grounded theory development 160
group discussions *see* focus groups
group norms 168–70

Health Belief Model (HBM) 4, 57–8, 59,
    206, 244
health education interventions 13–14
    assessment 199–216
    community project 179–98
helplines 207, 211
hesitations in HIV counselling 73, 74, 75
heterogeneity
    focus groups 170–1

prostitutes 114–16
hidden populations 7–8
    prostitutes 8, 111–22
high-risk behaviour, groups practising
    6–7
indigenous workers 7, 97–109, 249
    combined research methods 12
    data validity 10
individualist fallacy 59–60
induction, analytic 89
infiniteness, sexual acts 62
informed consent to research
    prostitutes 120
    young women 229
institutional settings *see* agency-based
    studies
intentionality, sexual acts 62
interrupted time series design 3
interviewers
    indigenous 7, 97–109, 249
        combined research methods 12
        data validity 10
    support 5, 104, 231
    training 5, 7, 105–6
interviews
    focus groups 162, 166–73
    longitudinal cohort-sequential designs
        32
    problems 126
    prostitutes' clients 154
    and questionnaires 10
    and sexual diaries 130, 136–8
    telephone
        continuous data collection 39, 41–2,
            53
        data validity 10
    young women 223, 227–35

jokes 165–6

key informants 98
knowledge about AIDS
    continuous data collection 50
    cross-national comparisons 214
    focus groups 162–73
knowledge, attitudes, beliefs and practice
    (KABP) surveys 200, 206–7, 213

language
    ambiguity 62, 248
    changes 31
    indigenous interviewers 103

questionnaires 9–10, 43
    polarity of statements 45–50
lesbians 165–6, 168
longitudinal cohort-sequential designs 3,
    25–38
longitudinal surveys 25–7, 42
    polarity of statements 49
lower bound estimates 6, 34

mainstreaming of research 15, 243–51
mark/recapture studies 8, 112, 113–14,
    121
marked acknowledgements (MAs) 79, 80,
    82–3
mass media education campaigns 14
    evaluation 199–216
    focus groups 160
measurement of data 8–13
    longitudinal cohort-sequential designs
    31–2
media analysis 211
medical self-management 250
men
    gay
        analysing sexual behaviour 61–3
        focus groups 164–5
        response to HIV/AIDS 123–48
    prostitutes' clients 154, 155–6
    reported sexual behaviour 51
    response rates 33
morale, community education project
    187–8
multiplier effect 204

naturalistic interviews 230
negotiation of sexual practices 220, 223,
    226, 233
network analysis 145n.7
networking, community education project
    186–7
non-participant observation 11
non-response to surveys 33–5
    *see also* response rates

objectives, preventive strategies 201–2
objectivism 86
objectivity of evaluation 180, 181, 193–4
observation 11–12, 125–6
    of focus groups 174n.2
    of illicit drug use 98
    by indigenous interviewers 103
    of indigenous interviewers 102

longitudinal cohort-sequential designs
    32
of prostitutes 151, 153
organization, community education
    project 188
orgasm, and risk 139–40
Orton, Joe 129
outcome evaluation 200–11
output analysis *see* volume analysis
outreach services
    indigenous workers 108
    prostitutes 113, 119–20

participant observation *see* observation
participants in sexual sessions 64–6
participation rates *see* response rates
partners, sexual
    numbers 126
        changes 50–1
        and risk 165
    semantics 65
payment
    indigenous interviewers 107
    prostitutes 154
peer education 14, 180, 183–97
periodicity of data collection 31–3
personal events 30
perspective of client 71, 79–84
pilot studies
    AIDS-preventive strategies 212
    continuous data collection 41
    KABP surveys 207
    longitudinal cohort-sequential studies
    30
polarity of statements 45–50
preference organization 75
preferred answers 75, 90n.1
probit analysis 46–9
process evaluation 199
prostitutes
    hidden population estimation 8, 111–22
    social science study methods 149–57
publicity, community health project 188

qualitative research 12, 69, 86
    feminist methods 226
    prostitutes 150
    reliability of data 88
quantitative research 12, 69, 85–6
    diaries 129
    feminist methods 227
    prostitutes 150

questionnaires 9-10
  continuous data collection 40-1, 43-9
  and diaries 127
  drug users 101
  focus groups 161-6
  longitudinal cohort-sequential designs
    32
  prostitutes 150, 151-3, 156-7
    clients 156
  response rates 33
  young women 227
questions, research 4-5, 69-90

rational choice concept 223, 225
rationality
  health behaviour 245
  and safer sex 60-1
recidivism, and safe sex 245
reciprocal sessions 139
recruitment
  of evaluators 195
  of indigenous interviewers 105
  of peer educators 187
relapse, and safe sex 59, 245
relational modality 131
relationship-type, and high-risk behaviour
    142-4
reliability, data 8-13
  diaries 134-6
  indigenous workers 100-3
  interviews 126
  KABP surveys 207
  longitudinal cohort-sequential designs
    32
  naturally-occurring data 88-9
  prostitutes 151-7
repertory grids 190, 193
representativeness of samples 5-6, 34, 247
resistance to advice 79-80, 82-3
response rates
  continuous data collection 41
  cross-national comparisons 213
  general population surveys 5-6, 33-4
  high-risk behaviour, groups practising
    6
  longitudinal cohort-sequential designs
    33-4
  prostitutes 113
responsiveness, evaluation 194-5, 196
risks
  of HIV infection 51-2, 126
    anal intercourse 138-44

categories 248
  focus groups 162-5
  perception 51, 58-9
  women 219-22, 224-5
  of researching prostitutes 118
romantic fallacy 60-1

safe and unsafe sex
  feminist perspective 220-2, 233-4
  traditional accounts 57-61
  see also condom use
sampling 5-8
  continuous data collection 41
  focus groups 161
  indigenous interviewers 102
  KABP surveys 207
  longitudinal cohort-sequential studies
    28, 32-5
  naturally-occurring data 85
  stakeholders 189-90
  young women 226-8
self-efficacy 58, 59
self-management, medical 250
self-reported behaviour, drug users 100-1
Senegal 151
sequential surveys 25-7
sexual acts 62-3
  diaries 130
sexual identity 66
sexual individuals 66
sexual sessions 63-6
  diaries 131
sexuality
  romantic fallacy 60
  young women's 14-15, 219-39
sexually-transmitted diseases (STDs) 207
SIGMA project 61-6, 126
  diaries 127-8, 130-44
societal events 30
sociology of health 250-1
spirituality and sexuality 60
stability, knowledge about AIDS 44-5
stakeholders, evaluation 182-3, 189-96
stepwise entry, advice-giving 79, 80, 83-4
stimulants 152
story-telling 166-8
stresses, fieldwork 104
subjectivism 86
  women's experience of sexuality 222-3
supervision, indigenous interviewers 106
support
  for interviewees 230

for interviewers 5, 231
   indigenous 104
for peer educators 188, 191
surveillance, ethics of 120-1

telephone interviews
   continuous data collection 39, 41-2, 53
   data validity 10
theoretical frameworks 4, 58-68
theory of action 181-2
   elucidation 183, 187
time of measurement effects 36
time series design, interrupted 3
time trend analysis 49
timeframes
   of counselling sessions 83
   of research 30-1
      continuous data collection 52
timing
   evaluation process 192-3
   sexual sessions 64
traditional accounts, safer sex 57-61
training
   of counsellors 71-2, 79-84
   of interviewers 5
   of peer educators 184, 185-6
transsexuals 66

unmarked acknowledgements 79-80, 82
unsafe sex *see* safe and unsafe sex

utility of evaluation 182, 187-8, 196

validity, data 8-13
   continuous data collection 45
   diaries 134-5, 136, 144
   focus groups 173
   indigenous workers 100-3, 106
   interviews 126
   KABP surveys 207
   longitudinal cohort-sequential designs
      32
   naturally-occurring data 88-9
   prostitutes 116, 151-7
   young women's sexuality 233
variables, types 42-9
violence, street prostitution 118
volume analysis 140-4

weighting of data 34-5, 247
women
   lesbians 165-6, 168
   prostitutes
      hidden population estimation 8,
         111-22
      social science study methods 149-57
   reported sexual behaviour 51
   response rates 33
   sexuality 14-15, 219-39
Women, Risk and AIDS Project (WRAP)
      14, 219, 221-2
word associations 167

Printed in the United States
by Baker & Taylor Publisher Services

Printed in the United States
by Baker & Taylor Publisher Services